*H*aving *B*abies

The Patients • The Doctors
• The Dramas and Joys •
Nine Months Inside an
Obstetrical Practice

THOMAS CONGDON

SIMON & SCHUSTER
New York London Toronto
Sydney Tokyo Singapore

SIMON & SCHUSTER
Rockefeller Center
1230 Avenue of the Americas
New York, New York 10020

Designed by Deirdre C. Amthor
Manufactured in the United States of America

1   3   5   7   9   10   8   6   4   2

Library of Congress Cataloging-in-Publication Data

Congdon, Thomas.
Having babies : the patients—the doctors—the dramas and joys—nine months
inside an obstetrical practice / Thomas Congdon.
p.   cm.
1. Obstetrics—Popular works. 2. O'Driscoll, Robert, Dr.—Career in
obstetrics. 3. Bonamo, John, Dr.—Career in obstetrics. 4. MacGregor, Susan.
I. Title.
RG525.C688   1994
618.2—dc20   94-4616
                                        CIP

ISBN: 0-671-76708-9

This is a work of nonfiction. I have changed some names. The following are
pseudonyms: Grace Findley, Lois Geller, Deirdre Kerry, Beth and David
Keyser, and Maria and Antonio Ramirez.

To the well-named
Constance,
and to our babies,
Pamela and Elizabeth

I was molded into flesh in my mother's womb.
For nine months I was compacted in blood.
I, too, breathed in the common air,
Was laid on the earth that bears us all,
And my first sound was a wail, like everyone else's.
No king is born differently;
For there is just one way into life, and one way out.

—Solomon, *The Book of Wisdom*

Prologue

Smellie

Everything seemed designed to win him ridicule. His name, of course, William Smellie, made him the target of jokes, but it went beyond that. A big, lumbering, raw-boned redhead with unfashionable clothes and plain manners, he had come from the provinces with an idea that in the early 1700s struck many Londoners as absurd, not to mention indecent and outrageous. He wanted to enter a profession that for thousands of years had been reserved almost exclusively for women. It was work that, scandalously, would bring him into intimate physical contact with the opposite sex, and work for which he seemed particularly ill equipped, considering that it required delicacy. William Smellie's hands were enormous—"fit only to hold horses by the nose," a rival sneered, "or to stretch boots."

Easy to dismiss when he came to the city, by the time he died William Smellie had changed his world and become one of humankind's great, though generally unknown and unsung, benefactors. Every modern woman who somehow must squeeze a baby's body through the narrow, twisting, bony hole at the base of her spine would be in his debt.

Smellie began his career as a doctor in Lanark, a village in the Scottish Lowlands. In those days, the early eighteenth century, physicians considered themselves much too grand to bother with childbirth. That nasty business was left to the midwives. Some midwives were skilled and sensitive, but some were ignorant and filthy, drunken and brutal. When a baby started coming out in the wrong position, they shoved it back up into the uterus for another try. When that failed, they dismembered it and extracted the parts. They killed as many as they saved.

Smellie was gripped by compassion for childbearing women and unable to forsake them. He began to deliver babies. But from the start he did something much more remarkable than taking pity: he took notes. Observing closely and thinking hard, he tried to learn from every delivery, and he kept careful and systematic records, so that one woman's tragedy might yield knowledge that would spare another.

Learning from experience, basing principles upon actual data— it was something that would never have occurred to most of his predecessors. But Smellie was a man of his times, and his times were the Enlightenment, when a fresh, inquiring spirit was sweeping aside the superstitious certitudes of the Middle Ages. He soon discovered that when he got right down into actual bodies, most of the medical pronouncements of the ancients, the theories of Aristotle and Hippocrates and the others which the Middle Ages had taken on faith, didn't hold up. Real women, real babies—they weren't the way Smellie's dusty old textbooks said they were.

For example, accepted wisdom said the birth canal was pretty much a straight shot, a chute connecting the uterus with the vagina, down which the baby dove. Smellie, however, found that the birth canal curved this way and that as it made its way through the architecture of the pelvis; the baby, as it descended, pivoted to conform to the changing contours, its head and body turning almost independently. In due course, after years of observation and measurement, Smellie created a detailed map of the birth canal. At last, thanks to Smellie, after eons of working blind, those attending a birth could know the course the baby had to take and could effectively assist its passage. Even more important, he brought science to the act of childbearing. William Smellie was not a "male midwife," as he was contemptuously called. He was, one could say, the first obstetrician.

Hungry for more knowledge, he went to Paris but found to his disappointment that he knew more than the doctors there. He went on to London with the same result. In London, Scots were considered buffoons, and "male midwives" were a scandal. Women were so mortified at the idea of a man in attendance that the kindly Smellie, doing what he could to spare their feelings, covered his hulking self with a flowered calico gown and his head with a bonnet tied with pink and silver ribbons. Despite all obstacles, he succeeded. Women who would have died lived; infants who would have been lost were rescued. His big hands proved an advantage; his long fingers deftly guided the baby. At first his patients were mainly the poor, those who couldn't afford midwives, but in time women of all classes came to him.

Once regarded a clown, he became a celebrated teacher. There were midwives who wanted to learn, and physicians too, more and more all the time. Eventually his disciples fanned out all over Europe and even to colonial America. Wherever they went, the new medical specialty of obstetrics became established. Standards began to rise, and babies' chances for survival improved.

They kept on improving. For two and a half centuries doctors, researchers, and inventors kept doing what Smellie taught them to do: look thoughtfully at real bodies and take notes. Throughout the nineteenth century and into the twentieth, advance followed upon advance. Time after time some danger or agony that had always been supposed a permanent part of the human condition was eased or erased.

As the twentieth century draws to a close, pregnant women are being given powers that not only would have dazzled Smellie but would have been considered impossible even a few brief decades ago: They can find out what sex their fetus is; learn whether or not it has inherited the family disease; peer into their own womb and watch their unborn baby and have its picture taken. In recent years the truly unthinkable seems to have been accomplished. Labor pains, the most notorious aspect of the biblical curse "In sorrow thou shalt bring forth children," have been lessened significantly. A new anesthetic technique allows a mother to be alert and almost pain-free throughout most of labor, if she chooses to be, able to chat or read through even heavy contractions yet fully able to push her baby out when the time comes.

Marvels, of course, become taken for granted. In one generation patients have gone from merely hoping for a perfect baby to expecting one as a right—and suing if their doctor fails to produce one. Confronted with those expectations, obstetricians can only shake their heads and say that though most of the time things work out beautifully, nothing is certain. For all the magical machines and for all the knowledge and skills accumulated by the heirs of William Smellie, childbirth is still an adventure.

One question that technology fails to answer is perhaps the most compelling: what is that adventure like? Women try to inform each other, but when those who have given birth tell the newly pregnant how it was for them, the accounts sometimes grow sensational; as with veterans swapping war stories, the purpose can be to impress, or appall. The pregnancy manuals, on the other hand, are instructive but impersonal.

Recently, in the spirit of Smellie, an inquirer spent nine months in one of America's 23,000 obstetrical practices, taking notes, chronicling the adventure. During the time it took a young patient of that practice, Susan MacGregor, to conceive and bear her first baby, he watched as, with the help of two doctors and their nurses, several hundred women made their way along the pilgrimage path that is childbearing.

Most of the pregnancies, if not idylls in pink and blue, were safe and satisfying. Sometimes the experiences would have been grim if they'd occurred in another era but, thanks to modern medicine, turned out well. Other times sad things did happen. The technical advances are blessings, but the human body remains variable and tenaciously complex, and childbirth is an intricate process with series upon series of steps and interplays that must come off exactly right. Even the sad experiences, though, were inspiring, as heartbreak summoned from families strengths they never knew they had.

One change in obstetrics, the craft that William Smellie helped make into a profession, would certainly have caught his eye: the role of women. He and the other "male midwives" had to force their way into the field, overcoming entrenched female opposition. They succeeded too well. Obstetrics became dominated by men; women were out. But now, 228 years after Smellie's death, the pendulum was once again swinging. Not only were the midwives he'd sought to help now skilled and respected but women in large numbers were becoming obstetricians. A radical change in the balance of the sexes was in prospect.

Would the time come again, Dr. Smellie might have wondered with a smile, when male obstetricians would need to dress like women to be permitted into the birthing chamber?

1.
Storks

To the locals, of course, there was no confusion, but there must have been times when drivers from other parts of the country, barreling across northern New Jersey on Route 280, had done a double-take at a large green sign spanning the highway. "The Oranges," it said, as if down the road a mile were a sign saying "The Bananas" and, after that, "The Apricots." William of Orange, the cold, unsmiling seventeenth-century Dutch sovereign after whom the towns called the Oranges—East, West, South, and Central—had been named, would not have been amused. For that matter, he wouldn't have been much charmed by downtown West Orange, into which an exit ramp from Route 280 issued. It had become seedy, its village charm nearly gone, its commercial vitality drained off by big new malls outside town.

On the edge of West Orange, a little farther from the urban difficulties of Newark and a little closer to expensive preserves like Short Hills and Upper Montclair, things were sprucer, more prosperous. The main streets were lined with two- and three-story buildings—banks, the headquarters of small companies, medical and dental offices of recent construction—each surrounded by parking lots full of late-model automobiles. One such building was 95 Northfield Avenue, a pleasant, red-brick structure with white, New Orleans–style ironwork. In the spring, white azaleas bloomed around its door, but now the blossoms were gone; it was mid-October, and the maples along Northfield were brilliant red.

For passersby, Number 95 was just another suburban commercial building, nothing to catch the eye. There was no way to tell that within its conventional walls, great happinesses and griefs were experienced and intense human dramas, concerning matters of life and sometimes death, were played out. This was an obstetrical practice, the work place of Robert O'Driscoll and his partner, John Bonamo. Their trained hands, during their combined forty years in obstetrics, had guided the births of perhaps ten thousand human beings.

The offices were not designed to impress. No polished granite, no sleek modern furniture, no designer colors. But there was one brilliant touch of decor. On the walls of the narrow corridor leading from the reception room of the practice to the three examining rooms in back were five bulletin boards the size of card tables. Each was paved with hundreds of tiny photographs of babies, given to the doctors by the patients. The photos dated back to 1973—squinting, red-faced newborns, most of them. Some had names written on them: Jennifer, Jaclyn, Christie, Brian, Tara, Rebecca, Chien Mei, Kevin, Kerry. The bulletin boards caused traffic jams all day long as the nurses tried to squeeze past pregnant women enraptured by the pictures.

"People love their child's picture on the wall," Dr. O'Driscoll said, "more than I ever could have imagined. For years afterward they visit the child's picture as if it's a shrine."

"The 'baby' may be fourteen years old now," Dr. Bonamo added, "but if we don't have him up there anymore, they want to know why. 'Where's the picture?' What I enjoy is when they bring the youngster in and say, 'Now look, honey, *there's your picture!*'"

The photographs had a power. They announced that the product of this little business was not doughnuts or cement but something truly extraordinary: human life.

Elsewhere on the walls were needlepoint samplers made by new mothers for their doctors. "Happiness," declared one, "is being delivered by Dr. Bonamo." Another showed a stork flapping across a starry sky with a baby in its beak and a doctor's bag in its claws; on the bag, in the jittery graphics of needlepoint, was the legend "Dr. O'Driscoll." Still another displayed a line from Carl Sandburg: "A baby is a sign of God's opinion that the world should go on."

Rod O'Driscoll (his nickname was an acronym made from the initials for Robert O'Driscoll), himself the father of six, was the senior doctor in this two-man group practice. He was just what one of his patients said an OB-GYN should be: nice-looking but not handsome. He was not short but not tall, not really thin and not really plump; he wore glasses and at fifty-four still had some of his hair, which was gray. He dressed in natty tweed sports jackets.

Rod's style fascinated the people he worked with; it was a topic often discussed. They marveled at his knack for calming patients without saying a word, at his uncontrived appeal, at his blend of strength and modesty. He was an old pro, the kind who made it all look easy. He was a top professional, truly learned in his craft, yet had a personal connection with every patient. A colleague at the hospital called him a state-of-the-art country doctor. "Rod," Jack Bonamo said, "doesn't have to spend a lot of time with a patient to make her comfortable. He doesn't have to talk her into it. His confidence relaxes her."

Making obstetrics—with its long hours and its urgent phone calls in the middle of the night—look easy was quite a stunt. According to one study, it was the busiest of the medical specialties. What was more, Rod had duties at the hospital, St. Barnabas, a thriving medical center in nearby Livingston that had been founded by Episcopal nuns but had become nonsectarian. He was chief of its entire medical staff of a thousand doctors, the person who arbitrated their disputes and championed them in encounters with the hospital administration. It was a big load on top of a job that was already exhausting.

Rod had ways of recharging his batteries. "Rod can sleep anywhere, anytime," his wife, Joan, said. "I have actually seen him sleep standing up. He puts his back against the wall and bends his knees and puts his head back and takes a little nap. If he's waiting in a line somewhere, the supermarket or the movies, he'll take a nap. He can fall asleep instantly and wake up totally coherent." Joan had seen him do it thousands of times at night, when he got a phone call. He'd get out of bed and answer the phone and sound just as he did at midday. He always seemed to remember, in the middle of the night, just who the patient was and what was supposed to being happening to her next.

Every now and then, however, perhaps once a year, he'd flub. Joan, lying in bed and trying desperately to ignore the call—she was the type who, once awake, stayed awake—would realize that Rod's responses were all wrong. Once he took a call from a woman who was well along in labor, and she heard him say, "Well, why don't you have a little something to eat and come by the office some time tomorrow?" After he hung up, Joan told him what he'd said. "Oh my God," he gasped. "I'd better call her back."

Another time, he'd been on call all weekend and had half a dozen deliveries. He was wiped out with fatigue, and when he got home he and Joan went right to bed. Hours later he got up and went into the bathroom, and she called and asked him to bring her a glass of water. He returned to the bedroom, came to her side of the bed, and turned on her night light. He put the glass of water on her bedside table, pulled the covers down, palpated her abdomen, and said, "I'm going to have the nurse give you something for pain. You'll feel much better in the morning." He pulled her covers back up, went around to his side of the bed, got in, and went right to sleep.

Throughout his career, Rod had been a solo practitioner. But in 1987, when he passed his fiftieth birthday, he began to think about bringing in a partner. He was talking one day with Jack Bonamo, a bright young physician who had come through the residency program at St. Barnabas. Jack was in his seventh year of solo practice. Rod knew Jack very well and admired the way he worked; he was the star of his generation of OB-GYNs at St. Barnabas, as Rod had been the star of his. Rod found himself saying, "Hey, we ought to join practices."

Jack Bonamo was in his late thirties and tall, an inch over six feet, with a waistline just beginning to expand. His complexion was olive, his brow prominent, his eyes black-brown behind his glasses. So densely seeded was his black, silver-stranded hair that it rose from his forehead like the bristles of a brush. His manner was classic Italian—warm, attentive, enthusiastic—though his voice was soft. His wit was quick and he loved to tease the people in his life, but when he was serious his composure was entire and his focus acute.

He had grown up on Staten Island in a traditional old-world family; his mother's people were Neapolitan, and his father's were from the Bay of Salerno. Altogether he had more than sixty first cousins. A half dozen of them had the same first name as Jack, so they were identified by their jobs—John the Dentist, John the Teacher, John the Doctor. Of his thirty-two Bonamo cousins, twenty-six of them became college graduates, though none of their parents were.

His mother was the classic Italian matriarch; love was expressed through food. "The family still talks about her cooking," Jack said. "If one of her brothers was sick and the sister-in-law was busy, my mother would be knocking on the door with the frozen sauce and the frozen meatballs. When my mother died, she left ten frozen meals in the freezer, which my sister still keeps. She calls them 'the religious articles.' It's a joke. I keep saying, 'Are you ever going to throw that food out of the freezer?' But she never does."

Jack's wife, Suzanne, a tall, trim blond, was German American. "Her family is so different from mine," he said. "Low key. Not at all ostentatious. I have a Mercedes, a little Mercedes. She drove it once—around the block—and when she got back she said, 'I felt so silly.' She never drove it again. When she needed a car, she got a Ford station wagon."

Since boyhood, Jack had known he wanted to become a doctor. His parents had little money, and to save for med school tuition he went to a state university. From his first exposure to obstetrics as a medical student, he knew it was for him. In his fourth year he took some elective time in the OB-GYN department at St. Barnabas Medical Center. He got along well, and when he applied for a residency there he was accepted. "I knew Rod then," he said. "He was a very popular obstetrician. Three words described him: pleasant, lucky, concise."

After residency he decided to take a shot at being in practice for himself. His first patient came through one of the nurses he'd befriended at St. Barnabas, who called him at home and said, "Look, there's a woman here with some problems and she doesn't have a doctor. Would you like to take her on?" Jack had no office, no instruments, no tables, no equipment—he couldn't afford them—so he arranged to use another doctor's office a few hours a week, and he hired a young woman, Barbara Valente, the wife of a school principal and mother of two daughters, to come in and be his staff. Some days he'd have only two patients. To make the patients think he was busy, he'd schedule the two appointments back to back and make the patients wait ten minutes.

Soon the nurses themselves were coming to him. He needed more office time for them, but the doctor he was subletting from couldn't spare any. So Jack rented and equipped a little office of his own. The problem was that he didn't feel he could charge the nurses; they were his friends, and there was such a thing as professional courtesy. After office hours he'd come out and ask Barbara, "How much money did we make today?" Barbara would say, "You saw eight patients: four nurses and two doctors' wives, and two paid."

The nurses, however, began to recommend him to their sisters and their sisters-in-law and their next-door neighbors and their cousins. And these patients did pay. As the practice grew Jack needed some-one to help out Barbara at busy times. The budget didn't yet permit more staff, so Suzanne became his secretary. In the office, he didn't want her to be The Wife. She had to be The Employee. He knew pa-tients would view her differently if they knew she was The Wife or was close to the doctor in some special way. They might not open up to her, or they'd say different sorts of things to her. She wouldn't be able to do her job. Suzanne was a good sport and put up with it for the two years he needed her.

Being there during Jack's work day gave her a perspective few ob-stetrical spouses ever get. She was amazed at the pace he kept. He'd be in with a patient and then answering the phone, and then all the phones would be going off at once, patients with questions. And all the while the patients were being moved in and out of the examin-ing room. "I wouldn't have understood that intensity," she said, "if I hadn't seen it. So naturally, when he came home, he'd lie down on the couch and wouldn't move. But now I understood that it was okay. He had to have that time, he just had to sit and not worry about peo-ple or questions."

One of his early patients was Eileen Schulte, a labor-and-delivery nurse at St. Barnabas. Nurses in Labor and Delivery see obstetri-cians up close, through informed eyes, and for a veteran labor-and-delivery nurse to entrust her pregnancy to a particular obstetrician says a great deal about him. "I've seen doctors who make mistakes," Eileen said, "and doctors who treat their patients almost as if they hate women—rough, almost abusive. When the women are in labor they don't spend time with them; they act as if they don't believe they're in pain. They're not into it; it's just a job for them. Dr. Bonamo is very gentle; he's kind; he spends time with you." It took her time to get pregnant, almost five years, and she had one miscar-riage. When she finally got pregnant, she saw that it seemed to mean almost as much to Jack as it did to her.

With Suzanne at home and Barbara Valente at the office, Jack was bracketed by affection, patience, and constructive candor. Having been with Jack since the beginning, Barbara could say things to him that no one else in the office could have gotten away with. Her par-ticular gift, crucial to an obstetrical practice, was taking phone calls from patients. With her soft, comforting voice and long experience, she was just the person a woman wanted to talk to if this was her first baby and bewildering new things were happening. She was an expert at the delicate game of solving problems without actually practicing medicine.

•   •   •

Joining practices is a consequential and ticklish matter for doctors, involving complex financial arrangements as well as work habits and professional attitudes. Rod O'Driscoll and Jack Bonamo were very different men, but as characters they proved complementary, and they were in harmony on all the essentials. The marriage worked, except for one nagging little problem.

By agreement Jack and his assistant had moved into Rod's offices at 95 Northfield. It was cramped, but someday, Rod had said, when the practice had grown, they could expand. The waiting room was small, and the space between the secretaries' desk and the bathroom door, a high-traffic area, was the scene of constant jam-ups. The corridor leading back to the examining rooms wound this way and that, like an alley in a medieval village. It could be a tight fit when two ninth-month mothers-to-be tried to pass each other.

Rod had been in these offices for fifteen years. They were made for a solo practitioner. There was no way to give Jack an office of his own, and he was obliged to do his paperwork on a nondescript metal desk in the bookkeeper's office. When he wanted to talk to a patient in an office setting—for example, when something serious had to be discussed—he had to use Rod's office, a cozy, dark-panelled cubbyhole with photos of Rod's wife and kids on the shelves. That room became the consultation room for both doctors. When they both had patients to speak to in private, they would shuttle them in and out of that office, taking turns.

None of this bothered Rod; he was entirely comfortable. If things were clean and serviceable, that was good enough for him. But to Jack, as much as he loved working with Rod, the partnership in one sense was flawed. If there was one thing Jack cared about as much as function—and he cared about *that* very much—it was appearance. Born with an eye for style, Jack was remarkably sensitive to how things looked: what people wore, the line of a chair back, the pattern of wallpaper. What many would have scarcely noticed—the imitation-veneer plywood on the walls, the mismatched carpets and curtains, the general-issue office furniture—was a daily distress for Jack. But he was too good-mannered and too respectful of Rod to make a fuss. He never complained or derided; his true feelings showed only in the occasional glance, the rare fragment of unguarded remark. He bided his time, inwardly feasting on dreams of an elegant office he would someday himself design. And slowly, unobtrusively, unthreateningly, he worked at converting Rod to the eventual need.

·   ·   ·

On this particular October evening, the waiting room looked a little like a clown convention. There were five young women dressed in brightly colored stretch clothes, each of them, it seemed, with a beach ball under her top. It was Thursday evening obstetrical hours.

Thursday evenings, the only late hours for O'Driscoll-Bonamo obstetrical patients, were busy. Some of the women brought husbands; some brought children. The seats were always filled. A source of never-ending amazement for the staff was the men who, on a crowded night, failed to yield their seat to a pregnant woman. How otherwise perfectly nice men could sit there like clunks, oblivious to the woman standing in front of them with eight months' worth of baby freighting her body, was something they could never comprehend. This was one of those nights. A conspicuously pregnant woman came in and hung up her coat. The seats were all occupied, so she stood.

One of the secretaries, Eleanore Steel, got up from her desk and went to the waiting room door. A rounded woman in her sixties, Eleanore had the face of a general or a nineteenth-century industrial titan, an effect her puffy ash-blond hairstyle was at pains to dispel. "Would one of you gentlemen," she said, pausing for effect, "please get up and let this pregnant lady sit down?" Three young men gaped at her and then, like scolded schoolboys, lumbered to their feet. The young woman took a seat, and Eleanore went back into the office and returned to her desk. "Way to go, El," the other secretary, Mary Jo Ward, said under her breath.

"I did it in a nice way," Eleanore said. "Have you ever seen Bea do it?" Bea Perez, the nurse on duty, was not known for her timidity. "When Bea does it, they *shoot* to attention."

Mary Jo herself was no stranger to the art of command. A part-timer, she worked days as a first-grade teacher in a tough public school in Jersey City. Her technique, however, was humor rather than terror. "Settle down, boys and girls," she would say to a noisy class.

"Now just for that commotion, you're not going to have recess . . ."
(groans) ". . . not until you say the magic words." And the class,
smiling but earnest, would chant, "Miss Ward is young, thin, and
beautiful." "That's right," Mary Jo would say. "Let's have recess."

Not precisely thin or young, Mary Jo, with her blue eyes and head
of white curls, was lovely in an ample, maternal, Irish way. Few of
the patients knew that she was in fact a nun. She wore regular
clothes and lived outside the convent. Once a young gynecological
patient came into the office with an infection that had lasted months.
As she left, she stopped at the door and said with great annoyance,
"Do you know how long it's been since I've had sex? It's been so
long that I feel like a nun."

"I know the feeling," said Sister Mary Jo.

A woman sitting on the waiting room sofa was reading a picture
book to two little blond girls. Her third child, a boy, had escaped the
waiting room and was headed for the lollypop supply in the secretaries' area. "Colette," she murmured to her older girl, "go tell John
to sit down or he's dead meat." The girl ran to the door and joyfully
shouted, "John, you're dead meat!"

"I love my children," the woman said dryly to the other patients.

A woman in a dark blue knit maternity suit came in and gave her
name to Eleanore, who instantly buzzed the intercom for Bea. "Margaret's here," she said. A half hour before, Margaret had called and
told Eleanore she had nausea and cramps and was afraid her baby
was coming. Her last child had been three weeks early, she'd said.
If she was really going into labor now, this baby would be five weeks
premature. Eleanore had put Dr. Bonamo on the phone, who'd asked
her how she felt. "I feel like a time bomb," she'd said.

Bea appeared and took Margaret by the arm. "Come on, honey,"
she said. "You don't have to wait. Dr. Bonamo wants to see you right
away."

A woman of about forty arrived and went to the desk. "I'm twenty minutes early," she told Eleanore. "I'm going down the street to
pick up my dry cleaning. Can I leave my specimen here?"

"Sorry, Pam," Eleanore said. "The front desk can't accept urine
samples. To avoid mixups, they have to be given to the nurse at the
start of your appointment." Pam rushed off, carefully carrying her
urine specimen.

Rod O'Driscoll came down the hall with a woman who looked
twelve months pregnant. "Lizzie's in labor," he whispered to

Eleanore. "Here, I mean. *Right now.*" Rod tended to whisper big
news. "And she wants to try for a V-BAC." V-BAC, pronounced
"vee-back," was short for vaginal birth after a previous cesarean delivery. Years ago it was thought that once a woman had a cesarean—
a childbirth in which the fetus is lifted out of the womb through an
incision in the lower abdomen and uterus—the only safe thing was
for her to have cesareans on all subsequent deliveries. As recently
as ten years before, only about 4 percent of women with previous
cesareans managed to deliver vaginally, usually over the strong ob-
jections of their doctor. But gradually the old once-a-cesarean-
always-a-cesarean view began to change. Doctors saw that there often was no problem, as long as the complications that arose during
the first labor and delivery didn't recur. Now the percentage of V-
BACs was up to ten. Rod and Jack and the nurses and staff all encouraged women to try for V-BACs.

"Oh my gosh," Eleanore said. "I just scheduled Lizzie's repeat
cesarean." She picked up the phone and dialed. "Hello, this is Dr.
O'Driscoll's office. We're sending in a lady whose repeat C-section
was scheduled for Monday. . . . Right. She's in labor. . . . No, she's
going to go for a V-BAC."

Bea Perez came down the hall and hugged the woman, trying to
ease her tension. "So Liz—you're going to have an October baby,
huh? How exciting!"

Lizzie asked Eleanore if she could use the phone. "I probably
won't be able to get myself to the hospital for another hour," she
said. "My husband's at work so I'll have to drop Justin off at my
mother's, if she's there." She pointed to the husky three-year-old at
her side, the first C-section. She punched the buttons on the telephone and waited impatiently for an answer. "Oh, Mom," she said
at the phone, "will you *please* answer!"

Justin was waving gaily to the room with a hand encased in a floppy rubber glove that reached his elbow. Rod looked at the glove,
then looked at Bea. "I gave it to him while Lizzie was being examined," she said. "That was to keep him from brushing his teeth with
the KY jelly."

Lizzie's mother finally answered, and after a hurried conversation with her, Lizzie grabbed Justin and led him out the door. "Good
luck to her," Eleanore said to Bea and Mary Jo. Lizzie would be on
her mind, she knew from experience, until she heard how the delivery went.

Margaret, the woman afraid she was in labor, came down the hall looking relieved. "I feel okay now," she told Eleanore and Mary Jo.

"Your mind is at ease," Mary Jo said. "You've seen the doctor."

"At home I was so crazed. I don't know. . . . I'm more worried this time than I was with my first one. The first time you don't know anything; you just do it. Now I know."

•   •   •

There was a puff of cool evening air as a young couple came into the waiting room. One seat was free, and the woman, who was slender and pale and had rich brown hair, sat down. Among the blatantly pregnant women around her she looked out of place. They were chatting with each other, but she was quiet and solemn. Her husband, a broad-shouldered young man in a business suit, holding a briefcase, stood next to her. He too was quiet and kept fidgeting.

During the next twenty minutes, Bea Perez came to the door again and again, summoning patients for their examinations. The young man seemed too nervous to sit. At last Bea picked up a violet file folder and read out the name written on its tab. "Susan MacGregor," she said. The young woman rose to follow Bea, and the young man came right behind her. "Just the patient," Bea said pleasantly, but not so pleasantly that it masked her wish to be obeyed.

Susan MacGregor stepped forward, and Bea led her up the crooked corridor, past those hundreds of pairs of brown and blue eyes staring from the corkboards, to an examining room. She weighed Susan, took her blood pressure, gave her a throwaway paper gown to put on, and asked her to sit on the examining table. Then she departed, leaving Susan to wait for the doctor. Over Susan's head, suspended from the ceiling by a thread, was a stuffed, white satin stork.

2.
Happy Hour

I t was the beginning of her senior year and Susan Sprague was dissatisfied, but not with Lynchburg. Lynchburg was the small college from heaven, or Hollywood: white-columned Greek Revival halls around green quadrangles set in the Blue Ridge foothills of Virginia's Shenandoah Mountains. But lately she'd become slightly fed up with the company she'd been keeping.

For three years she'd been part of a campus elite that was the envy of outsiders—best-looking, best-dressed, most athletic, most cosmopolitan. Lacrosse was the center of their lives. For Susan, who had come to Virginia from a small New Jersey suburb, acceptance into this social aristocracy was exciting. She had fit right in. She was convivial and poised, and she was pretty, with fair skin and abundant brown hair that looked red in the sun.

Lynchburg was more than merely social. The education was good, and Susan had done well in her courses. She'd majored in business administration, art, and history; had joined a service sorority, Gamma Sigma Sigma; and had tutored children in a nearby orphanage. Over her first three years she had grown. She had, in fact, outgrown her crowd.

This registered at the start of her senior year, when she found herself attracted to a boy outside her circle. He was reasonably athletic, a strong-bodied six-footer but by no means a jock. He wore glasses; had sandy, disorganized hair; and was obviously not preoccupied with clothes. He was handsome in a way that was new to her, not so much feature by feature as for the qualities she saw in his face. He wasn't rich—he worked in the campus post office; he belonged to no clique; and he lived in an unstylish dorm. None of that seemed to bother him, or, to her surprise, her. The thing about him that came through most arrestingly was that at an age when many are desperate conformists, he was his own man.

She'd gotten to know him slowly. For a year or more she'd seen him in the post office almost daily; they'd become casual acquaintances. In the first days of their senior year, when both acted as orientation leaders for the incoming freshmen, she'd seen him in a different setting. At some point, aware she was doing it, she began to observe him, and she detected a purposefulness underlying his friendly way and his offbeat humor.

One evening at a big campus party she looked up and saw him on the other side of the room. He was wearing striped pink trousers—very preppy, the kind of thing that just months before would have made her shudder—and he was standing alone surveying the scene. She crossed the floor and went up to him. Cupping her hand at his ear and shouting over the music, she said the first thing that came to mind: "Nice pants."

"As I crossed that room," Susan said years later, "I felt I was taking a big step. I was kind of moving beyond my old thing. Something was telling me to." Anthropologists wouldn't have been mystified—a routine example, they'd say, of the biological procedure called mate selection. For three years this female had casually consorted with the young males of her tribe, but now she was twenty-one, and some instinct was tugging her toward this sensible guy with the intelligent expression and nice smile who looked as if he'd be steady, good for the years, an effective companion in raising the children she did not yet realize she wanted.

"Nice pants." Those two little words would take her, in due course, up the front path of a small, gabled house with blue shutters, up the stairs to a room under the eaves occupied by an early-nineteenth-century four-posted brass bed with a floral cotton chintz comforter. There, on a clear, warm September evening, by a process whose intricate workings were the culmination of eons of human development, two genetic complexities would merge to produce a third, one that was both of them and yet in many ways neither. The human race was preparing to perpetuate itself.

The young man was named Tracy MacGregor. He'd been well aware of Susan for some time and been attracted to her, but he'd assumed she preferred to run with that other crowd. Standing there in his pink pants at the party, concealing his excitement, he said, "Oh, hi, Susan." They began to talk, and they talked all evening. They saw each other twice the next week; not dates exactly, more like making sure that they both would show up at the same party. For a while they saw other people too, but that came to an end.

After graduation, Susan got a job with the Coach Leatherware Company—which made trendy leathergoods sold then by catalogue and through a chain of retail outlets—as assistant manager of the Coach outlet in Hackensack, New Jersey. Tracy, meanwhile, had become a management trainee at AT&T headquarters in Parsippany. He lived in Warren, twenty-five miles from Maplewood, where Susan lived with her parents, and whenever their work schedules allowed, he'd drive over to be with her. Tracy was also going to graduate school at night, but they saw each other as much as they could, and the feeling that had blossomed in the special environment of the college campus continued to thrive in the outside world.

Tracy had grown up in Broomhall, a suburb of Philadelphia. He'd gone to public school and played in Little League. While he was in his teens his parents divorced. After Lynchburg he had wanted to go on to law school but lacked the money, so he started studying nights for a master's in business administration.

Susan's parents, Betty and David Sprague, took to Tracy immediately. He quickly became a member of their household, completely at home, one of the family. They were particularly touched by his attention to his grandmother. When she was living alone in Pennsylvania, he'd not only visit her but vacuum her apartment and clean out and restock the refrigerator. When she moved into a nursing home, he'd call a nearby hair salon the day before his visit and make an appointment for her. At the home, he'd help her dress, drive her to her appointment, then take her to lunch.

"He's wonderful," Betty Sprague said to her husband, David, who replied, "You know, any man who's that thoughtful is going to be wonderful to his wife."

His wife. It became clear to the Spragues that Tracy loved Susan, but when was he going to propose? Susan wondered too. They'd been going together for more than two years since graduation. Once, after a party, Tracy mentioned the ring a newly engaged woman was wearing and asked Susan how she liked it. Susan was caught off guard. The topic made her nervous. "The stone is microscopic," she found herself saying, in a lame attempt to sound cool. So at least rings were being discussed. But months passed, and no proposal was forthcoming. "Is this thing leading somewhere?" she asked herself. "Or is it levelling out?"

Both Susan and Tracy had Scottish roots. He was a MacGregor, of course, and she, through her mother, a McLeod. It was an ethnic link that meant something to them. Tracy suggested they take some vacation time and visit Scotland. It occurred to Susan that Tracy might be intending to propose during the trip. But as they drove through the English countryside, heading for Edinburgh, registering in hotels as Mr. and Mrs., she began to have misgivings. Had she read the signals wrong?

When they arrived at Grassmere, in the Lake District, she saw that he'd booked them into a beautiful inn, with antiques in every room and handmade quilts on the beds. The first night, after dinner, they took a moonlit walk by the lake. Tracy took Susan's hand—her right hand, as it happened—and tried to work a ring onto her fourth finger. He asked her to marry him. She was stunned. He had to ask her several times because she was speechless. There, halfway down her finger, was a diamond in a Tiffany platinum setting: a fairly significant stone. She said yes and burst into tears. Later Tracy said he had been planning to propose months earlier, but when Susan had declared her preference for a larger ring, he'd had to wait until he'd earned enough money to buy one. Susan was mortified to learn that thanks to a careless, tossed-off remark, she'd postponed the proposal.

They were married in a tiny, early-nineteenth-century church in Bernardsville, New Jersey, on a bright autumn day in October, 1988—a storybook wedding. The story had begun with two little words, "Nice pants," and ended with two more, "I do." Now a new story was beginning.

The recession had started and real-estate prices were way down, and they realized that with their savings and their two salaries and some help with the down payment from both their families they could buy a small house. Susan was now manager of the Coach shop in Princeton, and Tracy had been moved into sales and marketing at AT&T. After three months of hunting, they found a white, gabled house built in the 1920s, only eight blocks from Susan's parents' place. It had dormer windows and blue shutters and was nestled between a large hemlock and an enormous beech with a massive, twist-

ing gray trunk. Early each weekday morning they got in their re-
spective cars, rolled out onto New Jersey's snarl of superhighways,
and sped off in different directions.

On a Thursday in mid-September of their second year of marriage, Tracy phoned from work and asked Susan if she'd be off the
next day. She said yes, and he said he'd take the day off too—the office would be quiet, and he needed a break—and maybe they'd go
to the movies. On Friday afternoon they gardened together and then,
because the recession had set in now and become real to them, they
decided to save some money by going to the Twilight Special at four-
thirty at the AMC Tenplex over in Morristown—tickets for two dollars apiece.

They got out of the movie at six-thirty. It was a nice evening, clear
and warm. Their arms around each other's shoulders, they strolled
down to the other end of the mall and went into a publike restaurant
for half-priced happy-hour beer and appetizers. It was dark by the
time they got home. They decided not to watch TV. They went upstairs and got into their antique brass bed with the rose-strewn cov-
erlet. And there, having gone to the Twilight Special and happy hour
to save money, they did something very expensive.

Afterward they lay there and both, as it turned out, had the same
thought: *Something happened.* They had the thought, then dismissed
it. There couldn't be a baby just now. They were too busy; there was
too much going on.

One evening soon after the movie date Susan got home late from
work to find that Tracy had dinner almost ready. While he was setting the table she went upstairs to change out of her business clothes.
Suddenly she heard him summoning her in a voice that seemed un-
characteristically stern. "Susan," he said, "come down here, please.
Right now. You'll never believe this." When she got to the kitchen,
there was Tracy with her birth-control pills in his hand. Tracy had
opened the earthenware crock to get matches to light the dinner can-
dles, and there he'd found Susan's pills.

"Oh," she said. "So that's where they went."

The month before, some unexpected guests had dropped by, and
Susan, seeing her birth-control pills on the kitchen counter as she
hastily tidied up, had tossed them in the earthenware crock they kept
keys and matches in. The next day they went away for the weekend.
When they came back, she couldn't find her pills. But there was
nothing to worry about, she told Tracy. From time to time in the

past, she reminded him, the pill had made her sick to her stomach. She would go off the pill for a while, and everything would be fine. "It's time for another pill break," she'd thought when the pills got lost. She knew her body, her rhythm.

Early in October, she felt weak and tired and a bit nauseated. She sensed something wasn't right, but she had a new regional manager, so she thought it might be stress. Tracy thought it was a stomach virus. In just a few days they were scheduled to leave on vacation. He'd been dreading that one of them would get sick and mess things up. He insisted she see her doctor. "You've got to go," he said. "We're going to be overseas for three weeks. If it's flu, maybe he can give you a shot or something."

As many women do, Susan used her gynecologist as a general practitioner as well. Five years before, her GYN had retired and referred her to a younger doctor he thought a great deal of, John Bonamo. Susan had liked him immediately and felt completely comfortable with him. Now she phoned his office and spoke to Barbara Valente, one of the secretaries, who suggested she take an over-the-counter pregnancy test.

For the thousands of years before the development of the modern techniques of determining pregnancy, women groped for ways to relieve their uncertainty. In rural France in the nineteenth century, some maintained that the saliva from a pregnant woman would make a goat vomit. Others said that if a gold ring suspended over a woman's belly spun rapidly the woman was pregnant. Hippocrates, the great physician of ancient Greece, suggested a method based not on data but on his imaginative understanding of female physiology. A woman's body, he thought, was a tube, open from mouth to vagina. A woman wondering about pregnancy should therefore place a clove of garlic in her vagina before bed, and if her breath smelled garlicky the next morning, that would mean there was no baby inside her to obstruct the tube. Sweet breath would prove conception.

Not until 1931 did women have a simple, reliable way to confirm pregnancy. Dr. Maurice Friedman of the University of Chicago discovered that injections of urine from pregnant women would cause a reaction in rabbit ovaries. In the 1970s his technique, which inevitably became known as the "rabbit test," was surpassed by a simpler, quicker test. At first only medical people performed it, but in the 1970s it was made available for use at home. Even the most reliable test, though, was worthless unless the test-taker was open to its findings. When Susan took it, the pregnancy dot turned twice as blue as the control dot. "I'm not sure I did this right," she said to Tracy.

"We'd better go in and see the doctor," he said.

•   •   •

"So," Jack Bonamo said to the young woman sitting under the satin stork as he entered the examining room, as if he were continuing a conversation already under way, "you took the test and you couldn't believe your eyes."

When Jack was first practicing obstetrics, women suspecting pregnancy usually didn't see their doctor until they'd missed two menstrual periods. Now, with the over-the-counter pregnancy tests, it was different; obstetricians saw women within two to four weeks after the first missed period. They came in not so much to find out if they were pregnant but to have pregnancy confirmed. Susan Mac-Gregor, however, seemed to be in another category: she'd come expecting some entirely different explanation. "I don't think I did it right," she said in a dry little voice.

"Well, let's see." When a patient was new to the practice, Jack would begin with a get-acquainted chat in the doctors' office, which was called the consultation room, with both the prospective parents. But Susan was a regular and he knew her well, so he jumped to the second step: the pelvic exam. That procedure, he felt, was just between the patient and her doctor, and so unless she requested otherwise, her mate was customarily parked for the moment in the waiting room. "What was the date of the start of your last period?"

"September first."

Jack wrote the date on a printed form. "Okay," he said, "let's see how that date matches up with the internal state of things. Would you just lie on the table and bring your knees up and put your feet in the stirrups?"

Despite the existence of sophisticated tests for detecting pregnancy, doctors still rely on the traditional means of confirmation: looking and feeling. One indication, Chadwick's sign, is the bluish violet hue that the cervix takes on during pregnancy. But the main sign is the size and feel of the uterus. A pregnant uterus has a soft, rubbery consistency. It is also swollen and what OB-GYNs term "globular." With experience an obstetrician becomes adept at "sizing" the uterus—gauging its size with his or her fingers—and can tell from the maneuver almost exactly how many weeks pregnant the patient is.

In the O'Driscoll-Bonamo examining room the nurse was always present during pelvic exams. Bea Perez helped Susan lie out on the examining table, flat on her back, knees bent, and guided her feet into the metal stirrups that would hold them back and up. Jack put on rubber gloves and lubricated two gloved fingers of his right hand. He put his hands under the paper gown and slipped the lubricated fingers into Susan's vagina, advancing them until they touched her cervix. He gently pushed the uterus forward, and with his left hand he pressed her lower abdomen. The uterus was now between his hands. He moved his fingers, pressing in one place and then another, coordinating the movements of the two hands so that between them he could feel the entire length of the uterus: a distance of three or four inches.

If the uterus of a woman who had tested positive felt normal, non-pregnant, Jack would know that the fertilized egg might well be growing outside the uterus. If, for example, one of Susan's fallopian tubes felt unusual, that might mean the fertilized egg had imbedded itself there—an ectopic pregnancy. If Susan was having an ectopic pregnancy, she would soon be feeling severe pain. Jack would put her in the hospital and remove the growth; delay could bring rupture, hemorrhage, death.

Sometimes, for one reason or another, a doctor would decide against surgery, and the displaced pregnancy would end by itself during the first month or two. But there had been rare instances of overlooked ectopic pregnancy in the fallopian tube, the ovary, or even the abdominal cavity that had actually lasted nine months and resulted in the birth of a living child.

Jack withdrew his fingers and removed his rubber gloves. "I think I've got the answer," he said affably. Bea helped Susan sit back up.

"It must be written all over my face," she said.

"No," Jack said, "all over your uterus. It's huge."

"You mean . . . ?"

"I mean, congratulations," Jack said, smiling widely. "You are most definitely pregnant."

Susan gasped and gulped and began to weep.

"All right?" Jack asked her.

"It's wonderful!"

"Okay, let's go into the consultation room and call in your husband and give him the news."

Tracy looked anxious as he came into the small, dark-panelled room. He started to ask a question and then halted. The radiant expression on Susan's streaked face, a mixture of awe and happiness, told him everything.

"We're *pregnant?*"

"Yes!" Susan said and threw her arms around him.

Absolute bewilderment. Tremulous joy. They blinked, they sputtered, they laughed, their eyes filled with tears. They held each other and happily cried.

Jack shut the door and sat them down and began his customary introduction to that Oz called childbearing.

"The first thing you should understand," Jack said, "is that you're not sick. You're pregnant. Pregnancy isn't an illness; it's just a condition. If you're nauseous, it probably isn't because you're sick but because your hormones are functioning normally for your condition." Rod and Jack were amazed and depressed by the number of OB patients who insisted on being treated like invalids, demanding medicines and expecting severe restrictions on diet and activity. Women who'd had pregnancies elsewhere sometimes complained about the relaxed approach of the O'Driscoll-Bonamo practice. Previous OBs had laden them with do's and don't's and insisted they pamper themselves. Rod and Jack wouldn't play that game.

"Try to lead your normal lives," Jack said. "If you've been exercising, keep exercising. If you're a vigorous exerciser, that's fine, but just keep your pulse under 140. And you should continue to enjoy your sex life. It's an old wives' tale that it might damage the baby." Sometimes, he said, women felt a bit of discomfort during intercourse and got on the phone and said they were afraid they'd hurt their baby. But the fetus lay behind stout defenses—amniotic fluid, the thick uterus, the bowels lying over the uterus, the interior abdominal wall, and the skin. "It's protected in so many ways that you really couldn't hurt it by making love. So please, just put that right out of your minds."

Next Jack launched a preemptive strike against one of the obstetrician's prime annoyances. Having hired a doctor for medical advice, patients were constantly citing the contrary opinions of distinctly nonmedical authorities—their mothers, for example, their sisters, their best friends. When patients began with something like "Well, my cousin had a baby, and she says . . . ," obstetricians' eyes would dim and their spirits plunge. "Every pregnancy is different," Jack told the MacGregors. "The experiences of other people you may talk to may have nothing at all to do with your pregnancy, yet they can worry you, or mislead you.

"Even when you yourself have a second or third baby, your experiences this time may be irrelevant. People who had a nice healthy birth or two before, when they experience a different set of symptoms, they think, 'It wasn't like this before. This must be a bad sign.' It probably isn't. You may feel very different than you did the last time, or than your sister or cousin did and yet both pregnancies are fine.

"My advice," Jack said with a smile, "is, don't take advice from anybody . . . except us. We're in the office six days a week, and we're available twenty-four hours a day for emergencies. Our nurses are obstetrical nurses and they've been doing this for many years. There's rarely a question that we haven't answered before."

He picked up a small white plastic wheel with numbers on it; it was a circular slide rule designed to make it easy for obstetricians to calculate the EDC—"estimated date of confinement." Confinement just meant going to the hospital to have a baby, but the word had a dark nineteenth-century quality about it: the feeling of banishment, of being taken out of active society and put away to do something slightly shameful. Jack turned the dial on the wheel. "Don't schedule anything important for next June seventh," he said. "You're probably going to be otherwise engaged." Only about 4 percent of babies are born on their due dates, he added, but most of the other 96 percent arrive within a week on either side of it.

For Tracy and Susan, the specific date gave their condition sudden reality. This wasn't a movie or a dream; this was something that was going to *happen*. Tracy swallowed, and Susan squeezed his hand.

Jack began to explain how the obstetrical calendar works. Since ancient times, he said, humankind has known that a woman normally gives birth ten "moons"—ten lunar, twenty-eight-day months, or 280 days—from the first day of her last menstrual period. Though antique, the system actually works and has become part of obstetrical practice. OBs start their count at the first day of the last menstrual period, or LMP. They know that ovulation generally takes place two weeks later. "You know you conceived on September 15th," he said, "so you probably think you're four weeks pregnant. But to me, you're six weeks, because I count from the LMP. You're two weeks further along than you might think you are."

OBs measure the progress of a pregnancy not by months but by weeks. Calendar months are unreliable, he said, because they vary in length, from twenty-eight to thirty-one days; weeks work well because they never vary—they're always seven days long. Another problem with months is that they're too gross a measurement; in pregnancy, important changes occur week by week. One way to tell the first-time mothers-to-be from the veterans was that while the former counted in months, the latter had learned to count in weeks.

The MacGregors by this time were slightly dazed, but Jack pressed on. He knew that in their present state—excited, over-whelmed—they'd absorb only about half of what he told them. That was all right; he'd be telling them again along the way, adding information he now was skipping. He talked about medications; on their way out they'd get a list of the ones Susan could take and the ones she couldn't. Tylenol was okay, for example, but not aspirin, which can impair the development of the fetal heart. He took a brief medical history of both Susan and Tracy to check out the possibility of hereditary disease. Did either of them have health problems? Did anyone in either family have inherited diseases—Down's syndrome, spina bifida, diabetes? Neither MacGregor knew of any. For some of the conditions there were tests that could be performed beginning about the sixteenth week of pregnancy. The tests, when parents chose to have them, often enabled a prenatal diagnosis to be made, so that if the baby was in fact affected, the parents would not be surprised later on.

One important query was whether or not Susan had had German measles. German measles during pregnancy, especially early pregnancy, brought a 50 percent chance of fetal birth defects. Like six out of seven women, Susan had immunity to the disease. In the appropriate spaces Jack recorded the results of the pelvic exam he'd just done. She'd had a Pap smear a few months before, so there was no need for another. As federal law required, he tested her for syphilis. "If you wear contact lenses," Jack said, "you may find they get uncomfortable as your pregnancy develops." Along with much of the rest of the body, the eyes retain more water during pregnancy, changing their contours. Not knowing this, women often buy new lenses, unnecessarily.

Visit after visit, Jack and Rod and Bea would tirelessly add to these sheets of data, making Susan's folder bulge in tandem with her own expanding girth.

If Susan had been a new patient, Jack would have asked another question: what name she wanted the doctors to call her by. The typical patient, asked that question, gave her first name or nickname.

Jack would write it down on the chart, and that was how she'd be called from that point on. Only a few, mainly very old women, said "Mrs. Smith." A few younger ones gave their first name but from then on called him "John," which was okay with Jack, though it was a name no one else used for him. His general finding was that during the experience they were embarking on together, which was something of a partnership, and especially during hard labor and the throes of delivery, patients wanted the person with them to be both doctor and friend.

One patient said, "What I'm doing in childbirth is so intimate— I'm laid wide open, with a baby coming out of me—that I want my doctor to be more friendly toward me than a tradesman would. Yet I want to call him doctor, because I want a doctor there."

"And now, do you have any questions?" Jack said, knowing he'd probably anticipated most of them.

"When will I start to show?" Susan asked, reflexively looking down at her board-flat stomach.

"People usually show, oh, somewhere between fourteen to eighteen weeks. It's according to your build and the way you're carrying the baby." Susan and Tracy both laughed at the very thought.

"When can we tell people?" Tracy asked.

"It's up to you," Jack said. He knew that many women, when they come to have a pregnancy confirmed, have already told other people; in that case, if the outcome is unfavorable, they have a lot of painful explaining to do. He would have loved to save them from that, but it was their affair. "It's a personal matter. I generally tell people it's good to keep it private for the first twelve weeks, just in case things don't go as well as we hope they will. But it's up to you."

"I've got a question," Tracy said, his concern apparent despite his light tone. "What's this thing going to cost?"

"You'll talk to the ladies at the desk about that. That's their department. They'll help you review your insurance. They know the particulars, and they'll be available for all types of questions like that. It keeps changing and I really don't keep up with it. My job is to keep up with the medical changes and theirs is to keep up with the insurance changes. That's some job, believe me."

Jack was wrapping it up now. "You'll be coming in for an exam every month at first, then more and more frequently toward the end. You'll meet my partner, Dr. O'Driscoll, at some point. We both know all of each other's patients so that if one of us has the flu or is on vacation the other can fill in and the patient won't be encountering a stranger."

He stopped and looked closely at Susan. She was sitting there numbly. "You're not hearing a thing I'm saying," he said affectionately.

"I can't believe I'm pregnant!" she said. "I've never even held a baby!" She thought of her new job, so hard won and so prized. She began to sense the cataclysmic changes that would flow from this unexpected development.

"It really never occurred to us she was pregnant," Tracy said. "I mean, we knew *something* was wrong. But all we could think was she's sick and there we were, just about to go off on vacation."

"Nothing's wrong," Jack said reassuringly. "Something's very right. This is a wonderful thing—one of the most wonderful things that will ever happen in your life. You should go on that vacation and have a fabulous time, and four weeks from now, after you get back, come in for your first monthly OB visit."

As many times as they'd seen freshly revealed mothers-to-be come down that corridor, stunned and starry-eyed, and as late as it was and as tired and eager as they were to go home, Bea Perez and the two secretaries that night, Eleanore Steel and Mary Jo Ward, exclaimed when they heard the MacGregors' news and rejoiced with them.

"You're so lucky," Eleanore said. "So many people try so hard and never do get pregnant. And you've got great medical insurance."

Tracy thought of the financial implications of all this. The mortgage for the little house they'd bought in Maplewood had been a stretch, but they'd gone ahead because they both were bringing home salaries. Would there still be two salaries when Susan had the baby? He'd just been promoted to executive assistant to one of the AT&T directors, but the pay increase would go only so far. What about all the expenses that health insurance wouldn't cover, like a stroller, a crib, and a diaper service, not to mention college tuition? The budget had just gone out the window.

It was worse than he could have dreamed. The average amount parents spend just on medicine in the first year of a child's life is $396. Government economists calculated the minimum cost of raising a child born in 1991 to adulthood as $297,000.

Eleanore fished in her desk and came up with various items for Susan, among them the list of medications Jack had mentioned.

There were free samples of baby lotions and shampoos and other products that manufacturers were eager to introduce, such as remedies for nausea. And there were things to read: copies of magazines aimed at expectant parents; a small, pink book called "A Doctor Discusses Pregnancy," which Susan would find useful and refer to often; pamphlets on feeding the baby by breast or bottle, on exercise during pregnancy, on diet; and, for expectant parents caught in indecision, a booklet offering hundreds of possible baby names. Eleanore put them all into a pink plastic bag provided by still another manufacturer and handed the bag to Susan. Then she got out her appointment book and made a date with Susan for the first obstetrical visit, exactly one month from that night.

"It's amazing," Susan said in the car going home. "It's as if the finger of God pointed at us."

"Instead of at the pills in the crock," Tracy said.

Susan looked over to see if he was complaining, but he seemed cheerful and content, enjoying his joke.

"What really got me," Tracy continued, "was Dr. Bonamo's reaction. He was so happy. I said to myself, 'Wow, is this guy ever involved in his work.' "

"How about you, Dad?" Susan said. "Are you happy? You think you're up to this?"

"Well I'll tell you, Mom," Tracy said . . . and then they both had to laugh about the Dad and Mom thing, the newness of it, the touch of comedy in a lover suddenly playing the role of parent. "Let me tell you, Mom," Tracy went on. "I couldn't be happier. I'm knocked off my pins, but I couldn't be happier."

Sitting silently beside her young husband in the darkened car, Susan was beginning to absorb an astonishing fact. She was going to have a baby. A *baby.* Deep inside her, without her conscious initiation, an insistent, undeniable process had begun, and it would move steadily forward, almost of its own volition, putting her through a drastic regimen. Her stomach would swell, her body would open, and a human being would come out. It was all so improbable, and all so certain.

That night, as they lay in bed reflecting on their news, this day seemed the beginning of everything. But in fact that beginning had occurred more than a month before, in that same bed, and in the time since then astounding things had already happened.

It had started with a marathon, a six-hour obstacle race through vagina, cervix, and uterus. The contestants, some 360 million of them, each wearing the MacGregor genetic tartan, were microscopic cells with pointed heads and long, hairlike tails. By the time they reached the fallopian tube, the duct where Susan's newly released egg lay, only about two thousand were still in the running. One plunged headlong into Susan's egg and, wriggling furiously, was the first to penetrate. The race was over. From that moment on, the egg rejected all others.

The fertilized egg was a mere fleck, weighing only one-twentieth of a millionth of an ounce; all the eggs that had produced all the world's current population could fit in a top hat. Yet that one-celled egg, in combination with the sperm, carried all the genetic information needed to build the MacGregors' child, a creature that would contain trillions of cells. More than ten billion nerve cells would be required to build its brain alone.

Susan and Tracy had drawn down this genetic data from an immense archive. Like everyone else, they each had two parents, four grandparents, eight great-grandparents, and so on. Extending that progression back a thousand years, which is to say thirty-two generations, one could calculate that from that period alone the breeding of some 4.3 billion ancestors had contributed to the genetic instructions that would shape this baby. Of course, the progression did not stop there; one thousand years is just a flicker in humankind's million-year existence as a species.

Each of Tracy's billions of sperm had gleaned from that genetic data bank in a slightly different way, and so each would have produced a different baby. If the MacGregors had gone to a late movie instead of an early one, altering the time they went upstairs, a different sperm would have reached the egg, and the result would have been a different child: blond instead of brunette, perhaps, stocky instead of slender, an artist instead of a mathematician.

The newly fertilized egg had quivered, then slowly divided into two new, identical cells. This was the very first of an almost limitless number of cell divisions, the start of a complex process of development that would continue many decades, maybe a century, until this new MacGregor died. That first division, which occurred as the egg inched its way down the fallopian tube toward the uterus, took a day. The next happened just twelve hours later. By the end of three days, there were thirty-two cells; by the fourth, 128. So it went, faster and faster—a whole human being to build.

As it slowly tumbled down the fallopian tube toward the uterus, this ball of new cells was using up the last of the food supply the original cell had contained. Its urgent need now was to get another food source. One was waiting.

Every twenty-eight days or so since Susan was thirteen, her reproductive system had begun a new cycle. For the first fourteen days it produced the hormone estrogen, whose main job was to thicken the lining of her uterus. This was a preparation for the moment when, on the fourteenth day or thereabouts, one of her ovaries dispensed an egg from the limited supply she had carried with her since her earliest days in her mother's womb. The ovary secreted a second hormone, progesterone. Along with the estrogen, the progesterone made the lining what obstetricians called "succulent"—soft and ready to be implanted with the egg-of-the-month once it was fertilized.

For the fourteen years that Susan had had menstrual cycles, the eggs had gone unfertilized. At the end of each cycle the neglected egg had dwindled, and the progesterone it secreted had ceased. Without progesterone, the lining had deteriorated, and the uterus, by means of the contractions that most women experience as menstrual cramps, had gotten rid of it. On that warm Friday evening in September, however, the scenario for Susan had changed. This time, when her ovary offered an egg, there had been eager takers. This time the egg hadn't dwindled but flourished, and the ovary had pumped out progesterone, and the progesterone had made the uterine lining lush.

It was this luxuriant uterine lining toward which the cell cluster, on the fourth day of its existence, was drawn. It had to reach the uterus and embed itself in that lining, with its bountiful supply of nutrient-rich blood, before its own food ran out. But there was a danger of ectopic pregnancy. The cluster might embed itself too early, before it arrived in the uterus, perhaps to the wall of the tube.

On Friday, the nineteenth of September, as Susan drove to work, as she waited on customers, as she ate her dinner, as she slept, the cluster drifted down toward the uterus. It was propelled by tiny hairs in the tube, which waved rhythmically, fanning it along. And then, at a highly significant moment of which Susan was unaware, it tumbled out of the duct and into the uterine cavity, a speck wafted into a vast scarlet cathedral.

The cluster had become a sphere with two distinct layers of cells surrounding a fluid center. Soon every one of the cells would be given a specific mission. The ones in the outer layer would be directed to create a brain for the MacGregor baby, and a spinal cord and nerves and skin. The inner layer would be told to create the lining of the baby's digestive tract, from its throat down through the stomach, liver, intestines, and anus. Later a middle layer of cells would develop, commissioned to produce its skeleton and muscles and some of its internal organs.

All this specialization would be directed by chemicals that carried the genetic information from the Sprague egg and the MacGregor sperm. These were the nucleic acids, and one of them, DNA, was especially influential. They would keep on directing events, making Susan and Tracy's child what its genetic heritage meant it to be. In response to their commands an infinity of physical structures, ranging from large to minuscule, would appear at the right time, in closely sequenced stages, and grow to the right size unless external influences—disease, for instance, or alien substances such as alcohol, lead, or mercury—gave the cells pernicious counterinstructions.

Lolling free in the uterus, the sphere of cells had undergone another change: a number of cells had congregated on one side of the ball, thickening it. On Sunday, the twenty-first of September, or thereabouts, this mass of cells, whose name, *embryo,* came from the Greek for "swelling," touched against the wall of the uterus, near the top, and started to dig in. At first the wall tissues reacted with antagonism, trying to envelop the invader. But the resistance turned to welcome, and the uterus rushed nourishment to the site. At last the MacGregor embryo had found its food source.

By its eighth day the embryo, though no bigger than a dot, barely visible, was busy. First it made itself an enclosing membrane—the amniotic sac, or bag of waters—and into it began secreting amniotic fluid to float itself in. And then it began to make perhaps the most brilliantly designed mechanism in the whole extraordinary apparatus of pregnancy, the placenta.

While the fetus's stomach and kidneys and lungs and so on were still under construction, it would need a way to get food and oxygen and dispose of wastes. Nature's answer was to let the baby use Susan's organs, through a link with her circulatory system. The service Susan would provide her child would be far more profound than mere garaging; she would eat for her baby, breathe for it, receive its wastes, and eliminate them. It would all be accomplished through a shared circulatory system. The blood vessels of the baby and the mother couldn't be hooked up directly. For one thing, babies often had blood types different from their mothers', and mixing them could be catastrophic. For another, if the link was direct, the baby would catch every virus its mother carried, be affected by every drug she took.

The alternative to direct hook-up was the placenta (Latin for "flat cake"), a disk-shaped organ that would serve as an indirect link between mother and baby. It filtered out certain viruses and some drugs, but it was more than a shield. It was an organ, one with biochemical functions to perform. It took chemicals from the mother's blood and broke them down into usable fuels for the baby.

The embryo made its own placenta. First it ruptured blood vessels in Susan's uterine wall. Then, into the pools of blood that resulted, it sent tiny projections called villi, minute extensions of the baby's circulatory system. The villi mingled with Susan's capillaries but were not joined to them. From that point on, the embryo absorbed food and oxygen from Susan's pooled and processed blood. Whenever the concentration of nutrients in the embryo's blood was lower than in Susan's, nutrients would automatically diffuse into the baby. Whenever the concentration of stale air and wastes was higher in the baby's blood than in Susan's, those substances would diffuse into Susan's circulatory system for her to exhale and excrete.

The embryo, soon to become the fetus, would feast greedily on this source from now on, its hunger always taking precedence. If nourishment ever became scarce, the baby would feed first, taking its fill from the mother's bloodstream, leaving her the leftovers, if any . . . a paradigm for mother's love, and for nature's law of survival.

The placenta, which was connected to the embryo by a long flexible cord made up of two arteries and a vein, would be strictly selective about the substances it would allow to pass through it to the baby; to a great degree it would bar harmful ones. Many of Susan's disease immunities, however, would pass through the placenta to the baby. They would last for about six months after birth, giving the baby temporary resistance against many serious ailments.

Over the next few weeks, through the end of the first month, the MacGregor embryo continued to map out the being to come. The nervous system was given the highest priority because—as the rest of the body developed—the nervous system would have to run it. In no time these new strands of neurons would be controlling the baby's movements. The first step was to establish the embryo's vertical axis, the line along which the spine would be laid. A bulge formed along the length of the embryo, the so-called primitive streak; it became the neural groove, a channel that, closed over, would become the spinal cord. Initially the groove was open. If all went well, the groove would close over the cord at the end of the month. The situation in which the cord failed to close is called spina bifida; it happens to some degree in 5 percent of babies, and there is a test for it.

Once the cord was closed, the brain would begin to form at the top of the tube and nerves would begin to radiate from the brain and cord to all parts of the embryo. As the spinal cord formed, thirty-three pairs of primitive vertebrae would start to sprout along it, the basis of the spinal column. The column would end in a tail, a remnant of our evolutionary ancestry. Unless the MacGregor baby was among the 6 percent who are exceptions, the tail would disappear during the pregnancy. If it failed to, the condition could be treated surgically after birth.

The heart also began as a tube, in due course it would develop four chambers. Just above the heart a large mouth appeared, one end of still another tube: the early digestive tract. It took three tries to form a kidney. The first effort would resemble the kidney of a primitive eel, the second would look like those of frogs and fishes, and finally a true human kidney would appear.

As the first month ended, the embryo was a quarter of an inch long, coiled in a tight semicircle like a shrimp. Eyes were forming on the sides of its large, nodding head, and soon they would start drifting around to the front. The whole foundation for its ineffably complex nervous system had been established. Its arms and legs were beginning to sprout, and forty-four pairs of muscles had been set up.

All this work, the origination of a human being, had been going on in September and October, entirely unknown to Susan and Tracy MacGregor, who went to the doctor because they thought Susan had the flu.

•   •   •

At 95 Northfield Avenue the staff put things away and got ready to go home. "That's one of the things I love about this job," Eleanore said as she shut down the computer.

"What is, El?" Bea asked.

"It's so touching to see couples after they've just found out, the husband and wife together, and both of them just so truly excited."

"Not every couple," Mary Jo said. "Some fathers are too macho to show emotion. And some people are just too bland to have much of a reaction at all."

"But most couples are wonderful," Eleanore insisted. "Like the MacGregors. They were so excited they didn't know how to express themselves. And they looked at each other so lovingly, and they were *laughing* with each other. They just couldn't believe it. They kept looking at each other and smiling."

Jack joined them. "Part of the charm," he said, "was that she really didn't know she was pregnant. She didn't have to spend months and months taking her temperatures and timing her sex life. She just suddenly *was*."

"I remember a patient whose period was very late," Bea said, "She had herself convinced that she had ovarian cancer. This was about ten years ago. She was sure she was very sick and was dying. She said, 'I haven't had my period.' And I said, 'Well, could you be pregnant?' She said, 'Pregnant? I've tried so many years to get pregnant. If I'm pregnant, I'll buy you a bottle of your favorite perfume.' I said, 'That's a deal.' I tested her and said, 'Let me give you the name of my favorite perfume.' And she said, 'You're kidding. I'm pregnant? My husband's not going to believe it. I brought him with me today because I was sure I was going to get bad news. They were gonna tell me I was gonna die.' I said, 'At the moment, my scent is Ralph Lauren's "Tuxedo." ' And she bought it for me. She still remembers. She had a little girl.

"She was sure she was dying. I told her, 'You're not dying, you're pregnant.' But you know," Bea added with her wry, seen-it-all smile, "sometimes it seems like the same thing."

•   •   •

Rod had already left, not for home but the hospital. The next morning he'd bring the staff the good news: Lizzie, the young woman who'd gone into labor right there in the office and deposited her son Justin at his grandmother's, had had her V-BAC. "An eight-pound girl," he said. "Popped it right out."

3.
Queasy

It was as if on the last day of Creation, as an afterthought, God had divided the pregnant of this world into two tribes. Some of the women were blessed with tranquil stomachs. But most were condemned to reel through bilious first trimesters, forever wistful because He hadn't left well enough alone.

Susan MacGregor, apparently, had sat at God's right hand. Throughout her pregnancy her stomach would be steady. Linda Cohen, however, another O'Driscoll-Bonamo patient, must have sat at the left. It was the third week in October, and she was three months pregnant, and nearly every day of those three months had been a trudge through billowing nausea. A whiff of someone's cigarette smoke could set her stomach heaving, or the sight of meat frying, or the taste of a vegetable she'd always loved. There was no safe time, no hour she could depend on for reprieve. Nausea might strike at any moment, instantly draining her strength, her stability, her control.

Linda and her husband lived in West Orange, but she worked in Manhattan, which meant that twice a day she had to ride rolling, pitching buses through stop-and-start traffic and a fume-choked tunnel under the Hudson River. Often at work she felt dreadful and wanted just to go lie down. But she couldn't. She was a travel agent, constantly on the phone. Her job took the composure and diligence of a short-order cook.

She hadn't planned to tell her boss about the pregnancy until she started to show, but the matter was taken out of her hands the week before. It was a Monday morning. She was three blocks from her office, crossing the street, when all of a sudden she was bending over vomiting. Two strangers gave her tissues and took her by the elbows and guided her to the curb. She recovered enough to walk to the office, but when she got there her face was white. Her boss, a sensitive and sympathetic woman, knew immediately; ever since Linda's wedding she'd been anticipating the day when Linda would come in and say she was pregnant. She helped Linda as much as she could. She dealt with a man in the next office who insisted on smoking. ("In Finland," she admonished him, "it's against the law to smoke near a pregnant woman." "This isn't Finland," he of course replied; but he obliged.) She even started planning an office baby shower for Linda.

"I feel awful," Linda told Rod O'Driscoll. "Sometimes I think I can't stand it another day."

The lamentations of the nauseated were a familiar litany in the obstetrical office. The doctors and staff heard it all day long.

"I can't even eat," Marion Todaro said to Jack Bonamo. Marion was a nurse for another obstetrician. "I've always been able to eat, no matter how I feel. But not today. Crackers, ginger ale, all those things I always tell women on the phone—nothing works. My mother, she's had six babies. She says to me, 'I never had a single pain with any of them.' But I feel awful."

"I spend all my time in 'B and B'," said Pat Becker. "That's bed and bathroom. Either I eat and get sick or I don't eat and get sick. It's like the worst possible hangover."

Morning sickness has baffled humankind since the beginning, but in this one category the ancients did manage to make some fairly good guesses. As today, diet was thought to play a role. The Greeks said the problem was salty foods; not only would they sicken the mother, said Aristotle, but shorten the child's life. The people of the Middle Ages believed peas and beans, which cause flatulence, should be avoided but that capons and partridges were helpful, along with lettuce, spinach, sorrel, and borage. Three hundred years ahead of her time, the seventeenth-century French author Madame de Sévigné said attitude was a factor. "Avoid gloom," she wrote to her ailing pregnant daughter. "You know that one cannot always be laughing," she said, "but try to be merry and gay. Be careful not to make any black bile."

To this day, no one knows for certain why four out of five women experience nausea during pregnancy. The most commonly cited villains are the hormones that regulate pregnancy, particularly human chorionic gonadotropin, or HCG. In the first trimester, HCG production booms, but by the start of the second three months, the layer of cells that produces most of the HCG has disintegrated, and the HCG supply drops off. As HCG fades away, so does the nausea. Another theory is that the intestines slow down during the first trimester, allowing acids to back up in the stomach. Some researchers believe that women with diets high in protein and low in carbohydrates and vitamin B6 are more susceptible to nausea while pregnant.

Although silent on the black bile question, most present-day experts agree with Madame de Sévigné that a woman's attitude makes a real difference. Anthropologists long ago noted that in primitive societies where women aren't raised to anticipate sickness in pregnancy, they usually don't get sick. In 1908, Aleš Hrdlička, a physician and explorer who visited hundreds of native American tribes, wrote that "pregnancy in its earlier stage generally interferes in no way with the woman's habits of life and occupation in any of the tribes. . . . Functional disturbances and diseases of pregnancy are much less frequent and serious than with white women." In 1938 a scholar named William Holden, studying Yaqui Indian women of Sonora, Mexico, wrote: "Pregnancy is a pleasure because [the Yaqui woman] experiences its stimulating and exalting effects and little of the nausea and illness so common with white women." One purely physical explanation for the lack of morning sickness in many third-world societies, if there is a lack, is that foods common to them such as yams, plantains, cassava, cornbread, tortillas, and rice and beans are not only excellent sources of complex carbohydrates but also easily digestible. (Another explanation may be that investigators sometimes romanticize the peoples they study and attribute superior virtues to them, particularly hardiness.)

There are other signs of a subjective aspect to morning sickness— a misnomer if there ever was one; doctors prefer the term pregnancy sickness. When women suffering from nausea are removed from the stresses of their daily lives and put in the calming atmosphere of a hospital, they often recover completely without treatment. Some studies show that nausea is more probable among women with unplanned pregnancies. Others indicate that women prey to morning sickness tend to be easy to hypnotize and are unusually susceptible to suggestion, presumably including their culture's implicit suggestion that if you get pregnant you get sick.

Whatever the theories, Linda Cohen and Pat Becker and Marion

Todaro, all of whom were ecstatic about their pregnancies, felt terrible. "I keep thinking my body's a mess," Linda said to Rod. "It's as if nothing inside me is right, everything's wrong. It's hard to believe that anything healthy and normal could be in there. I mean, these are the symptoms of sickness. I worry about the baby."

There is very little a doctor can tell a woman with morning sickness. ("You're going to feel better," Rod said to a patient. "That," she replied, "is what all the men say.") But when a woman expresses fears for the health of her baby, afraid that her sickness might affect it, doctors have news that is specific and encouraging.

"Your baby is fine," Rod told Linda. "In fact, women who have nausea and vomiting are likelier to have healthy pregnancies. Statistically, the sick mothers are likelier to keep their pregnancies and carry them all the way through."

Some biologists feel that morning sickness is one of evolution's brilliant accomplishments, meant to safeguard the baby. Mothers get sick so their babies will be healthy. "Pregnancy sickness," according to Margie Profet of the University of California at Berkeley, "is an adaptation that evolved to protect the embryo against toxins that cause malformations or abortions. Toxins that are extremely easy for an adult to handle can be dangerous for an early embryo." When embryos are in formation and are particularly vulnerable to chemical assault, Profet suggests, morning sickness forces pregnant women to avoid foods that contain natural toxins—including many vegetables and spices and some fruits—and instead choose bland, low-toxin foods like cereal, breads, and cheese, which are less likely to sicken them. She points to studies that found women with little or no morning sickness have two or three times the rate of miscarriage of women who do have nausea.

A researcher once made a comprehensive list of all treatments known to have been tried at one time or another. One was to immerse the woman in ice water or pack her in snow. Others included injecting her with honey or with her husband's blood or with some of his testosterone. In the absence of any approved remedy, doctors simply repeat the conventional advice: Don't eat three big meals; eat five little ones. Lie down for fifteen or twenty minutes after each meal, if you can. Have some crackers and milk before you get up in the morning and keep on lying there for another quarter of an hour. Have a snack when you go to bed; drink plenty of liquids but not in large quantities all once. Sip ginger ale; buy some natural ginger capsules at the health food store.

Another measure that some O'Driscoll-Bonamo patients tried was acupressure. Traditional Chinese medicine maintains that pressure applied to the "Nei-Kuan" acupuncture point, located on the inner wrist just above the hand, relieves nausea. Some Western practitioners believe that Nei-Kuan pressure reduces nausea after surgery or chemotherapy. In recent years sailors and fishermen have tried the technique on sea sickness and found it often works. A manufactured device helps them apply the pressure correctly. It consists of a pair of elastic bracelets, each with a protruding metal button sewn to its inner surface. Users are told to position the band so that the button presses between the two tendons on the inside of the wrist, about three finger-widths above the crease where the wrist meets the hand—the Nei-Kuan point. When the button presses against it for short intervals during the day, the company says, the nausea of pregnancy is usually eliminated or much reduced.

In 1988, a team of researchers in Belfast, Ireland, reported that among 350 nauseated pregnant women, the 119 who pressed the Nei-Kuan spot—for five minutes four times a day for four days—had "highly significant" improvement in their condition. In 1989 a smaller study was conducted in Baltimore and another in Connecticut and Oklahoma; both found wristbands effective on at least two-thirds of women involved.

Newspapers and women's magazines heard about these investigations and ran features on wristbands. Pregnant celebrities such as television newsperson Maria Shriver said they'd used wristbands for morning sickness and felt better. But most obstetricians remained hesitant. The U.S. Food and Drug Administration, which closely controls the claims that can be made for any medical device, had not yet approved wristbands as a treatment for the nausea of morning sickness, and doctors were reluctant even to appear to be prescribing them. Rod and Jack gave them a try. "They're like chicken soup," Jack said. "They couldn't hurt." Some patients were helped; others weren't.

Acupressure, however, was making its slow way into medical orthodoxy. During the same weeks and months that Linda Cohen and Pat Becker and Marian Todaro were going through their daily ordeal, sixty pregnant and nauseated Italian women were taking part in a study at Bologna University. The Bologna study used Sea Band, elastic bracelets sold in a variety of outlets including pharmacies, luggage shops, sporting goods and health food stores, dive shops, and marinas. It found that wristbands were effective 60 percent of the time. There had been other studies, of course, but this one was so carefully designed and executed that its findings were published in *Obstetrics & Gynecology,* the prestigious technical journal of the American College of Obstetrics & Gynecology. At last the use of acupressure for morning sickness was brought to the serious attention of the profession.

For Linda Cohen, unaware of acupressure and worried that nausea and vomiting might mean something was wrong with her baby, the best remedy came in the form of a sound. From the day that Rod O'Driscoll's sonar probe first found her child's heart and the examining room filled with the strong, vital thumping of the amplified beat, Linda felt a world better. "When I heard that heart," she told her mother on the phone that evening, "suddenly I realized that everything was right."

Pregnancy brings another gastric riddle—the sudden, intense cravings many expectant mothers develop for certain foods or drinks. Often they begin even before the woman knows she's pregnant, and to the alert they are a tip-off to her condition. Like morning sickness, they are thought to result from pregnancy's hormone jamboree: new chemicals sending bizarre messages. In some parts of the world, though, they are said to be the child's own wishes for special foods and are treated sympathetically and carefully indulged. In India the most common cravings are for sour fruits and vegetables such as green mangos and plums; in Malawi, grain husks and crab; in Thailand, powdered chalk.

When the cravings are for nonfood substances, the phenomenon is called "pica," from the Latin for magpie, the bird that eats anything. Parkland Memorial Hospital in Dallas questioned all the recently delivered women in its postpartum wing on one particular day. Many confessed to eating an amazing variety of substances including laundry starch, clay, flour, baking powder, baked dirt, and powdered bricks. Several women spoke of eating the frost that had formed in their freezers.

"No one knows why some women have these cravings," Jack said, "but some of them make good sense. Women crave starches, complex carbohydrates—pasta or rice or bread or potatoes—because they make them feel better. They neutralize the gastric juices. Women also have food loathings. One thing they dislike, for some reason, is chicken; a lot of women say that. They can't eat it. It nauseates them even to look at it."

Pica is fairly rare, but food cravings are common. Linda Cohen

had the classic American yen for pickles and chocolate ice cream,
though not together. Susan MacGregor's craving, too, was so ordinary it would never have landed her on Parkland Memorial's list:
cheeseburgers. She did not give in to it.

•   •   •

Judy Lombardy felt spherical. She stood just five feet tall, and during the five months she'd been pregnant she'd gained considerable
weight. Because she was small, the extra weight was clearly apparent. It troubled her, but another statistic worried her more—her age.
She was forty-three. Whenever there had been any sort of problem
during the pregnancy, she'd been quick to connect it to her age and
to the notion that in trying to have a baby at her stage of life she was
violating some principle of nature.

Obstetricians all over the country were seeing floods of older
mothers-to-be. For one thing, there were a great many more women
in the over-thirty-five age bracket than there used to be; the baby-
boomers, that immense generation born in the decades after World
War II, were now in their late thirties and early forties. Another reason was that large numbers of these women had done something that
masses of women had never done before: put off childbearing to
pursue careers. But now, with their so-called biological clocks winding down, many were delaying no longer. Births to women in their
thirties more than doubled during the 1980s, and births to those in
their forties increased 50 percent. The labor-and-delivery wings of
America were awash in what the medical establishment unchival-
rously called "elderly primagravidas"—older women having their
first babies.

Since girlhood Judy had dreamed of the day she'd have a baby.
She had eleven nieces and nephews, and she was like a second
mother to every one of them, a ready babysitter, happy to feed or
change or wheel any tot who needed tending—"a Mary Poppins figure," as she put it. But in college she'd developed another passion:
psychology. After college she worked full time as a school psychologist and at night took courses leading to a master's degree. As she
was finishing her degree the college, Seton Hall, added a doctoral
program, so she went on for her Ph.D. To pay for it, she held two
jobs. "I worked all day in the schools," she said, "and most nights I
taught psychology. Every other minute I studied. When the weekend came and most girls were out dating, I stayed home with my

books. I didn't allow myself that social part. I made my profession my priority. One thing just kept leading to another. I had to do a residency. Had to write a dissertation. Had to defend it. Two years of postdoctoral study. And so on. It went on forever. My career became enveloping. It just took me over. I loved it, but one day I looked up and I was forty."

She'd grown up knowing a boy named Michael Lombardy. Like Judy, he was Italian but as dark as she was fair. He got married in his mid-twenties, but after his wife gave birth to a little girl she died of cancer. It changed his idea of what was important in life. He wanted his daughter to have the attention of a loving woman, and his own mother was eager to give that attention, so he quit his job as an executive of the New Jersey Turnpike and sold his house and moved in with his parents. He went to work at the family gas station so he could be close to home.

"One day I happened to pull into Michael's gas station," Judy said, "and from that day on, whenever I came in, he was very friendly. He asked me out on a date, and we went dancing and stayed out till four. We got engaged a year ago Valentine's Day and married five months later."

Judy wanted a child, but Michael, having already lost one wife, was apprehensive. He was afraid that because of Judy's age something might happen to her. "We have to talk to a doctor," he said. "We have to make sure there's no risk."

Judy's parents were worried too, and Judy herself was concerned. She'd been raised with the assumption that an older woman courted many dangers when she became pregnant. The leading one was Down's syndrome—mongolism, mental retardation. The older a woman got, the greater her risk of having a baby with Down's syndrome. In mothers up to the age of thirty the risk of giving birth to a live infant with Down's was less than one in eight hundred, but the risk increased to about one in a hundred by age forty and one in thirty-two by age forty-five. The rates of other fetal afflictions, too, were thought to be dramatically higher in pregnancies of older women. All things considered, late-in-life babies were viewed with hesitation.

Judy's doctor had stopped practicing obstetrics to concentrate on gynecological problems. He referred her to three other doctors, one of whom was Rod O'Driscoll. Judy and Michael immediately liked him. "He had a soft way about him," she said. "He was very consoling. I'd always had menstrual problems, and he was so understanding and helpful. He gave you all the time you needed. He became like a friend."

Rod talked to Judy awhile and thoroughly examined her. Then he took her back into his office. Her age didn't worry him, he said. His practice was full of older mothers. "Monday morning, I delivered a woman forty-four years old. She never blinked an eye. On Wednesday Dr. Bonamo delivered one who's forty-two. Couldn't have gone better." In short, he said, things had changed. Women past forty who became pregnant weren't mocked anymore for engaging in sex past the "appropriate" period of life, no longer embarrassed into lying about their age. They were given psychological support, not scolded for playing Russian roulette with their babies and their lives.

Parallel to the revolution in women's roles that made some want to delay childbearing, there had been a revolution in technology. New tests—notably amniocentesis, which involved taking a small sample of the fluid surrounding the baby and analyzing it genetically, and CVS, another genetic sampling procedure, which could be performed as early as the eighth week—now made it easy to detect Down's syndrome, the most formidable threat. Women with good results on their tests had no greater reason to fear Down's than had women in their twenties. And women with unpromising results now at least had a choice. "With these tests they have today," Rod said, "what you do is, you follow the pregnancy closely and make decisions as they come up."

That wasn't all. A study of more than half a million births in British Columbia indicated that except for Down's, an older woman really doesn't have a greater risk of having children with defects. The woman's health is the key thing. People are of course increasingly likely to suffer from disease the older they get, and some diseases—diabetes, for example, and high blood pressure—can cause birth defects as well complications that can threaten the lives of both babies and mothers. But if a woman is healthy, her chances of having a healthy baby are the same as any woman's. In fact, the British Columbia study found that children of older mothers actually had less of three birth defects: dislocatable hip, a narrowing of the stomach, and a heart problem called patent ductus arteriosus.

Not that the experience of childbearing is the same for an older woman as for a twenty-year-old. For one thing, there is a difference in muscle tone. The uterus of the younger woman usually does a better job of pushing out the baby. But the older mother has her advantages. In some ways her age works for her. Her financial circumstances may be better, and she may be more secure in her career. Her maturity and her depth of experience in life work in her favor when she faces the trials of bearing and rearing a child.

To Rod, childbirth at Judy's age was distinctly "doable," but he did have one concern. Older couples, he said, often had trouble conceiving. The Lombardys had only a little; after six months of trying, it happened. A month later Judy had an ultrasound; a technician sent sound waves into her uterus and produced a moving, X-ray–like image of its contents. The fetus looked fine. Two months after that she had an amniocentesis. When the results were ready, she made Michael come with her to hear them. Rod immediately told them there was no evidence of Down's syndrome.

"I'm in my fifth month now," Judy said as she waited to be called into an examining room, "and my biggest fear is that something still might go wrong. Of course Italians are great worriers. We're both from Old World families, and they can be morbid. Superstitious. A woman in the supermarket says, 'How cute,' but an Italian will think she might be giving the baby the evil eye. It's called 'overlooking' the baby, wishing the evil eye on it. So you've got to say God bless. But not just God bless. God-bless-God-bless-God-bless. My grandmother, she taught us all the special prayers you can do. It's funny. I'm a social scientist, I have my doctorate, but when it comes to something I really care about, all that doesn't matter. I say the prayers."

Rod examined Judy and gave her his findings. "The baby's fine, but his mama, she's something else. Your blood pressure is still high."

"It's the anxiety," Judy explained. "We're very happy, but at the same time there's a sort of negative excitement around this whole birth experience—not really knowing what to anticipate, the fear I won't be able to stand the labor."

"I understand that," Rod said. "Everybody goes through these things. But I'll tell you what I think it really is. You're not really taking it easy, the way I told you. Am I right? When are you really and truly going to cut back on your work hours?"

Once again Judy promised to slow down her practice, to start discontinuing patients.

"Except for your pressure," Rod said, "everything is great. But," he added with fatherly authority, "you've got to ease off on your practice. You have too much invested in this to take the chance."

4.
Legacies

On the brisker November days, such as this one, the patients were wearing coats again, jamming them into the small coat closet at 95 Northfield Avenue and causing the familiar traffic problems in the hall. The woman who appeared in the reception room this evening for her monthly OB visit avoided all that; she kept her car coat on, huddling in it on the sofa. She was very thin and though only thirty-four looked older. Her skin was pallid, her complexion lifeless, and as she spoke to the secretary her voice was dull and indistinct. Her first child, a two-year-old girl in green corduroy overalls, clung to her leg, ignoring the colorful toys scattered around the room.

That morning, seeing the woman's name on his daily appointments list, Rod O'Driscoll had shaken his head. "She's a poor soul," he'd said. "An alcoholic. Comes from one of those families that's full of alcoholics. She won't let you say anything about it." Then he'd paused. "What really upsets me," he'd gone on in a softer voice, "is her child. I just don't think she's all right. The shape of her head. Her expression. Her listlessness. She doesn't seem right to me. And I'm worried about the one she's carrying."

There was a chasm between that woman, who was drinking heavily while pregnant, and the woman sitting across from her, Gail Bryan, the most moderate of social drinkers.

A few minutes later, as Gail sat on the examining table waiting for Rod O'Driscoll to come see her, she told the nurse, Bea Perez, about an episode that was still bothering her. The week before, she and her husband had gone to a luncheon. Pregnant with her second child, three weeks to go, she was seated next to a young man whose wife was newly pregnant with their first child. The hostess offered wine, and Gail took a glass of red.

"This man was appalled," Gail said. "He said to me, 'I can't believe you're drinking. Haven't you read the articles on fetal alcohol syndrome?' "

If the man had expected Gail to burst into apologies and pledges to reform, he had picked the wrong woman. She was a self-assured thirty-seven-year-old banker's wife from the wealthy New Jersey suburb of Upper Montclair, who, because of her marriage to an Englishman and several years of living in London, spoke with a trace of British accent. She wasn't easily cowed. And her tormentor couldn't have picked a worse moment to accost her. She was thoroughly fed up with gratuitous intrusions by the aggressively well-meaning, and fed up with the load of guilt that was being dumped on pregnant women.

"I gave him my coldest look," she said to Bea, "and I told him, 'Listen. I didn't have cocktails. I'm having just one glass of wine. My obstetrician said that an occasional glass of wine won't hurt. I am going to have this glass of wine no matter what you or anyone else tells me.' "

The young man had come right back at her, full of certitudes. She began to feel tormented by his lecture. It was as if a perfect stranger had walked in off the street and told her she was voting wrong.

Rod came into the examining room and examined her. A few minutes later, talking with Bea down the hall at the secretary's desk, Gail picked up her topic again. "The more you read about what they think is toxic," she said, "the more you think you probably shouldn't ever eat or drink a thing throughout your entire pregnancy. But the worst part is the thought of hordes of people watching what you're doing and being judgmental. In the past, people looked at a pregnant woman as healthy and blissful and believed that she'd just naturally do what made sense to her. Sometimes I think the bliss has gone out of it entirely."

If she had a cup of coffee somewhere, she would find herself bracing in anticipation of the comment "You're drinking *coffee?*" The intruders were aware of the early cautions about caffeine and pregnancy, but they apparently weren't aware of the authoritative recent studies reporting that normal amounts of caffeine were harmless to babies in the womb. But their favorite topic was alcohol.

She was just as concerned about the health of her baby as any mother, and she took the scientific findings and the doctor's warnings seriously. But there was something about the way people went after pregnant women that seemed less like compassionate concern and more like harassment. It made her angry.

Fifteen days later, Rod O'Driscoll delivered Gail's baby, William. He weighed seven pounds three ounces and seemed in all ways flawless. To Gail, that appeared to prove something, if only that people zapping pregnant women ought to improve their manners along with their information.

•   •   •

Until several decades ago, women seldom made the connection between what they put into their mouths and what happened in their wombs. Then came a massive tragedy that laid the groundwork for enlightenment. In the 1950s, twelve thousand women who had taken the drug thalidomide as a sleeping pill gave birth to severely deformed children. The scandal horrified the world. It provided a dramatic example of how poisonous substances can pass from the mother's blood, via the placenta, into the baby, and of how poisons can affect fetal development. The thalidomide horror ushered in a new era of toxic consciousness.

Many researchers set out to expand this hard-won truth. Some were on the faculty of the University of Washington, which they soon made into a center for studying the effects of drinking on pregnancy. In 1973, two Washington researchers gave a name to a pattern of defects that seemed to afflict children of mothers who drank heavily. They called it fetal alcohol syndrome, or FAS. FAS children tended to be poorly developed. They were usually small; their growth in the womb was hampered. Their heads were undersized, and their faces were misshapen: Their faces were flat, their noses short, the bridge of their noses low, their upper lips thin. Their hearts could be defective and their nervous system impaired, and they usually had trouble learning.

In the mid-1970s Ann Streissguth, a developmental psychologist at the University of Washington, and others published reports that children born to heavy drinkers (five drinks or more daily) were much likelier to be blighted. Streissguth followed FAS children over a number of years and found they had trouble in school; their IQs were low; they learned badly; their attention span was short. She and her associates estimated that five thousand babies a year were born with FAS, with another thirty-six thousand less severely but still badly affected. In 1981, prompted by these findings, the Surgeon General of the United States declared that "women should not drink alcoholic beverages during pregnancy because of the risk of birth defects." Eight years later Congress ordered that the labels on containers of alcoholic beverages advise pregnant women of its dangers.

Streissguth had also been studying the possibility that lesser levels of drinking might also affect fetuses. Large, well-conducted studies repeatedly confirmed that pregnant women who drank in moderation—defined as just two drinks a day—hurt their babies. These women were more apt to miscarry or to deliver prematurely than women who drank no alcohol. The studies demonstrated that social drinkers' children had more birth defects, lower IQs, and more learning problems. Alcohol use by pregnant women was revealed as the leading known cause of mental retardation in newborns. Even when social drinking was stopped early, as soon as a woman learned she was pregnant, there could still be a long-term impact on the IQ because so much crucial development takes place in the fetus's first two months.

"The effect on children," said Dr. Streissguth, "occurs even at the social drinking level. The women in our study did not see themselves as having alcohol problems." The report noted that some of the heaviest drinkers in the study, and thus the mothers whose children were most at risk, were the most highly educated professionals. "Many career women," Dr. Streissguth said, "assume the drinking habits of professional men—a few glasses of wine at dinner, some drinks over lunch or at a cocktail party."

In 1990 Dr. Streissguth uttered the words that rocked female revelers from coast to coast. "We recommend," she said, "that women who are trying to become pregnant or might become so do not drink alcohol at all." "Might become so" meant that unless she wanted to take chances with the health of her future children, a sexually active woman of childbearing years should not drink. Period. This was a staggering notion in a country where 55 percent of women over seventeen drank moderately.

Soon other reports confirmed the findings. One said that at the consumption level of one to two drinks *weekly,* the chances of miscarriage increased. Another noted that the distinction pregnant women made between beer, wine, and liquor was a fantasy: The standard serving of each contains about the same amount of absolute alcohol—half an ounce.

The reactions were predictable—denial, guilt, intense concern, all three of which were displayed in early 1991 in a trivial incident at a Red Robin Restaurant in suburban Seattle. A pregnant woman ordered a raspberry daiquiri from a twenty-two-year-old waiter named G. R. Heryford.

G. R. Heryford was dismayed. He asked another waiter, twenty-one-year-old Danita Fitch, what she thought. She thought it was terrible, and she went over to the customer and asked her if she really wanted that drink. The customer, distressed, emphatically replied yes, she really did want the drink. Danita Fitch then found a beer bottle and showed the woman the Surgeon General's warning. The customer blew up, and the manager came over.

"We just tried to inform the woman," G. R. Heryford said.

"They tried to make me feel like a child abuser or something," said the customer, "and they were just plain rude."

"I was a week overdue," the customer told the newspapers afterward. "I had been very careful throughout the whole pregnancy, and I thought it would be safe to have just this one drink, which I ordered with dinner. I went there to eat, not to drink."

The two young waiters were fired. They promptly launched an unsuccessful campaign to get the state's liquor control board to allow restaurants and taverns to refuse to serve liquor to pregnant women. A week after the fracas at the Red Robin, the customer gave birth to a healthy baby boy.

There was another kind of reaction. In a piece in *The New York Times,* Jean Mager Stellman, an associate professor of public health at Columbia University, and Joan E. Berlin of the American Civil Liberties Union asked why women were being made to bear the whole responsibility for producing healthy babies. There were studies showing that chronic drinking in men, too, could cause genetic mutations or other changes in sperm that could cause defects. "How," they asked, "could only women be responsible for producing perfect children?"

Some studies indicated that fathers who had more than two drinks a day had smaller-than-average infants. There were signs that fetuses fathered by drinkers were more prone to miscarriage. Researchers pointed out that sperm are easier to damage genetically than eggs are. It is when cells divide that they are most susceptible to genetic damage. Eggs don't divide at all—when a woman is born, she comes equipped with a lifetime supply—but the cells that produce sperm cells are champion dividers and therefore all the more vulnerable to the devastations of toxins. On the other hand, as *The New England Journal of Medicine* pointed out, if a man and a woman of similar weight drink the same amount of alcohol, 30 percent more alcohol will enter the woman's bloodstream because women have less of a certain stomach enzyme that digests alcohol.

One baby in every fourteen is born with a birth defect, physical or mental. Some are not severe, but other are serious flaws that might affect a child the rest of its life—missing limbs, major heart problems, cleft lip and palate, and spinal and brain irregularities that could cause paralysis. There are thought to be over 900 toxic substances that can cause defects. One common source of those substances is drugs; a tenth of pregnant women in America take illegal drugs. But the major source is alcohol. And from what their studies reveal, it has become clear to many scientists that like a drinking mother, a prospective father who drinks is increasing the odds that his baby will be defective.

So the point seems made at last. Women, though not absolved of responsibility, are no longer alone in bearing it. Both parents, in a world in some ways increasingly hostile to fetal health, have to do what they can to protect their babies. For male or female, the task can prove punishingly hard.

To the staff at Rod and Jack's office a particularly stirring example was the battle that one of their patients had waged to have a healthy baby. Sitting in the reception room that evening, wearing casual suburban clothes and nothing much in the way of makeup, Beth Keyser immediately registered as an exceptionally handsome woman. Her hair was dark brown, her dark eyes were deeply set, and her eyebrows were arched like those of a 1930s movies tragedienne. Her voice was husky and she spoke rapidly, with a Brooklyn accent and a trace of ironic, self-deprecating Brooklyn shtick. Beth's manner, slightly bossy, was the sort that usually didn't go over too well with the staff at 95 Northfield. She seemed like the kind of patient who would soon be phoning with imagined complaints or off-the-wall questions like which outfit she should wear to the hospital when the baby came. It would have been normal for Bea, no long-sufferer, to be aloof with Beth, but Bea clearly liked her.

"She knows who she is and what she is," Bea said.

Whenever the subject of Beth came up, someone would say, with sympathy and admiration, "She's been through a lot." What Beth Keyser had gone through to have a child was a struggle against a triple addiction: bulimia, drugs, and alcohol.

Beth had been brought up in a kosher Jewish family in Brooklyn. Her father was a "garmento"—he owned a manufacturing company in Manhattan's garment district. "Nobody in the family drank, as a rule," she said, "but once or twice a year, on special occasions, my father would open the liquor cabinet. I was ten or eleven years old, and I just started to drink, to get attention. Just a few sips, but it would get me drunk. Everybody thought it was cute, and after a while it even began to taste good. As soon as the bar was opened, I'd immediately head for the Southern Comfort and the Wild Turkey. Great names, but boy, what they did to me!"

Her mother was forty when Beth was born. Although Beth loved her, they never could connect. She had four brothers, one of whom was her twin, but no sister to ally with or model herself on. To make matters worse, her twin brother was a star, always excelling, and Beth felt she walked in his shadow.

"I was very spoiled," she said. "I had my own car before I had my driver's license. I always had what I wanted. But no one ever told me how to deal with setbacks. As I grew up, if something was bothering me, I went right to the alcohol or, later, the drugs."

A bright child, she entered high school two years early and had a hard time finding her spot. "One day, I'd go to school and rehearse with the cheerleaders," she said. "I got to be captain of the pom-pom girls. But the next day I'd cut classes and fix my hair some wild way and put on my worn-out jeans and go down to Greenwich Village to hang out and smoke pot. By the time I got to college—I was just sixteen—I was doing a pretty steady diet of pills. I discovered that Black Beauties, uppers, were good for diet control."

She nevertheless made the dean's list at college, then entered the training program for a chain of department stores. In just two years she was promoted to buyer. She married and six months later learned that her husband, a salesman who traveled a great deal, was seeing other women. "I didn't know how to live through the pain," she said, "so I did drugs and started with cocaine. I used to go out with my friends after work, go to bars, and drink and do coke."

She got divorced and started working for her father. She created her own division of his company, featuring loungewear. Soon she was making a lot of money. "I worked in the showroom, and when customers came in I would get very, very hyper. So between customers I would go into the bathroom and snort coke."

She'd developed one more problem along the way. When her husband had turned to other women, she'd decided there must be something wrong with her, and she became obsessed with losing weight. She became bulimic: She'd gain twenty-five pounds or so and then, instead of vomiting it away, as many bulimics do, she'd exercise fanatically. She'd spend at least an hour and a half a day on her stationary bicycle, a frantic, lonely peddler, then do calisthenics, then climb onto her rowing machine. Sometimes she'd exercise four hours a day. Her job, her social life, everything was made to work around her exercise schedule.

This went on for several years, until she met a young orthopedist named David Keyser. He was kind and steady, qualities she was hungry for in a man, and she fell in love with him. Not wanting to lose him—he didn't know she had a drug problem—she tried to tone down her act. Right after they were married there was an incident that gave her extra incentive. "We were living at Fifty-fifth Street and First Avenue," she said. "One morning I went downstairs to get some groceries. I got down to the corner and couldn't remember where I was. I finally got back to the apartment somehow, and I said to myself, 'No more coke.' " She stuck to it.

Beth and David wanted a baby, but she couldn't get pregnant. "I'd stopped doing cocaine," she said, "but I was still doing pills, and I was still crazy with the exercise, to the point where I had absolutely no body fat and would lose my period for months at a time. Every month I wanted so badly not to get my period because I wanted to be pregnant, but I'd dread not getting my period because I knew I had taken all these pills. I'd say to myself, 'If I *am* pregnant, what am I doing to my unborn child?' "

She and David went to Rod O'Driscoll to see if he could help her conceive. He did some tests and told Beth to quit her job and to try to relax. She tried, and the next time she saw Rod he told her she was pregnant. He asked her the routine questions about the medications she was using. At that time she was taking Valium and Librium and Xanax and odds and ends. She didn't tell him about the heavy stuff, just the odds and ends. She didn't think of it as lying.

In her view she didn't lie; she just left things out.

But she did stop using drugs altogether and stayed off them all the way through her pregnancy. Nothing—not even an aspirin. When she was seven months pregnant, she and David went to a doctors' party at his hospital, and she took one sip of wine. The baby began to kick hard, which terrified her. That was that; no more. It was her only lapse.

"When the baby was born," she said, "I was so afraid it would be wrong somehow. But when they put her in my arms, she just looked up at me and sighed and went to sleep next to me. My little Lisa. She was perfect. Six pounds, fourteen ounces. Twenty-one inches long. Just the sweetest little thing. I loved her. I didn't know how to change a diaper, I didn't know from anything."

The delivery had been ordinary. Like many women, she'd had an episiotomy, an incision from her vagina toward her anus to widen the vaginal outlet and avoid haphazard tearing of the flesh. The night of the birth a nurse came in and asked, "Do you want something to help you sleep?" To the addict in Beth, that seemed like a great idea, and she accepted a Percocet and some Seconal. "Pretty soon I'm on cloud nine, just flying around the hospital, and I'm not feeling any pain, and everything is wonderful and beautiful." Four hours later she got more, and more after that, and she took some home from the hospital.

"As usual, I didn't want to face things. Here I was, thirty-one years old, wanting a kid more than anything else because that was the next step in life, but I still hadn't grown up, and I didn't know what the hell I was doing with the kid."

She did know enough to know she should not breastfeed. "I was taking all those chemicals," she said. "I couldn't feed my baby that stuff." When she got home from the hospital, her breasts swelled enormously, and she was in severe pain. That meant more pills and an all-out return to addiction.

David hired a practical nurse. Four days after the birth, Beth was back on her exercise equipment, and the nurse took care of the baby. Beth would get up in the morning, do her exercises, visit the nursery, take her pills, and be in her cloud for the rest of the day. After two weeks, the nurse left, and then she was a mother. She didn't know how to manage. It was overwhelming.

As strong as her dependence on pills became, they weren't the most important thing in her life. "Exercise was number one, pills were number two, and Lisa was up there with them, kind of, sort of. It hurts to say it, but I took care of Lisa out of guilt most of the time, and I really resented her because she kept me from doing my exercises when I wanted. We're talking about heavy addiction. But I never did anything to hurt her, and if she had a dirty diaper, I'd say, 'Oh, fuck,' and get off my bicycle or rowing machine and change her.

"I've got a lot to be thankful for, because it could have gotten a lot worse. I never abused her, I never hit her, I never did anything like that. But I wasn't there for her. I hugged her, I kissed her, but I would rather have been someplace else. Thank God for my husband. He was so good with her. He'd get up with her in the middle of the night when I was too stoned. I can't believe he didn't even know what was wrong with me. Or maybe he knew that there was nothing he could do. An addict has to hit bottom herself."

And then something happened. It was eight on a Monday evening, and she had gone through four powerful pain pills since four that afternoon. She became nauseated and paranoid, and she began to see that it wasn't fun anymore. The pills were ruling her life, putting her on edge, making her impatient with Lisa. Two of Beth's brothers were staying with the Keysers, and sitting with them and with David she burst into tears and admitted her addiction.

She had been going to a therapist for several months for her bulimia and her exercising mania. He had been treating her with aversion therapy, putting her exercise on a schedule she had to follow, and he'd started to work on her low self-esteem. Now she called the therapist and said, "I need your help."

The therapist told her to come right over, and after she had blurted it all out, he said, "You have three choices. One is to get into AA. The second is to kick it yourself. And if you don't do one or the other, I'm going to put you away for a month."

"I'll kick it myself," she said.

But it didn't work. The pill-taking continued. "And all this time," Beth said, "Lisa went on her merry way. The only reason she's a normal kid—I can say it in one word: David."

At a family celebration a few months later, David took a Polaroid picture of Beth. She looked at it and was horrified. Her face was so thin. There were bags under her eyes. She looked like a drug addict. On the way home she said to David, "I don't want to be like this anymore." She went back to the therapist. He wanted to put her in a rehab. She said no and phoned a close friend, someone who'd been through her own hell, and that friend took her to AA. She started going to meetings every day.

Withdrawal was a nightmare. She'd had no idea what it would be like. Coming down off pain-killers, as many as ten a day after five P.M., she was racked by anxieties and paranoia. She heard voices. Her heart pounded. Sometimes she ran around the room like a mad person, one step from diving out the window. After five weeks she was still a wreck, but gradually she regained control.

"That was a year ago," she said, "and I haven't had a pill or a drink since. The bottom line is, the reason I finally did it is because I didn't want to pass this legacy on to my daughter. One day Lisa came to me and said, 'Mommy, I don't feel so good, give me a Tylenol.' That really pushed a button with me. I didn't want her to start, even with Tylenol. I said to her, 'Sweetheart, medicine doesn't make you feel better. You don't take medicine unless you're sick.' I went through a whole big thing about it. And I told her food doesn't make you feel better, either. I said, 'Sometimes the best thing is just a hug from Mommy.'

"Months later we were in Florida, and she said to me, 'Mommy, I don't want to be a junkie when I grow up. Drugs kill.' She'd seen it on TV. I said, 'I know.' We had a whole discussion about drugs. At first my heart broke because this child was not even four years old. But this was something that she had to start being educated about.

"I've tried so hard to build her up and give her self-esteem and tell her that she's wonderful. I want to make her love herself, because I think that was my problem. I just don't want what happened to me to happen to my children."

•   •   •

Lisa was four now, and Beth was still holding her own against her addictions. She had to. This appointment at 95 Northfield Avenue was not routine gynecological. It was obstetrical. In May, Beth was expecting her second child.

5.
Friday

It was a routine obstetrical Friday in early November. In the last few minutes before office hours, the four women on duty that day— Bea Perez, the nurse; two secretaries, Barbara Valente and Genevieve Collins; and Eleanore Steel, who handled collections— were having a second breakfast in the tiny room at the far end of the crooked corridor. No one had ever said so, but the room was understood to be reserved for the staff; if one of the doctors came in, he came on sufferance and tended to stand near the door rather than sit. There was a microwave and a refrigerator and an old sofa, useful for those moments when things up front got impossible and one of the staff felt like lying down.

Someone always came with pastry, and this morning Eleanore had provided a gooey coffee cake. As they ate it they talked about diets, as they always did when they ate rich food. Then they had their usual Friday morning conversation about last night's episode of *L.A. Law*.

"That was luscious," Genevieve said when she finished her cake. She wiped her fingers on a paper napkin, taking care not to get crumbs on her white trousers.

"Better than sex," Barbara said. The remark made heads spin, and Barbara laughed and looked mischievous. "My husband and I," she explained, "like to make lists of things that are better than sex."

"From what you've told me about Bob," Bea said, "it must be a short list."

"Fairly short," Barbara said, "and everything on it is edible."

Bea looked at her wristwatch. "Nine A.M.," she said, rising. "Man your positions, ladies. Let's do it to them before they do it to us."

As the registered nurse, Bea ran things during office hours. She was the top sergeant, the majordomo, the commanding figure at the center who kept the patients moving in and out and the doctors co-ordinated. She had curly auburn hair, big blue eyes that popped, and the sort of generous figure that Latin men are said to admire, which was fortunate because her husband, Oscar, was Cuban.

Bea herself was born in a tiny town above Edinburgh, Scotland, the daughter of a coal miner. When she was ten, her hair done in long braids that were doubled back and tied with big bows, the family sailed to America. Her father found work as a mechanic for a chemical company. Bea's mother had always wanted to be a nurse, and Bea set out to fulfill her mother's dream.

While still a nursing student, she met a young Cuban exile named Oscar Perez, who had fought against Castro and now worked as a maintenance man in the same hospital where Bea was apprenticing. He bought her a cup of tea, and as she sipped she noticed he had particularly well-shaped lips. Their first date they went dancing. Bea had been so nervous about the evening that she'd skipped dinner, and now, on an empty stomach and new to alcohol, she had several drinks, with the predictable result. She leaned toward Oscar. "You know," she said, "you have the most beautiful mouth." With that she slipped off her barstool. Oscar picked her up and helped her back onto her stool.

Immensely embarrassed, she was sure that was the end of the friendship. It wasn't. Cuban and Scot, Latin and Celt—they came from wildly different cultures, but though their marriage was frequently compared to the Lucy-Desi Show, it worked. They had a son, Adam. Oscar became a plumber. He was Rod's plumber, in fact, and also his friend. The O'Driscolls and the Perezes had often been in each other's home.

At Bea's prompting Barbara and Eleanore and Genevieve gathered up the paper plates and put their cups in the sink and went down the hall to their desks. Barbara phoned the answering service and told them that the office was in operation now and the calls should come through directly. The waiting room was already full.

Bea surveyed a handwritten copy of the appointments schedule. Every name meant something to her. There were women she liked and would be happy to see and women she would have to pretend to

like. There were women who were breezing through pregnancy and
women with reproductive histories that shrouded them like the epic
tales trailing the heroes of yore: a stalwart quest for motherhood despite a series of heartbreaking miscarriages, a pregnancy undertak-
en in the face of a risk to the mother's life, a pregnancy finally
achieved after years of infertility.

To the greatest extent that it could, the office kept the obstetrical
patients separate from the gynecological patients. "It's exceeding-
ly difficult," Bea said, "if you have suffered a loss, had a miscarriage, and you come to be checked, and there are three mothers
out there with brand-new babies. It's very hard if you're struggling
with infertility and can't conceive, and you come on a day with all
these bellies and all these kids crawling all over the floor. You may
be sixty-five and 'Enough of this already, I don't want to know from
young women, who only make me feel older because they're having
babies and I'm too old.' So there are times for the GYNs and times
for the OBs." All the women today were obstetrical.

The atmosphere varied according to which kind of day it was.
GYN days were quiet. The patients sat there matter-of-factly, some
of them looking as if they'd prefer to be anywhere else. They seldom
spoke to each other. OB patients, however, readily chatted, comparing experiences and swapping stories. The pace was different
too; the doctors handled three OB appointments every fifteen minutes but three GYN patients every half hour.

OB appointments went rapidly because nearly all pregnancies,
after a certain point, went well. "If I'm doing beautifully and there's
nothing to worry about," one woman in her seventh month asked
Rod O'Driscoll, "why do I have to come so often?" The reason was
that in the relatively rare situations when problems developed they
could arise swiftly, and prompt detection could make a great difference. The obstetrician's job mainly involved watching and checking and answering questions and making suggestions that had more
to do with comfort than with health.

Barbara and Genevieve were on the phones. "You have nausea?"
Barbara asked sympathetically. "That's the way it is sometimes in
the first trimester." She waited a moment while the patient talked.
"Listen," she said, "it sounds like you're really doing well. It'll be
over in the next few weeks. The second trimester is much nicer. I
can almost promise you it'll be over soon."

Genevieve was talking to a woman who thought she might be

pregnant and wanted a pregnancy test. "Yes," she said, "that's right. First morning urine."

Barbara took a call from a gynecology patient. "You can expect bleeding during the first week on those pills," she said.

"The only appointments left are Wednesdays," Genevieve was telling a caller. "No, we don't have any on Friday nights." Her eyebrows lifted in astonished indignation. "No, the doctors don't see people on Sundays! *Wednesday afternoons!*" The pressure for appointments, and for a few words from the doctors, was relentless.

"You'll love this one," Barbara said to Genevieve. "I just talked to Mrs. Davis. She said that the last time she called she'd spoken with 'one of the older ladies.' " Barbara and Genevieve both knew whom Mrs. Davis had talked to.

"Thanks," Genevieve said. Genevieve, just forty, was the youngest of the staff members, but her voice was a little deeper and her manner more formal.

"I told her we didn't have any older ladies here," Barbara said.

"Thanks again."

Once, at the busiest moment of the morning, a patient had asked Genevieve to fill out a complicated insurance form for her. "I can't do it now," Genevieve snapped. "Come back in an hour." When the patient came back, she brought an armload of gladiolas for her. Ever since, when flowers were delivered to the office, someone would say, "Oh, Genevieve was bad again," and Genevieve, still embarrassed, would put her hands over her face.

Until five years before, Genevieve had been a secretary to a hematologist at St. Barnabas, a job that involved seeing a lot of people get bad news about their blood tests. "One day I decided I couldn't stand death anymore," she said. "I looked in the paper for another job, and I saw an ad with a phone number. I said, 'I recognize that number.' It was the number of my own obstetrician, Dr. O'Driscoll, the guy who delivered both my babies. I called him up and he said, 'Get up here fast.' " She loved the job. In her time with the practice she had never taken a sick day. "I'd be afraid I'd be missing something," she once said, a humorous explanation that had some truth in it.

For Bea and Barbara, Eleanore and Genevieve, the office was a source of a loving female companionship that nourished their lives. It was also a continuing entertainment, a drama in which each of them, and the doctors as well, had been assigned a character to play—her own self slightly caricatured—and they relished their parts. Bea was outspoken and outrageous, Barbara sweet but mischievous, Genevieve tart of tongue but with a heart of gold, and Eleanore lovably ditsy. There was, of course, a great deal more to each of them. Bea, for example, though outrageous, was sensitive and much loved by many of the patients. Eleanore was adept at running the computer, tending the practice's finances, and collecting on overdue bills—none of it work for the ditsy. But there was enough truth in the exaggerations to make them fun. To be out a day would be like missing an episode of one's favorite soap. So no matter how they felt, they came to work, not just Genevieve but all of them. The sum of the combined annual sick days taken by the staff, a total of eight women, was seldom more than six.

Every five minutes or so, Bea would come to the door to the waiting room and summon another patient. "Nancy? We're ready for you. How you feeling? Okay? Good. Come on in." And five minutes later, more or less, Bea or one of the doctors would show a woman out.

"Genevieve," said Rod O'Driscoll, ushering a young, pink-clad, titanically pregnant woman back down the narrow hall, "I'd like Sheila to come again tomorrow so I can take her blood pressure."

Ten minutes later Rod came down the hall with a short blond woman they all seemed to know well. "You'll have to start watching your weight," he told her. "You've gained about twenty-seven pounds already."

"Where is it?" said the woman. "It doesn't show in my face."

"Don't worry, honey," said Bea, "it's right behind you." The patient laughed.

The phones kept ringing, and Barbara and Genevieve kept picking them up. The secretaries, who had had varying amounts of nursing training, all had abundant experience in talking with pregnant women and were fluent in the O'Driscoll-Bonamo approach. The patients all wanted to speak to the doctors, and the secretaries' art was knowing who really needed to and who didn't. They were masters of the understanding, legitimately reassuring, brief answer. They weren't doctors, more like extremely well-informed friends, and in most cases that was all the caller needed.

"You're still having some, uh, problems?" Barbara said to a caller with concern. "Did the medication help you last time? Can Dr. Bonamo call you in an hour? He's not in yet. Oh, you can't talk at work, right? Okay, I'll have him call you at home, then. . . . Right, and in the meantime, you won't worry, will you? It's not necessarily something to worry about, you know that. . . . Okay, dear, bye."

"You're coming in Monday, right?" Genevieve said to a patient named Karen. "Remember, at eight-thirty you drink the orange liquid."

Each staffer seemed almost unconsciously aware of when another was tied up and automatically filled in. When both Genevieve and Barbara were on the phones and something urgent came up, Eleanore, in the adjacent room where she and her computer kept company, would sense it immediately. She would drop whatever she was doing and dart into the main area, handle the exigency, and duck back into her quarters. At times the office seemed like an air-control tower or the Tokyo stock exchange.

While handling the phone, Genevieve was also making appointments, taking payments from patients, and giving them insurance receipts.

"I know I owe you," a patient said to her, "but I forgot my money. I'll get it next time, okay?"

"Okay," said Genevieve, whose expression suggested she'd heard that one a million times before. Some 6 percent of patients who didn't pay on the spot never paid at all.

Bea came down the hall with a first-time mother-to-be whose due date was imminent. "The doctor said I might want some anesthetic—an epi-something," the patient told her.

"Epidural," Bea said. "Great, you'll love it. It's the latest thing in anesthetics. Me, when I had my child, they gave me a bullet to bite."

"It's wonderful," Eleanore called in from her office.

"Of course, *I* always say," Bea said, "that they should start the anesthesia in the parking lot."

A very small boy appeared in the door and looked up at Bea.

"Hello, there," said Bea.

"I've come to help!" said the little boy brightly.

A patient was querying Genevieve. "How long does it take to get results from a Pap smear?"

"About a week," Genevieve replied, "but if you're not comfortable with that, call us."

The other patient had opened her purse and was rummaging through it. "I've got three different checkbooks," she said. "Let's see which one has the most money."

Overhearing, Eleanore, whose main job was keeping the books, dealing with insurance companies, and pursuing deadbeats, delivered an aside to Barbara: "She makes up for the last three patients who came without their checkbooks."

A pregnant mother arrived with her three daughters. The two-year-old, wearing a pleated tartan skirt with suspenders, took a lollypop and soon was banging it against her teeth. "Don't do that, Moira," said her mother. "If you break a tooth, I don't have time to take you to the dentist."

Moira's sister Jeanette, age six, sweet and shy, with one long pigtail, had her arm in a cast. The arm had been broken in a scuffle with her sister Rebecca. Bea turned to Rebecca, a four-year-old, with an angelic face surrounded by black curls, and asked in mock reproof: "Rebecca, did you break Jeanette's arm?"

"I'm glad I did it," Rebecca said.

A big, blowsy woman came back from the examining room. "Did he have any good news for you?" Barbara asked.

"Just, 'See you next week.' "

"When's your due date?"

"Tomorrow!"

"Well," Genevieve said, "I guess we can make another appointment for you. See you next week."

Genevieve picked up the phone and said, "Yes, Mrs. Maloney . . ."

Barbara exclaimed to no one in particular, "I can't *believe* she's calling again. It's the fourth call this morning, all of them billing questions."

A young pregnant woman and two little girls came into the reception room. Both girls wore T-shirts that said "We Love Our Dad." The woman had dark brown hair and a fresh complexion, olive with pink blushing through at the cheeks. She came to the sliding glass window, but before she could speak, Barbara and Genevieve greeted her in unison. "Karen," they cried, and Barbara said, "How *are* you?"

"We're just fine," the woman said, smiling a wonderful smile. She spoke to her daughters. "Girls, say hi to Genevieve and Barbara."

This was Karen McDonough. There were patients the staff was especially fond of, and then there were Favorite Patients. Karen McDonough was a Favorite Patient. For one thing, she had been employed at St. Barnabas for ten years as a unit coordinator, so she was a professional colleague. For another, she had a warmth close to ra-

diance. But now there was something else about her that mattered
to them: her courage.

Karen was married to Michael McDonough, chief operating offi-
cer of a hospital in Orange. In the late spring, returning to work after a business lunch, he had parked his car in the hospital lot and
opened the door, and as he was stepping out he grew dizzy and stag-
gered. Suddenly he was stricken with a full grand mal brain seizure
and fell to the asphalt, thrashing and raging.

The parking attendant saw him and sounded the code for emergency, and in moments Michael was on a stretcher headed for the
Emergency Room. A CAT scan seemed to show an abnormality, a
shadow in one region of the brain. But Michael was extremely com-
bative and moved during the scan, which could have created a blur.
To calm him the doctors had to administer 65 milligrams of Valium—a huge dose. Karen was summoned. She was devastated.
Michael was a strong man, an athlete. He swam a mile a day and ran
ten. He was registered to run the New York Marathon. Karen had
never seen him ill.

The next day at St. Barnabas he had an MRI, another kind of brain
scan, which confirmed the doctors' fears. Michael had a lymphoma
in his brain. The question then became whether or not the tumor
could be removed. It was lodged in the lower left rear section of the
brain, the area that controlled vision and speech. The operation
might result in horrendous impairment.

That night Karen, about six weeks pregnant, began to bleed vaginally. She was afraid the bleeding was caused by her stress. She worried that the stress might make her miscarry, that she might lose not
only her husband but her baby as well. She couldn't stop the dreadful thoughts. Would Michael ever come home again? Even if he
lived, would he be the way he'd been? She didn't sleep at all that
night. The next morning, the moment the office opened, she called
Rod O'Driscoll, but he was on vacation in Ireland. She spoke to Jack
Bonamo.

Almost every pregnant woman these days, sooner or later, said
something like, "My job is so stressful. Will it hurt the baby?" Most
of the patients were drawn taut, taking care of a family while holding down a job that just a few years before would have been divided between two people. The doctors were reassuring.

Some studies indicated that high levels of stress doubled the risk
of premature birth. Rod and Jack didn't trust those studies. How do

you define and measure a phenomenon as vague as "stress," and how do you isolate it from all the other factors involved in prematurity?

"You didn't bleed from stress," Jack told Karen. "It's probably a problem with the placenta, maybe something to do with its position in the uterus. This sort of thing happens a lot, and almost always things turn out well. Stress doesn't affect the baby. It just makes pregnancy a little harder for the mother."

The bleeding stopped, but the sleeplessness continued, and Karen's appetite dwindled. Over the next weeks she failed to gain weight as she should, which once again led to anxiety about the baby. Again she got reassurance. "You don't have to worry about the baby's going hungry," Rod said. "Babies see to it they get enough to eat. All the vitamin supplements and so forth we ask you to take, they're not for the baby, they're for you. The baby will take what it needs whether your levels are high or low, it matters not." Rod and Jack sometimes treated poor, pregnant young women, mostly from the depressed neighboring town of Orange. These girls typically lived on soda and potato chips, but their babies weren't malnourished at birth. The girls themselves would often be run down and anemic, but their babies were fine. "The mother is the host," Rod said, "and the baby is the ultimate guest. It gets fed first."

Michael came home again, to the McDonoughs' house in the woods near the top of a mountain. There to greet him was a large WELCOME HOME DAD poster, decorated with pink hearts and flowers and butterflies, painted by the little girls with their mother's help. In the following weeks he was taken to specialists at university hospitals in Manhattan, and the opinions were varied. The decision was to wait until after Labor Day and to repeat the MRI scan.

One Sunday in August, Karen drove over to her mother's house to pick up the girls, who'd been there for the weekend. She didn't like leaving Michael alone, but he was on Dilantin and not in great risk of a seizure. When she got back, she found him collapsed on the lawn. He'd had a bad episode. She called for an ambulance. Alarmed, the doctors said waiting was too dangerous; they must operate right away. On Tuesday, at a hospital in New York, neurosurgeons opened up Michael's skull and removed the lymphoma, or hoped they did.

Now it was three months later, and Karen had come to 95 North-field Avenue for her seventh-month obstetrical visit. Bea took her

down to one of the examining rooms, put her on the scales, squinted at the dial, and smiled. "Good for you!" she said. "Your weight
is right where it should be."

"It was my friends," Karen said. "They wouldn't let me starve
myself. They nearly force-fed me for a while there."

Rod came in and looked her over closely, then took her down to
his office for a chat. "How's Michael?" he asked.

"He's fine," she said. "Next month he gets the first of the follow-
up scans to see if they got it all out. So we're all doing a lot of praying.

"The Sunday before the surgery," she went on, "we went to
church. The place was packed. And at one point I looked over and
saw that the sun from a high window was shining right down on
Michael, no one else.

"Later that day we took the children for ice cream. We were outside, sitting on a bench, eating our ice cream, looking out over the
valley, not saying much. We looked up, and there was a rainbow,
from one horizon to the other. I said, 'Michael, just look. We're going to be all right.' "

At five minutes after ten, Jack still hadn't shown up, and Bea was
sending his patients to Rod. "Jack," said Barbara, who had worked
with Jack since his first day in practice, "has a tough time in the
morning." Once she had decided to speak to Jack's wife about his
punctuality.

"Suzanne," she said, "would you please tell your husband to get
in here at nine-thirty tomorrow?"

"He just can't help it," Suzanne said. "He's not a morning person."

Barbara, unwilling to accept that, confronted Jack. "You know,"
she said, with the kind of playful audacity that only an old friend
can hazard, "if you don't start getting in here on time, I'm going to
have to change your hours." And that is what she did, but without
his knowledge. She'd tell him his appointments started at nine-
thirty and in fact not have anyone for him until ten.

Fortunately, Rod was the epitome of the morning person. He'd
make his rounds—visiting all the O'Driscoll-Bonamo patients in the
hospital—at the crack of dawn, but he faded in the evening, when
Jack was still peppy. In this as in so many other ways they seemed
made for each other.

Jack appeared at ten-ten and, like any clever miscreant, entered
with a distracting anecdote. "My son Alex," he said, using a favorite

opener, "has successfully made it through one month of the first grade. But there were some rocky moments. The other day the class had to watch a movie, and Alex refused to. The teacher said he's aggressive. That's Alex."

Jack's lateness was a phony issue, and everyone knew it. In an office that loved to tease, it was mainly another thing to tease about. Jack worked not only hard but long.

"It's been some week," he said later to the four women of the staff. They were fixing lunch in their nook at the end of the corridor. The room had a door going to the parking lot, and he was standing on its step, just outside, sneaking a smoke and talking through the screen.

Jack's smoking was an embarrassment to him. In the baby business, the white box in the cigarette ads that tries to point out the sad connection between parents' smoking and fetal health has some immediacy. As a gynecologist treating cancer, he saw poignantly what smoking does to women; as an obstetrician he saw what it does to babies. If a father smokes, his semen is affected, making his child more susceptible to leukemia and immune-system cancers. Babies of women who smoke are more prone to have a low birth weight, suffer brain impairment, and die early. As female smokers' children grow, they have twice as many behavior problems as other children, problems as serious as those caused by divorce, poverty, or chronic illness.

Jack never smoked in the office or near patients. He was constantly trying to cut down or quit, but the tension of both his job and his personality made him easy prey to nicotine addiction. If, however, he'd ever had an excuse for a cigarette, the past five days had provided him with one of the better ones.

"You *have* had quite a week," Barbara said, egging him on, knowing he was ready to tell his tale, like a ballplayer in the locker room after a sixteen-inning game.

Encouraged, Jack recited the highlights of a week of piggybacked deliveries and procedures, long and late hours. "When I left the office last night," he said, wrapping it up, "I hadn't been to bed in a full day. But I slept last night and now I'm caught up." Finished with his cigarette, he came into the nook and, passing through, peeled a slice of cold cuts from the plate on the table.

6.
Knowing

For Susan and Tracy MacGregor, back from their vacation, seven long months of pregnancy stretched out ahead, full of awesome unknowns.

Already the larger questions were becoming compelling. Would the baby be all right? Would Susan? What would happen to the Mac-Gregors' relationship, to their finances? The big questions broke down into smaller ones. What did they need to buy for the baby? Where would the baby's room be? Their house was small, especially the second floor, where the slanting roof formed low ceilings. The other bedroom was down the hall, not close enough to their own room to hear the baby's little noises, not really convenient for late-night diaper-changing runs.

Tracy thought he could partition off the front part of the second-floor hall, right outside their bedroom door. There was about eight feet of extra space there, and a window looking out into the branches of the hemlock. He had been using the area for his home office, but he'd have to move, the computer would have to go elsewhere. A crib would be taking its place.

Nearing the end of her second month of pregnancy, Susan was receiving ever-stronger direct evidence that something was happening. For one thing, she needed to eat all the time. If she didn't eat she not only felt starved but got dizzy and sometimes cranky. Tracy tried to help. Every morning he laid out her vitamins for her. Then he packed her a lunch and some snacks she could eat during the day. Knowing how busy she could get at the store, he'd phone her every few hours and remind her to eat. "Liz, may I speak with

Susan, please? . . . Susan? Yes, it's me again. Did you have lunch yet? What did you have? Are you sure it was enough?"

They wondered how long it would be before Susan's coworkers caught on. Tracy's frequent calls were a tip-off; he'd never done that before. So was Susan's change of diet. She nibbled almost constantly, feeling very self-conscious about it and about the amount of milk—skim milk—she was drinking at the store, a quart a day.

"I hide the carton in a brown paper bag," she told Tracy.

"Maybe they think it's vodka," he replied.

When the staff went out to Burger King, she continued to have the salads she'd always had, but now her lust for cheeseburgers was getting ferocious. She held off. She was determined to eat as healthfully as she could, for the sake of the baby and also her figure. It was one thing to be pregnant but another to be fat.

Susan had a health problem that diet couldn't help, a condition that if left untreated could kill not only this first baby but all the babies she and Tracy had after it. In her grandmother's day, about 10,000 babies a year died from the condition; it had, in fact, killed two of Tracy's grandmother's children. Many other babies lived but were devastated by the jaundice, anemia, or heart disease it could cause. By the time Susan's mother had her three children a treatment had been developed, but it was drastic and hazardous. Only within Susan's lifetime had safe, easy prevention become possible.

The first signal had come on October twenty-second, six days after Susan's first visit to the obstetrician. On that day the Endocrine and Radioisotope Laboratories, in nearby Livingston, made its report on the blood samples Bea Perez had taken from Susan. Among its findings, under the heading "Blood Group Factor," was the notation "Rh negative."

As Jack Bonamo reviewed the newly-arrived lab report, that notation had set off an alarm. He had peeled a bright red sticker off a pad on his desk and applied it to the upper right-hand corner of Susan's prenatal record. *"RHminder!"* said the message that was printed on the sticker in bold, black letters. "This patient is Rh negative. Administer RH_O (D) Immune globulin Glamulin RH at 28 weeks."

Jack raised the matter with Susan when she came into the office on November fifteenth for her second obstetrical visit. Tracy came with her but she saw Jack alone. She'd wanted to establish a connection with him, patient and doctor, a woman and her obstetrician. Tracy could return to the examining room next time and be there all the visits after that. She was touched by his intelligent, well-meaning interest and grateful for it. He was the model of the modern, involved dad, and it was *his* baby too, after all. But where she tended to be fairly serene about what was happening, he sometimes got worked up, the dynamic young executive concerned about someone he loved. He was the one who was reading all the baby books, cramming himself with information, becoming what he humorously called "a subject-matter expert." He was getting into childbirth with the vigor he brought to new assignments at AT&T. Susan asked him if he'd mind if she talked to Jack alone, and after a moment of surprise he smiled and said it was a great idea.

At the end of her session with Jack, he told her that she and Tracy might have an Rh incompatibility. She was Rh negative, and if Tracy was Rh positive, as 85 percent of people are, there was a good chance the baby's blood would be Rh positive too.

"The problem," Jack said, "comes when the baby's blood mixes with its mother's. When we deliver your baby and the placenta breaks free of your uterus, some of the baby's blood will find its way into your veins. If the baby's blood is Rh positive, your blood cells would identify those positive blood cells as invaders and begin to form antibodies to destroy them. That wouldn't hurt the baby you're carrying now—the level of antibodies won't build up enough in time to cause any trouble. But if you and Tracy have a second baby, by then your level of antibodies would be high, and it would get higher with each subsequent baby. Those antibodies would pass through the placenta into the new fetus. If its blood was Rh positive, the antibodies would start killing its red blood cells, and it could become severely anemic and might even die. Fortunately, there's a way to prevent it."

The disease was described as early as the seventeenth century— "dropsy of the fetus," it was called—but doctors had no idea what caused it and could only stand by as the affected babies died in the womb or soon after birth. At last, in 1939, two American scientists, Philip Levine and R. E. Stetson, made a brilliant guess. They were trying to understand why a woman who had just given birth to a stillborn baby had a violent reaction to a blood transfusion. In the course of their investigation they identified an unusual component in the woman's blood. Maybe, they reasoned, with amazing vision, it was an antibody, one that had formed in reaction to some substance her blood normally lacked but had received from the father via the baby. They were right. The substance the antibody had formed in reaction to turned out to be the Rh factor. (The name Rh stands for rhesus; the substance was identified by comparing the patient's blood with the blood of rhesus monkeys.) The father and baby had it, the mother didn't.

Over the next quarter of a century scientists discovered a great deal about the Rh factor and its subtypes. But the treatments developed in response to this knowledge were extreme and somewhat risky. In 1968, a breakthrough was finally achieved. Researchers in England and the United States developed a serum that by tricking a mother's immune system cleared Rh-positive fetal cells from her blood, preventing her from developing antibodies that she might pass along to her Rh-positive babies. The commercial name for the serum is Rho-GAM.

"The lab report," Jack told Susan, "says your blood is fine. No Rh antibodies. But we want to be safe. In your twenty-eighth week we'll give you a shot of Rho-GAM—just in case a tiny bit of the baby's blood has leaked into your system—and you'll get another within three days after delivery."

"Does it hurt?" Susan asked.

"Nothing special," Jack said. "Maybe a little muscle soreness. But be grateful. Rh disease is one of obstetrics' happiest stories. It's one hereditary disability that can be prevented."

•   •   •

That same Thursday night, after Susan and Tracy left, Maria Ramirez appeared for her obstetrical visit. It would be one of her last. She was broadly pregnant and due to deliver in a few weeks. A young woman, no more than thirty, she had blue eyes, delicate, intelligent features, an ivory complexion, and softly curled brown hair. She was Polish and was married to an electronics engineer from Spain, Antonio Ramirez. With their three-year-old son, Peter, they lived in South Orange, a few miles from the O'Driscoll-Bonamo office.

Near the beginning of the year the Ramirezes had decided to have a second child. Peter then was over two and needed a sister or brother. Maria became pregnant in the spring. In July, during her fourth obstetrical visit, she told Jack Bonamo she felt different from the way she'd felt last time. She kept thinking, she said, that she might be having twins.

Jack said he thought twins were unlikely but if it would make her feel better she could be examined by ultrasound, the device that enables a specialist to look into the womb and see a fetus and watch it move. Maria scheduled an appointment for the following Wednesday. When the day came, she brought her husband along.

Nurse Bea Perez performed the ultrasound. "Well," she said almost immediately, "it looks like you're right. I've got two babies here." The Ramirezes gasped and smiled. Antonio took Maria's hand and kissed it.

Bea continued the examination. She moved the scanner up the little torsos, doing her routine check. What she saw confused her. She could identify two bodies but only one head. She moved the ultrasound sensor over the surface of Maria's belly, aiming it this way and then that, and looked and looked. "No," she told herself. "No. It can't be. The other one's just hiding."

Both the Ramirezes sensed Bea's anxiety. Bea felt she had to say something. "I'm just having a little trouble picking up this other baby's head," she said. The words hung in the air. "I see the one," she went on, "but I can't see this other one's head. It might be tucked under down here." She searched for another minute, her panic mounting. "You know," she said with false heartiness and false modesty, "Dr. Bonamo knows more about these machines than I do. Let me bring him in to take a look."

She called Jack out of another examining room. "Maria Ramirez," she said. "I can't find the second head."

Jack went in and searched. Then he stopped, finally raising his head and giving Bea a grave look that said, "You're right." He collected himself and adjusted his expression and turned to the parents, two stricken people who knew but didn't want to believe. As calmly as he could he said that they were having trouble locating one baby's head. "I think you should be scanned at the hospital," he said. "Their equipment is better. More sophisticated. You can get a better scan."

The scan took place later that day. An ultrasound technician took still images that looked like large photographic negatives. In an adjacent room a radiologist clipped the images to a light box covering most of a wall and studied them. One twin was perfectly normal, but the second twin was pathetically deformed. At the top of the spine, where there should have been a skull and brain, there was nothing. The child would have a face, the radiologist knew, but very little behind it.

The baby suffered from anencephaly, a condition affecting one baby in every 1,500 or so. As the fetus was developing and its neural tube was closing over and becoming a spine, something had kept a brain from forming at the upper end. No one knows exactly what causes the failure, although studies suggest that folic acid, a B vitamin contained in spinach and other foods, many guard against it. If its development followed the usual course, the Ramirez baby would survive a day or two after the birth, relying on its brain stem for breathing and primitive reflexes, but then it would die.

The radiologist, whose lot in life was so often to deliver dreadful news, informed Maria and Antonio. Maria burst into tears and ran from the hospital, Antonio running after her.

There was no discussion of trying to abort the afflicted baby by a process called selective reduction; at this stage, it could have killed the healthy fetus and might have endangered Maria as well. Maria had no choice but to suffer the ordeal of carrying the babies knowing that one would die. As her belly grew larger and larger people on the street and at the supermarket—wherever she went—would exclaim and ask if she was having twins. She had to endure their intrusive high spirits, had to listen to their twins stories and receive their twins advice, had to play the part of the happy mother-to-be, had to keep herself from screaming out the dark, heart-breaking other half of her truth.

"At first it was hard to believe it," Maria told Bea in the autumn. "We didn't want to believe it. We wanted to believe something was wrong, that they'd made a mistake. But after a while, we realized we would have to just accept it and go along with our lives, without the other baby. The thoughts are always there. It's been like that ever since. Up and down. Sometimes you think more, sometimes you think less. The only thing you can do is just pray and get some kind of strength from that. I think that's what keeps me going."

Now the first part of the ordeal, the carrying of a doomed child, was almost over. Her due date was December 10, just a bit more than three weeks away. Jack examined her and talked with her awhile, and then she came out and said good-bye to Bea and the others and left.

There were two more patients after Maria; they were in and out swiftly, without event, and the office hours were over. The women of the staff were unnaturally quiet as they tidied up. Then Barbara spoke. "Sometimes when I see Maria," she said, "I think she's just been crying."

Bea nodded. "She must cry a lot."

"Her eyes show it," Barbara said. "I just wish it could be over."

"What an awful thing," Bea said.

"What I don't understand," Genevieve said, "is if there's no brain, how does it live?"

"Lots of people live without a brain," Bea said. "Their brain is dead, you hook them up to a machine, and you can keep them alive. You don't need a brain to survive."

"Will she see the baby?" Barbara asked.

"They have to ask her," Bea said, "so she can turn that page in her life. Otherwise she'll never be able to resolve it. My mother had a friend who had twins, and one was stillborn. They'd asked the woman if she wanted to see it, and she said yes, but her eyesight was bad and they didn't give her glasses to her. She spent the rest of her life wondering what her baby looked like."

"If the mother doesn't see it, it's not final," Genevieve said. "A part of you doesn't believe that it really is over. Mothers can talk themselves into believing, 'They took my baby' or 'My baby is with somebody else.' They're told, 'No, it's here in the hospital.' And they insist on going to the morgue. It's terrible."

"They need to be asked, 'Do you want to see your baby, do you want to hold your baby?' " Bea said. "They may choose not to, but the decision is theirs. You can't make it for them. That's what they used to do, you know. 'Oh, just don't let her see it, and she'll get over it faster.' Well, she won't get over it faster. A mother wants to know, is it a boy, is it a girl? She wants to hold it and tell it, 'I'm your mother and I love you and I'm sorry you're not going to spend your life with me.' "

There was a silence, and then Barbara said: "I wish Maria didn't have to know . . . that there's something wrong with one of her babies. Six months of misery."

"She and her husband are just the nicest couple," Barbara said.

"Her family's in Poland," Bea said. "Her mother can't get an exit visa. All her mother and father know is that she's having a baby, nothing more. Nobody knows what she's going through, no one at all. I asked her, 'Do you have anybody you can talk to?' And she says, 'My husband.' I said, 'Well, he can't really help you, because your pain is his pain.' Neither one of them has any relatives here, no support system."

"When did we have those Siamese twins?" Genevieve asked.

"Three years ago," Bea replied. "Rod's patient, but he was on vacation, so Jack delivered them. They were attached at the chest. Two bodies but they shared major arteries, and they may have shared lungs. Four arms and legs. I remember when I did the ultrasound.

God, I couldn't get the images of the heads separated. I said to Rod—I'll never forget it—I said, 'What is the incidence of conjoined twins?' He said, 'So rare you wouldn't even think about it.'

"The delivery was cesarean. The resident couldn't get the baby out; there was something in the way. And Jack says to him, 'You gotta put your hand in.' And he was trying to but he couldn't do it. And then finally Jack did it. And he realized it was Siamese twins.

"I was on vacation at the time. I came back and I said, 'How's everything?' And Jack said, 'Don't ask.' "

"That's Jack's kind of luck," Barbara said. "The odds against having Siamese twins could be one in 300,000, but if there's a set of Siamese twins to be delivered, he'd get it."

"They say that if you practice long enough, you'll get a set. Well, we've had our set."

"They died quickly, didn't they, Bea?" Barbara asked.

"Yes. And the mother never knew until it happened, so she was saved all those months of misery. But here is Maria, going through hell, and then after it's over, there's more hell. What do you tell people who say, 'I thought you were having twins?' Terrible. Poor soul."

Bea wondered out loud the thing she always wondered: What does the mother do with the baby clothes she bought before she found out? Does she keep them or give them away? A small matter, really, but it spoke the whole.

For years Bea had given ultrasound tests every Tuesday, and nearly all of them had been occasions of joy—parents getting their first look at their baby, months before the birth, and falling immediately in love with the little creature as it wriggled or snoozed in its snug cocoon. But the happy occasions all blended in her memory. It was the others that stood out and persisted. The ultrasound told the truth, and if the truth was sad, it said so. Once in the back room after lunch she had talked about her experiences with the ultrasound more openly than ever before.

"The ultrasound machine," she'd said, "doesn't know anything about the patient. It just lets you measure the baby. The measurements may be appropriate for a twenty-five-week-old baby, and your patient may be only eighteen weeks pregnant, or she may be thirty weeks. But the machine just tells you what the measurements are. It's up to me to take that information and use it. Is this head too small? Too big?

"So you go to another bone. You take the thigh bone—the longest bone in the body—and you measure *that*. It's a very accurate indication of the baby's age. And you say to yourself, 'Well, the thigh is thirty weeks and the patient is forty weeks, but the head is only twenty-five weeks. Why is the head so small?' At that point, I send the patient to the hospital to be examined further.

"Ultrasound is fun. I like to do it. But not always. Lots of people want to have a scan done just to look at the baby. Well, that becomes a very expensive picture session—$150. You have $150 you want to spend on watching this baby move around? Hey, my time is valuable, you know? You scan people who are bleeding or whatever, not for the fun of it. The 'social scan'—I have a lot of trouble with them. They make me crazy, the people who want me to tell them what sex the baby is so they know what color to paint its room.

"Sometimes you don't find wonderful news on these scans. A woman who's bleeding, you find out she's had a fetal demise. Her baby's dead. When that happens, well, that's really something. Usually it's just me here, the doctors are gone. Hopefully she's someone I've gotten to know. You just can't tell them, 'Your baby's dead.' I sort of lead into it. Very often I'll wait for them to ask the significant question. They'll say, 'How does it look?' And I'll say, gently, 'Well, I don't really see what I expected to see. I don't see a heartbeat here. It doesn't appear to me that this baby's viable.' They'll say, 'Well, what does that mean? Do you mean my baby is dead?' And I'll say, 'Yes, I'm afraid I do.'

"I will only ever say that if there is not a doubt in my mind. That's not my place. But, you know, they're not stupid. They can read my face and they can *see* that something's not right. It doesn't happen very often, but it's happened often enough for me to dread it.

"Sometimes the women come here and they're already prepared for that verdict. Sometimes it's so far removed from what they ever thought could be wrong that it devastates them. It's like they've been hit by a brick. You try and comfort them as best you're able, and try to judge whether they're able, number one, to drive themselves home. Did she come by herself? Sometimes it's a family affair. She comes and she's got her husband and two little kids, and I think, 'Oooo, this is not so wonderful, you know,' and I say, 'Could we maybe have them sit outside before I do this?' Otherwise, it becomes a nightmare.

"And why do you want to tell little kids that you're pregnant, you're nine weeks pregnant, and then go out and have to tell them, 'Well, no, the baby died.' Kids don't have the capacity to understand a thing like that, but I see women do it all the time.

"I did have a patient one time who was at term. She was probably due in about two weeks, and she herself was a labor-and-delivery nurse; I'd known her a long time. And I was just answering the telephone—no patients here, no doctors, no nothing—and she came into the office and she says, 'You know, I haven't felt the baby move.' I said, 'Oh, well, come on, I'll scan you and we'll take a look.'

"So I scanned her, and the baby's head was like this, chin on chest, no heartbeat at all. So I think to myself, 'Oh, boy, what did you do this for?' Because there's no way out. So I said, 'Wait a second. I want to call Dr. O'Driscoll.' I was using a different ultrasound machine, not this one. It only had a small screen, way over here— she couldn't see it from where she was lying.

"Dr. O'Driscoll was on late delivery, and I told him what I had found. I said, 'What do I do?'

"He said, 'You have to tell her.'

"I said, 'Well, how do I tell her that?'

"He said, 'You have to tell her.'

"So I went back inside, and I straightened my shoulders and I started to cry, and I said, 'I'm sorry, I have terrible news.' And I put my arms around her and we both cried.

"When she'd left, I was all alone in this place, and I sat down and cried. I couldn't stop crying. I'd been so sure everything was fine. I was overwhelmed by the feeling that I just never again could let myself be the bearer of bad news. I couldn't stand it. But then I thought, well, she had to get the news from somebody, somewhere. Maybe it was better that it came from someone she knew. Maybe better here, in this room, in private, just the two of us, than in the hospital with a lot of strangers. And I knew that I would of course, in the future, do the same thing again, be giving that same bad news to other mothers.

"I had another patient who came in—the baby was due in three or four days—for a regular routine visit. As I was bringing her in from the waiting room, she said she'd just felt the baby move. I brought her in here, and as part of the routine Dr. O'Driscoll listened for the baby's heartbeat with the Doppler. Nothing. He takes me out of the room and he says, 'There's no fetal heartbeat. Take a look with the scanner.' And I did, and Dr. O'Driscoll had to tell her.

"And she says, 'That can't be. That can't *be*. I just felt it move.' Usually fetal demise occurs over several hours. But for this mother, sometime between when she was out there in the waiting room and when she got in here, her baby had ceased to live. She was convinced that what she'd felt in the waiting room was her baby's last movement.

"And then we had to call her husband, and we all sat and waited for him with her. Terrifically painful.

"On ones like that you never know why, you never know why. There's never an answer for some. It would be great if you could say, 'Oh, there's a knot in the cord; the baby didn't get any nutrients.' Or, 'The baby was so severely deformed it wouldn't have survived anyway.' But we're talking about beautiful, healthy babies who just die. You get nothing back on an autopsy, get nothing back from Pathology. Who's to say?

"At the hospital they induced her. They gave her a medication to start up her labor so that she would deliver the stillborn. And that's the way you have to do it. You don't do a cesarean for something like that. You only do a cesarean if there's a chance to save a child. A child that's alive. Otherwise it's too invasive. Better to deliver vaginally than to run the risk of surgery and anesthesia and all of that. You try not to do that for a dead fetus.

"Sometimes a woman can know for many weeks that her baby is dead but there's nothing that can be done about it. It's terribly brutal but for a number of weeks or months you carry that dead fetus. The pregnancy is too far along to abort and not close enough to term to make labor start, and you don't want to subject the patient to a surgical emptying of the uterus, which is a difficult and stressful procedure because the uterus isn't ready; so the mother usually carries until labor can be induced. So she's at the mall, and people say, 'Oh, when is your baby due?' Is she going to say, 'Well, my baby's dead and I just have to wait'? It's dreadful, just dreadful. We don't see it very often, thank God, but it does happen.

"What some women go through. By and large the rest of us are very lucky. We have very healthy, beautiful children. Except when it doesn't happen that way, and God, it's really such a nightmare, because you expect all of this wonderful stuff to happen, and sometimes it doesn't, and for some people it never does. The gals who keep getting pregnant and never have babies; they just can't carry them to term. Devastating.

"But such a small percentage of this job is tragedy, and there's so much joy associated with it, that that's what keeps you doing it. It's 99.9 percent happy. But that tiny percentage hits you so hard."

Ready to leave, Bea slipped into her car coat and picked up her bag and got out her keys. "Mostly, people are so lucky," she said.

"They come in and they complain about their this and their that, and in the end they have a perfect baby. I feel like saying to them, 'Listen, spend twenty-four hours in Maria Ramirez's shoes. That's it. You'd never complain again.' "

Rod had come out to the desk for a moment to leave a folder to be filed. "When it goes wrong," he said, "you hope you've got the right kind of person. Someone with a little faith. Not one of the 'Why me?' types. Or someone superstitious."

"Life stinks sometimes," Bea said. "But that's obstetrics for you. Not always sweetness and light."

"Those folks need a lot of reassurance," Rod said. "You've got to keep talking to them and reassuring them that it didn't happen because they did something wrong. They're always looking for a reason. What did they do? Or maybe, what didn't they do? That sort of thing." He went back up the hall.

"I'll never forget Maria's face as she left tonight," Barbara said. "On the verge of tears."

"The closer it gets," Bea said from the doorway, "the harder it gets."

Over the months, Maria had talked at length with both Jack and Rod. They'd told her how things would probably go, and she was prepared, as much as anyone could be. They talked about the nature and function of grief, and the professional support available through the hospital. It was clear to the doctors that she did have a deep maternal connection to the damaged baby. "I feel the same about both of them," she said. "I love them both." She told them she wanted to see the child. "Whatever it is, it's *my* baby."

This evening, in the examining room, Maria had said to Jack, "Whatever happens will happen. I have to live with that. I know there is nothing that can be done. Nothing is going to change. Still, it's always on my mind. I want the baby to be healthy, I keep praying it's going to be all right, but I know it's not going to be all right. In the end you have to accept it. Nothing's going to change. You know there are miracles and all those things, but . . .

"It's hard on my husband too. It's hard for everybody, I guess, to hold together. We depend on each other. More than anything, I think, our little boy helps us keep our spirits up.

"They say God never gives us a cross we're not capable of carrying. I hope I'll be able to carry mine."

7.

Bubble

When Karen McDonough arrived for her December check-up, Barbara and Genevieve were the only staff members up front, in the part of the office next to the waiting room. She came to the window to let them know she was there, and they both swung their heads to look at her. A few days before, they knew, her husband had gone to Manhattan for his first brain scan since his operation. It was expected to reveal whether or not the doctors had succeeded in removing the tumor that had devastated him.

Karen's face instantly told the whole story. She was smiling, and it wasn't a brave smile but a real one. "It went beautifully," she said. "The doctors say it looks like they got it all out. Not a trace." He'd have to go back for examinations every few months, she said, but she was sure he'd be fine.

Only one other patient was in the waiting room that afternoon, and her expression contrasted with Karen's. She looked wistful. She was gazing at Karen's three-year-old daughter, Jacqueline—adorable in a party dress, her hair drawn up and cinched into a little fountain on top of her head.

The patient, Lois Geller, had long, slightly graying brown hair, and she was dressed in a simple jumper. Except for the dark red Infinity she'd driven up in, there was no indication she was prosperous. She was married to an executive of a chemical company and lived in a handsome house in Short Hills, one of North Jersey's moneyed old suburbs.

Lois Geller was four months pregnant, expecting in May. She had three sons and had desperately wanted a daughter. Her question had been answered two weeks before, but she wasn't yet completely reconciled to the answer; she still looked at little girls like three-year-old Jacqueline McDonough, the image of little girlhood, with longing. Her reflexive thought was "After three sons I'm entitled to one of those. I'm missing something."

At first, when she learned she was pregnant again, the yen for a daughter was a mild thing, something to kid about in conversations in the bleachers at Little League. "If I get another boy," she'd say, "I'm throwing it to the crocodiles." Over the months the yen turned into an ache. She'd been a great mother to her boys; she loved them; she enjoyed their company. But just this once, she thought, this last baby, let it be a girl. She'd begun to dream about it, about dressing a little girl, playing dolls with her, having her as a female friend when she grew older. Let it be a girl, she'd kept saying to herself.

The baby's sex had been determined at the moment of fertilization, when Lois's chromosomes matched themselves up against her husband's and worked out their abstruse combinations. When the fetus had been about an eighth of an inch long, the embryo's yolk sac had given rise to about a hundred so-called germ cells, and these tiny cells had migrated a distance that compared with their own size was considerable. For a week they oozed along like amoebas, until they reached the places where the reproductive system was meant to form. There they began the task of forming ovaries or testes. As if in a slow-motion film of the blooming of a flower, the tissues at the bottom of the torso between the legs folded this way and that, according to their genetic brief, constructing the apparatus of sex.

For four months the fetus grew within Lois's womb, its gender thoroughly established but a secret unto itself. Then, two weeks before this office visit, Lois had a test that revealed, among other things, the baby's sex. The test was called amniocentesis. A remarkable procedure in wide use since the early 1970s, it provides for the first time something that doctors of the past would never have imagined possible: a safe way to invade the amniotic sac during pregnancy and check on the health of the baby. It is like entering a bubble without popping it.

Amniocentesis is performed around the sixteenth week of pregnancy. Though it identifies the sex of the fetus, its main use is to discover genetic problems—chromosomal abnormalities. It can't pick up some of the most common, such as congenital heart and cleft palate, but it can pinpoint Down's syndrome, the most frequently occurring of the genetic flaws, responsible for much mental retardation. And it can identify more than a hundred rare inherited metabolic disorders. Couples who fear they might have inherited certain genetic problems can find out whether or not they have. An amnio can also flag certain structural faults like anencephaly and spina bifida by measuring the levels of a protein substance—alpha fetoprotein, or AFP—in the fluid.

Lois was in her early forties, a time when certain fetal defects and disorders occur often enough to cause concern and when amniocentesis provides useful advance knowledge. Ninety-five percent of amnios give good news; as for the others, at least the parents can know and prepare. A favorable amnio doesn't guarantee a perfect baby—nothing can—but it lets parents rule out several problems. That kind of assurance means so much to many women that they choose to have the procedure, though Rod or Jack warns them that in something less than 1 percent of instances it prompts miscarriage. Those are national statistics, however. In their forty combined years of OB-GYN, Rod and Jack had had only one case in which an amnio caused a miscarriage. In that one instance the mother developed a case of chorioamnionitis, an infection of the membrane lining the uterus, a week after the procedure. There was no way of knowing why it happened to that patient and not to someone else; the technique they used was the same they always used.

A simple description of amniocentesis sounds like something out of a horror movie: doctor takes a long needle and inserts it into the belly of a pregnant woman. When childbearing women swap war stories, those who've had amnios tend to depict them as terrifying ordeals. The reality, however, is somewhat less lurid.

When Lois had reached her sixteenth week, Jack Bonamo had performed an amnio on her. The scheduled time for the procedure was eight-fifteen in the morning, but Jack didn't appear. Renée Dubiel, the young ultrasound technician who would work along with him, had him paged. Three times a well-modulated voice sent his name from the hundreds of speakers set into the ceiling tiles along the endless corridors of the vast hospital. No answer from Dr. Bonamo.

And then Renée received a call from him, over his car phone. He was late, he was sorry, he was on his way, he'd be there in five minutes. Renée told Lois. She smiled pleasantly, and so did her husband,

Mark, who was clutching his briefcase as if ready to dash off when the whole thing was over. He wouldn't be with her during the procedure; he'd sit in the waiting room. Husbands tended to wince and gasp, even pass out, when the needle went in, and that could be a distraction.

Jack arrived in a cloud of apologies. "My son Alex . . . ," he began, then backed up and began again. "My car's in the shop," he said, "and my sister is letting me use hers. I went to start it up this morning and the ignition key wasn't there. Suzanne and I looked all over the place. No key. It wasn't until about a half hour later that my son Alex—he's six—looked up from his cereal and informed us that yesterday he'd added the key to his key collection."

What makes amnios safe is the ultrasound machine. It lets doctors see into the womb and make sure the baby is in good position before the needle goes in. Lois's baby was crowded into the high end of the uterus, near the placenta, leaving a large baby-free zone into which the needle could safely go. The ultrasound machine would be scanning during most of the procedure. If the baby shifted or stretched out a leg just before the insertion, Jack could see and hold back.

Renée asked Lois to lie on a narrow padded platform, which Renée then elevated electrically. Jack took off his suit jacket but didn't put on a hospital garment; everyday clothes, instead of a surgical gown, helped patients relax. But he pulled on rubber gloves. Great care would be taken to keep things sterile at the place where the needle would go in.

Renée gently pulled Lois's pale blue hospital gown up, revealing the white globe of her swelling abdomen. She squeezed a large blob of clear electrolytic jelly onto the sphere to make a good contact between the patient's skin and the sensing device, as in an electrocardiogram.

"Ooh, it's so cold!" Lois said and laughed.

"Not for long," Renée said. She pressed the sensor into the jelly, and immediately a ghostly image popped onto the screen. To Lois the strange white forms against a black background were confusing at first, hard to read, but Renée's trained eye saw a baby about seven inches long lying in profile near the top of the womb, its limbs pulled in tightly and its head tucked down. Perfect position.

"The black area is fluid," Renée explained to Lois. "See the little arm there? Up by the side of the head? See? It just moved."

"Oh, how cute!" Lois said. "It's adorable."

"There's one leg," Renée said, "that white line."

"That's a leg?"

"And the other leg is this white line."

"Yes, yes, I can see," Lois said. "And do you see . . . anything else down there?" If this baby is a girl, she thought, I'm going to rent a billboard on Route 280 and tell the world.

The fact of the matter was evident to Renée, and with her help, Lois could see it too. There, plainly, between the legs, was something that stuck out like a windsock on a gusty day. As Lois later put it, it was either a third leg or a penis.

Lois's heart stopped for a moment. She was stricken by disappointment. But afterward Mark kissed and thanked her, and she saw how happy he was. "My husband," she told her friend afterward, "felt bad for me. He would have liked me to have a daughter, to please me, but he couldn't hide his relief. My own father felt the same way. I don't know what it is. Some sort of macho thing I can't fathom. My husband said, 'What more could I ask for than four sons?'

"That desire for a girl was a real thing to me; it wasn't just a preference. But once I got through that initial ache, it got easier. Now all I care about is I just hope he's healthy."

Jack and Renée were watching the ultrasound screen intently, noting the baby's pattern of movement and looking for the place where a needle could be inserted with the least risk to the baby. The baby was in perfect amnio position and hardly stirring. Jack pointed to a dark area on the screen, the largest baby-free pool of amniotic fluid.

Renée took a wooden stick that looked like a five-inch Q-tip with cotton just on one end, and she carefully touched the wooden tip to Lois's stomach at the precise point the ultrasound scanner had been. She held the stick vertically against the stomach and twirled it slightly, making a light, circular impression on the taut skin.

"Okay, I'm marking an area below her navel," Renée said to Jack. She made a measurement on the screen. "Four-point-eight centimeters." That was the distance Jack would insert the needle—the distance between the surface of the stomach and the place in the uterine cavity from which the fluid would be drawn. Calibrations were marked on the shaft of the needle, but Jack wouldn't use them; he had done so many amnios he could accurately judge the depth to half a centimeter.

A nurse had entered the room. She handed Jack a sterile package encased in cellophane. Jack tore the cellophane open and slipped out the package: a light blue plastic sheet folded around a syringe, a coil of slender tubing, needles, and some receptacles that looked like test tubes.

"I'm not going to watch," Lois said.

"No, don't watch," Jack said. "We're just going to chat a little before we begin." He turned to the nurse. "Is there a smaller needle?" he asked.

The nurse removed the needle from the end of the long thin tube and took another from the contents of the package. Then she sprayed rusty-red disinfectant at the marked point and dabbed up the excess. Lois lay with her head turned to the side, her eyes closed, her expression calm, her hands resting on her chest just above her breasts.

"First comes the Novocain," Jack said, "like you get at the dentist. It'll make a pin-prick and then that slight burning sensation."

"Yes."

"Then we wait one minute, and after that you won't feel anything as we put the needle through the skin. And then you feel a sharp cramp, like a menstrual cramp."

"I see."

"And that'll last a minute, but try not to move. Try not to lift your legs up. And it's better not to watch. Keep your eyes closed."

"I *will*."

"We'll tell you everything we're doing. But if you watch, the tendency is to tense up your muscles."

Lois's belly was now covered with the light blue sterile sheet that had come in the package. It had a circular hole in it about the size of a silver dollar, and the hole was centered on the spot where the needle would enter. Jack took a syringe containing Novocain and touched the needle to the skin. Then he pushed it in a short distance.

"Ouch," Lois said without much intensity.

"Okay?" Jack said. "Just burns a little bit, right?"

"Uh huh."

He withdrew the needle. The anesthetic raised a small welt at the point of insertion. "Okay, how's that? Not so bad?"

"No, it was all right," Lois said in a small but steady voice.

"All right. Now we're going to put the other needle in, and you're gonna feel dull pain for a minute, then a short cramp."

Jack made a mental note: Four-point-eight centimeters, straight down.

The amnio needle was five inches long; there were needles as long as eight inches for use on obese patients. It was extremely fine and looked delicate. To keep it from snapping as it penetrated the peritoneum—the dense, tough wall of the abdominal cavity—a stiff wire had been run down its core. Once the needle reached the right depth, the wire would be removed. Jack positioned the needle vertically on the welt raised by the Novocain needle and pushed down slowly. "You're feeling dull pressure," he said to Lois.

"Mm-hmm."

"Now sharp . . ."

"Mm-*hmm*."

"Sharp cramp . . ."

"Mm-hmm."

The needle descended, then stopped, not quite two inches in. The tip was through the amnion now, the filmy membrane of the amniotic sac. Jack withdrew the stiffening wire, and a pale amber liquid rushed into the transparent tube that led to a small glass reservoir.

"Okay," Jack said with satisfaction. "We have nice clear amniotic fluid. Looks like ginger ale, which is just what it's supposed to look like."

Lois risked a careful little laugh. "Glad you like it," she said faintly. "Just tell me when you're done."

"You all right, Lois?"

"Huh?"

"You okay?"

"Yeah." As she breathed, the needle rose and fell with the rise and fall of her abdomen. No one spoke as the nurse took three clear vials with black rubber caps and starting filling them with fluid.

"The worst is over," Jack said after a moment, to ease the silence. "The worst is that cramp when the needle goes through the uterine wall. Did you feel it as a menstrual cramp; is that how you felt it?"

"I thought the Novocain was worse," Lois said, her voice less tentative. "The big needle wasn't much of anything."

"That's good," he said. "The fluid's the exact color we want it to be." The most important thing about the color was that it wasn't red. Jack hadn't hit anything he hadn't wanted to, most notably the baby. Like Rod O'Driscoll he was particularly skillful with the needle. Neither of them, in all their years of performing amnios, had ever nicked a baby. Every OB nurse knows there are some doctors who aren't quite as meticulous. Malpractice suits for fetal death by careless amnio are not unknown.

"Are you almost done?" Lois asked.

The nurse was filling the third of the vials. "Almost done," Jack said.

"Hooray."

"Didn't hurt?"

"It didn't hurt. It's just the idea of it. I've always hated needles."

"We leave the needle in until the fluid is in the vials *and* the tops are on, in case one is dropped or anything like that. The most dangerous part of the procedure is putting the needle in, so we don't want to have to start all over again.

"One important test," he went on, "we do last: testing to see if it's really the amniotic fluid." The nurse took a narrow piece of pale yellow chemically treated paper and held it to the hub of the needle, where a few drops of fluid had collected. "If it's amniotic fluid, it will turn the paper blue."

The nurse showed Jack the moistened paper. "Show it to Lois," he said. "Is that blue?" he asked her.

"It's blue."

Jack slowly and smoothly lifted the needle up and out. "The needle's out," he said. "You're finished."

"Oh, wonderful! I couldn't feel a thing. It's just the thought of having the needle in me. So everything came out all right?"

"Yeah, it looks good."

Renée repositioned the ultrasound sensor on Lois's stomach while gazing at the images on the screen. "This is the very last step of the procedure," Jack said. "The technician looks to make sure the baby is fine after the amnio." He pointed to a spot on the screen the size of a pea. "See the little flicker? Can you see that? That's his heart beating." On the screen the little spot was rapidly alternating between black and gray.

"Oh, I see it now . . . his little heart!"

Jack wiped the electrolytic jelly from Lois's belly. Where the needle had entered there was a tiny red dot. "Your battle scar," he said. He stretched a Band-Aid over it. "You can take this off when you get home. It's just for the ride."

"All right," Lois said. "What do I . . . expect?"

"Just take it easy. No work. Off your feet. No grocery shopping, no laundry, no malls, no dancing. No intercourse for twenty-four hours."

"Okay."

"If you feel a little cramping, have a glass of wine."

Lois's eyebrows lifted. "I can have wine?"

"Yes, because wine relaxes the uterine muscle. If cramping starts, the wine will knock that right out."

"Well, well," Lois said, brightening.

Jack smiled. "Everybody ends up having that glass of wine. One way or the other, they manage to have that cramp. 'I *think* this is a cramp. I'm pretty sure this is a cramp.' " Lois laughed, making her belly rock. "All right, today you're basically off your feet. And tomorrow, back to normal activity."

Lois sat up and swung her legs over the side of the cot, then slid her maternity blouse down. Jack held her shoulders as her feet touched the floor, but she was steady. She went into the little dressing room next door to meet her husband, and they left.

Later Jack discussed the risks of amnio. "There was a time when this procedure was done blindly," he said, "without the benefit of ultrasound. Before a patient has an amnio she has to sign an amniocentesis consent form, which says that she understands that the baby may be punctured or perforated. That warning terrifies most patients, but unnecessarily. With ultrasound keeping a close watch on things, that almost never happens. But, along with a lot of the other complications listed on that form, it's there because it used to happen in the era of non–ultrasound-directed amniocentesis.

"I've drawn blood. Sure. Because even with the ultrasound, you still can wind up in the placenta. Sounds awful, but it's no problem. Lots of amnios go through the placenta, sometimes deliberately, to get to a pool of amniotic fluid. Not desirable, but not a problem, either.

"We don't scan with the ultrasound while the needle's being inserted. It's difficult, because both the scan and the needle are aimed at the same spot. There is a device that let's you do it, but the procedure is bulky and much more awkward, so we don't use it. While the needle is actually being inserted—a few seconds—the doctor is blind. The baby can change position. But we look at the general activity pattern of the baby. If we have a baby that keeps moving into a certain spot, we won't go near that spot. If we have a baby that's jumping all over the place, we won't proceed.

"The baby generally cooperates. There have been studies in which babies have been monitored while the needles are inserted, and these studies have shown that the baby actually moves away from the needle. The baby knows something is invading the cavity—and pulls away from it."

The nurse packed the vials of amniotic fluid taken from Lois to be sent to a laboratory. The fluid contained various substances—proteins, hormones, carbohydrates, enzymes, fats, and the baby's urine—and all these would be analyzed for clues to the baby's condition. The fluid also contained free-floating cells that had been shed by the fetus. These would be examined in the laboratory to see if the chromosomes, carrying the genetic instructions that would form this human being, were there in the right number and proper arrangement. This analysis would reveal whether the baby had Down's syndrome or any of a series of other genetic irregularities that might cause birth defects. It would also disclose the baby's sex. Knowing the sex was important if there was a family history of a sex-linked defect such as hemophilia or muscular dystrophy.

Amniocentesis isn't the only way to discover birth defects early. CVS, or chorionic villus sampling, can be performed at eight weeks or so, two months earlier than the time for amnios. If a woman is frightened about the possibility of a major fetal defect, CVS can allay that fear much sooner, and the lab reports come back in a few days, much faster than the two weeks required by amnios. That speed is a mercy. If the baby is gravely defective, and if the woman intends to have an abortion, CVS lets her have it well within the first trimester, when the rate of complications is lower.

There are two ways to do a CVS. In the transcervical method, the doctor, guided by ultrasound, slips a catheter through the vagina and into the uterus to take a small sample of the placental cells, the chorionic villi. The other method, the transabdominal, involves taking the sample by means of a needle through the abdomen. The choice between the two methods depends on the location of the placenta and the doctor's training. Either way the cell sample, when analyzed, gives a complete picture of the genetic makeup of the growing fetus.

Rod and Jack hadn't been trained in CVS. When one of their patients requested one, they referred her to a perinatologist at the hospital. None of their patients had ever had any trouble with it. Early word was a blessing for worried parents, and terminations performed in the first trimester were much easier on the mother than those in the second.

CVS had been expected to sweep past amnio in popularity. It was riskier—three out of every 200 patients had complications leading to miscarriage, versus amnio's overall rate of one out of 200. But, as these kinds of gambles went, those risks were generally considered acceptably low. In 1991, however, Italian researchers reported that babies of mothers who'd had CVS had detectably greater chances of being born with a deformed leg or arm. That finding made obstetricians pause before jumping from amniocentesis to the newer technique; what a pitiful irony it would be to cause a defect by trying to detect one.

Lois Geller chose amniocentesis. It was hard to balance these things off. She wanted to know, but the knowledge involved risk. She was running a risk to eliminate risk. She was convinced that if, God forbid, there was something really wrong, she would have to have an abortion.

"I don't feel that it's fair to the other three children," she'd told Bea Perez a few weeks before the procedure, "to knowingly bring a seriously handicapped child into the family. It would take so much of my attention, and my attention is already very divided. It would have to be divided three-quarters for the handicapped baby and only one quarter for the other three children. I just hope he's okay, so that I won't have to . . . I just hope . . . He looked awfully cute in the ultrasound, kicking away, and the arms were waving around. I just hope he's healthy.

"I know they don't do it," she'd said, meaning Rod, Jack, and abortions. "I'd have to find somebody else."

·   ·   ·

It was true. Rod and Jack didn't perform abortions. Two-thirds of the nation's OB-GYNs don't, though the vast majority of them feel that abortion should be freely available. The apparent contradiction between those two positions is explained by several factors, fear of harassment and violence from pro-lifers being high on the list. In Rod's and Jack's cases, it was personal. Both were Roman Catholics. Performing abortions ran too strongly against their upbringing, but they were not judgmental. They were always sympathetic. They were always ready to refer patients seeking abortions to competent colleagues who did them. Both quietly but firmly believed in choice.

It was a subject that came up often. Just over half of the six million pregnancies that occur yearly in the United States are unplanned, and of those a sizable number are unwanted. Half of all American women will have at least one abortion in their lifetime.

"Patients tell me why they want to have an abortion," Jack said, "and I tell them what to do, where to go. We literally set it up for them. We just don't perform it. In this business, you can't be so pro-life that you don't understand the other side. We can't function that way; we're just tied too closely to the patient and her well-being and her wishes. You have to understand people's *right* to make their own decisions. And if they decide to terminate, you want to make sure they have it done in a reputable facility; there are questionable little abortion places around that we make sure they don't go to. We want to make sure that if they choose abortion, at least they come out of it healthy. I think it's my medical responsibility to make sure that if that's what they choose, they have it done in a decent place."

Both doctors tried to keep their own views out of it. "I hate to give patients my own bend on the question," Rod said, "and I almost never do. But that doesn't mean you suspend your own judgment. When there are people you really think can't handle it—and a lot of patients, because of their upbringing or their situation or whatever, really can't—I make them stop and ask themselves, can they really do it?"

Eight months before, Rod had seen a patient of his, Deirdre Kerry, a pathology nurse at a nearby hospital. She had just had a cancerous kidney removed. She had come to see Rod because her periods were irregular and she was worried about it. "And Deirdre is not a worrier," Rod said. "This is a tough, hard-working girl." He tested her, and it turned out she was pregnant. She asked the doctors who were treating her cancer, and they said, in effect, "Forget it; terminate the pregnancy; you need to be followed with X rays and cystoscopies to make sure the cancer isn't in your bladder, and we can't do any of that while you're pregnant."

"She went home and talked it over with her husband," Rod said, "and she was going to have an abortion. She already had three kids. But there was something about the way she said it that troubled me. I was afraid she might be making a decision she couldn't live with. I didn't tell her what I thought, though. I had her talk to one of these bioethics people about her decision. They help people make decisions like that."

After several sessions with the bioethicist, she told Rod she still was going to have the abortion. And then one day she came in and said to him, "You know, I can't have an abortion. Who am I kidding? My name is Deirdre Kerry and I was born Deirdre Phelan, and I'm pregnant. When you're like me and you're pregnant, you have a baby. You don't have an abortion." Then she added, "The doctor says I might die of cancer. Okay, then I die of cancer and my husband raises four kids."

"Last week Deirdre had her fourth child," Rod said. "She did nicely and they're happy as they could be. And now they're going to start some intense testing to make sure everything is all right." He paused. "I knew she couldn't have an abortion."

•   •   •

Four miles west on Northfield Avenue was the practice of Dr. Sandra Fornwalt, a young obstetrician for whom Rod and Jack had great respect. She had come to St. Barnabas as the younger colleague of a St. Barnabas OB and had then gone into solo practice. They had seen her up close and thought so highly of her that they readily sent her patients when, for example, the daughter of one of their own patients decided she wanted a female OB-GYN.

Dr. Fornwalt performed terminations. "It's not something I seek to do," she said, "but if I have a patient who says this is something that she wants, then I do it. I feel abortion should be available, and I don't think it's my job to assess the responsibility of their decisions. I speak with them about their choices: 'If you feel that you can't terminate the pregnancy, you could continue the pregnancy for adoption.' I'm not their judge and jury. They need to know that whatever decision they make is okay with me. Because I don't think that if I were in that situation I would want someone judging my decision. By the time they come to my office, they've pretty well made up their mind.

"It's one of the worst decisions a woman has to make, because regardless which choice you make, each one has a consequence. Sometimes people who've had terminations come into the office a couple of years later; now they want a baby but they're having problems getting pregnant. Or even if they are pregnant again and this time are continuing the pregnancy, the new pregnancy brings it all back and fills them with guilt about what happened the time before. On the other hand, when they've found the right man and are ready to begin families, many women are even more convinced they made the right decision.

"I'm very conflicted about the possibility of minors having to have parental consent, or wives having to have husbands' consent. I don't know. But getting the government's consent is unthinkable. I get so angry, because I see people in Congress, their kids are all grown, they've never had to face that decision, they've probably never known what their own daughters went through. Yet they're making these rules and regulations for what I might want to do with my life."

Once, when abortion was being debated with particular heat, Dr. Fornwalt ran into one of the St. Barnabas physicians who operated his own termination clinic. She asked him what he thought of it all. "You know, it's very interesting," he said. "I see women who are demonstrating for pro-life, and then two weeks later they're in my office, wanting a termination."

"When the tables are turned," Dr. Fornwalt said, "all of a sudden one's values change. It's almost as if, by demonstrating, they've paid their dues and now they can go have their abortion. We all grant ourselves little exceptions. Who knows what any of us will do when we're faced with that kind of situation?"

Several years before, one of her patients had undergone an amniocentesis that indicated her baby had Down's syndrome. On her previous pregnancy the woman had had a termination, and Dr. Fornwalt assumed she'd choose to terminate again. "If you want me to," she said to the patient, "I can schedule the procedure. Why don't you think about it and give me a call?"

It was some time before the patient called. "I'd like to go see a genetic counselor," she said.

Dr. Fornwalt gave her a name. The genetic counselor reviewed the odds with the patient. She constructed a family tree to determine whether there had been some abnormality, where it had come from, and whether the gene for it was recessive or dominant. She laid out for the woman and her husband what their chances were of having a baby with an abnormality. Her work with the couple went far beyond anything an individual OB could do in an office.

Dr. Fornwalt didn't hear back from the patient, so after a while she called her and said, "You're getting to the point where we really need to go ahead and schedule this, because you're getting near the upper limit."

The woman was silent a moment, then said, "I don't know if I want to terminate this pregnancy."

Dr. Fornwalt was stunned, not by the woman's apparent choice but by what she perceived to be her own insensitivity. She'd automatically assumed that because the woman had had one termination, when confronted with Down's syndrome she'd have another.

"I'm really sorry," she told the patient. "I certainly will support whatever decision you make." Dr. Fornwalt saw the woman's husband and told him the same thing. The woman continued the pregnancy. Knowing the baby had Down's syndrome, she was prepared for it. Well before its birth she enrolled it in a special program.

When the woman gave birth to her Down's baby, another obstetrician asked Dr. Fornwalt, "She opted to continue the pregnancy? Why didn't she terminate?"

"Listen," she said. "I've learned my lesson. I will never try to figure out what somebody is going to decide when faced with that. Who knows what causes somebody to make that decision?"

Recently the woman had come to Dr. Fornwalt's office for a routine examination. Her husband, she said, had a hard time dealing with the handicapped child, and their marriage had fallen apart. With profound sincerity, Dr. Fornwalt replied, "I certainly respect what you're doing."

●　　　●　　　●

Sitting in the waiting room and watching Karen McDonough's three-year-old, who had a book on her lap and was pretending she could read, Lois Geller waited anxiously for her doctor to tell her the results of the amniocentesis. At last she was summoned into Jack Bonamo's office.

"Everything's great," he immediately said as she walked through the door.

"Oh thank God," she breathed. At that moment, in a clarifying rush, the matter of boy versus girl finally and permanently dissolved into one overriding concept: healthy baby.

8.
Boom-Boom

The second Saturday morning in December, Susan and Tracy MacGregor went shopping. When they returned and approached the back door, they noticed the screen door was ajar. Something was holding it slightly open—a package, a dark green Laura Ashley box. Tracy took it inside and put it on the kitchen table. Susan's name was on the envelope, in a familiar feminine script. She slipped off her coat, opened the envelope, and read the card. "We're so proud of you," it said. "Love you lots. Mom and Dad."

Susan set the card down gently and opened the box. Inside was a sailor dress in a navy and slate calico print. It was very full, with no waistband.

"Oh, it's cute!" Susan said. "But it's enormous!"

The first maternity dress was a gift with significance. More vividly than had any event until now, it made the whole thing abruptly real to Susan. "You," it proclaimed, "are going to have a baby." It was hard to ignore the message implicit in its billowing cut. "Your body," it said ominously, "will swell and swell until it fills this tent." But the dress was more than a graphic portent; it was also a recognition, the first tribute the outside world had paid to Susan's new estate: her status as mother-to-be.

Ever since she and Tracy had told her parents about the pregnancy, back in October, Susan had been mildly surprised that her mother wasn't more obviously pleased. Betty Sprague was a warm and expressive person, not reserved; without thinking about it directly, Susan had assumed she'd make more of a fuss when her only daughter announced she was carrying the Spragues' first grandchild. But there had been something restrained about Betty's enthusiasm, and Susan had been just a little disappointed. She'd even mentioned it to Tracy.

Now the mystery began to come clear. Betty Sprague was an experienced woman. She'd seen a good many pregnancies—her own, her friends', her relatives'—and she'd seen how many had miscarried in the chancy first three months, the first trimester. The statistics backed up her impression: roughly one out of ten known pregnancies miscarried. And that didn't count the many miscarriages that happened so early in the pregnancy the woman never knew she'd been pregnant; about half of those very early pregnancies failed.

All kinds of things can cause a miscarriage—a mother's smoking or drinking, for example, or the chemicals she is exposed to on the job. But far and away the most common reason is genetic accident. Either the egg or the sperm has the wrong number of chromosomes, and so, in the union, the match-up isn't correct. "Every normal male produces a certain number of bad sperm," Rod told patients who'd had a spontaneous miscarriage, "and normal women produce abnormal eggs. Usually they don't start a pregnancy, but when they do, Mother Nature steps in and says, 'Not this time.' "

People persist in thinking of miscarriage as the premature expulsion of a baby that would otherwise have survived. What did I do wrong? patients ask their doctors. Was it because I exercised too much or lifted a heavy package? To deal with that kind of heavy guilt, Jack would sometimes resort to harsh reasoning. "If it was as easy as that," he'd say, "women who can't get abortions wouldn't go to the awful lengths they do, the coat hangers and the turkey basters. They'd just run ten miles." You can't cause it, Jack would always say, and you can't prevent it. "If you'd stayed in bed from the time you conceived until the moment you lost the baby," Rod often said, "the outcome would have been the same." Which was not to say there was nothing that could be done if a woman miscarried repeatedly. Tests should be performed and examinations made. Sometimes steps could be taken to make birth likelier.

Betty had known how devastating those losses could be for the parents, particularly the mother, especially with a first child. She hadn't wanted to intensify Susan's pain, if the pregnancy went wrong, by having celebrated it too effusively. She wouldn't want Susan to feel that in losing the baby she had broken her mother's heart.

But now she could celebrate. The first trimester was nearly over. The chances of loss would drop dramatically now, from the one in ten of the first trimester to less than one in fifty for the remaining two trimesters. The week before, while shopping, Betty had seen a Laura Ashley shop, and instead of passing by she'd gone in.

Susan went to a mirror and held the dress against her body. Her eyes were glistening. "I'm touched," she said. "I'm really touched. She hadn't really—I mean, I'm sure she was excited, but she hadn't really let on."

"I didn't tell you," Tracy said. "I talked to her last night before you got home. She said she'd been a little bit cautious about being too overexcited, just in case. It was still early. But then she talked to you during the week, and you sounded so excited that when she saw the shop she thought, 'Oh, what the heck.' "

After lunch, they set up the Christmas tree they'd bought that morning. The ceilings of the old house were low, so they'd chosen a small plump tree, one that would fit beneath the living room's hewn oak beams. Most of the tree decorations were from a collection Susan had been building for years, including some tiny wooden puppets from Germany; if you pulled the string, they danced. "Next year there'll be a baby crawling around the tree," Susan said.

Their two previous married Christmases, they'd gone to the Spragues for Christmas Eve, but this year, they'd decided, they'd spend the evening alone, in their own home. "Just the two of us," Susan had said. "It'll be the last time like this, just the two of us." She hung another star and then said, "Sometimes I'll be doing something or other, and suddenly the thought will just cut right through, that in six months I'll be the mother of a little baby!"

"I know," Tracy said. "I know. I just can't believe . . . Just today, this morning, it hit me. It's so hard to believe. Hard to believe, but great hard-to-believe."

"It's next June. I think, 'That's not far off,' and then I think how I'll be off for the summer, having a little infant to take care of, and how different things are going to be."

"It's amazing," Tracy said, "how when this thing happens to you, your focus changes just ever so slightly. You start to think about stuff that you never thought about. Like, maybe we need life insurance? More than we have—whatever it is that we have. I don't know. Maybe we should talk to somebody. And maybe we should be saving more money. I mean, it's serious. We're going to have to put this kid through school."

"Yeah, now that we're parents, we've got to get up on all that stuff." Susan laughed to herself as she picked pine needles out of the sleeve of her sweater.

"What are you laughing at?" Tracy asked.

"I was thinking, we're real grown-ups now."

"It's real enough for me."

"It's official. This is really it. I'm not nauseated, I'm not showing, but when someone gives you a maternity dress, there's got to be a reason for it. Someone must know something."

There was a silence, and then Tracy said, "I can't wait till you start to show." He meant it—he couldn't wait. Things couldn't happen fast enough to please him. Every new development, though savored, only filled him with eagerness for the one after that.

"Well, it won't be long," Susan said. "When I got dressed this morning I realized this was absolutely the last time I'd be able to get into these pants. Some of my slim clothes are getting slimmer. Things are fitting me differently."

•   •   •

Five days before Christmas Susan had her third obstetrical visit. It didn't start well. After drawing Susan's blood Bea Perez showed her to the scales for the monthly weigh-in. She squinted at the calibrated balance arm and read off, "One-thirty-four."

"One-thirty-four!" Susan exclaimed. "That's impossible."

"That's what it says," Bea said. "But here, let me check." She moved the small weight along the balance arm a few inches, then tapped it back again until the arm leveled. "Nope. It's right. One-thirty-four."

"But it can't be. I weigh one-twenty-eight at home." Susan was somewhere between anger and tears.

"Well, now, look," Bea said consolingly. "One-thirty-four isn't so bad. What I wouldn't give to weigh one-thirty-four."

"It's this sweater," Susan said as if pleading for clemency. "It weighs a ton."

"So next time you won't wear that sweater and you'll think you've lost weight."

"Susan really doesn't want to get fat," Tracy explained.

"I know she doesn't," Bea said. "That's fine, as long as she's eating well, which I gather she is. But she's a long way from getting fat."

"I'd better be," Susan said.

The doctor on duty was Rod O'Driscoll. Susan hadn't yet met him, but Jack Bonamo had prepared her for the day he'd be examining her and for the possibility that when her time came, Rod would deliver her baby. A few minutes after Bea had signalled him that Susan was ready, he popped into the examining room, a portion of floral necktie visible between the lapels of his starched white cotton jacket. "I'm the other guy," he said, and the MacGregors laughed. "How are you doing?" he said, looking at Susan's chart. "Hey, you're into your second trimester. Almost sixteen weeks. That's great. I'll bet you're glad. But you've had a pretty easy time of it, right?"

"I guess I have."

"Chart says you've put on a couple of pounds, eh?"

"That's not right!" Susan erupted, half amused, half furious, surprising the doctor with her passion. "It's this heavy sweater."

"Can I explain something to you?" Rod said supportively. "Sometimes when you're pregnant you put on weight faster than you used to from the same amount of food, especially cookies, cake, any of the high-fat foods."

"How much weight am I supposed to gain?" Susan asked. "Is Chinese food okay?"

"As far as what you eat," Rod said, "the key thing is, everything in moderation. At this point in your pregnancy, an occasional glass of white wine . . . Chinese food, don't eat it every night. You've got to watch the buttered bread, the cookies, the crackers. That's what really seems to put on the weight when you're pregnant."

Everything in moderation—such a reasonable stance, yet it had taken obstetricians a long time to get there. Medical advice on the subject has varied widely over the years—weigh more, weigh less—and succeeding generations of women, ever obliging, have stuffed or deprived themselves, their bodies swelling or wasting as they tried to accommodate.

For a long time, doctors thought it important that pregnant women gain plenty of weight to make sure the baby was nourished. "Remember, you're eating for two" had been the standard counsel since ancient days. But in time it was discovered that babies in the womb have first call on the available nourishment, demonstrating the truth in the old proverb "The first morsel goes to the child."

Amplitude became suspect. A big weight gain was thought to cause complications during labor and delivery. Studies found that the more a woman gains during pregnancy, the more weight she retains afterward, and that the more she retained, the unhealthier it was for her. Some physiologists believed, in fact, that very obese women need not gain any weight at all during a pregnancy if they were eating the right things. Excess weight also tended to raise a woman's blood pressure; it was estimated that just ten extra pounds increased the length of the capillaries through which the heart must pump by about six miles. High blood pressure was bad for the baby, too. Billowing flesh made pregnant women awkward and prone to accident, and it multiplied their aches and pains. By the 1950s doctors were telling their patients that fifteen to eighteen pounds was the right gain. Some doctors said ten.

Science, however, kept poking into the question. By the time Susan was born investigators had concluded that fifteen to eighteen wasn't enough—not enough, for example, to support the growth of the fetus and the placenta and the amniotic fluid. It also found that women who didn't gain enough weight, especially in the first three months, were much likelier to bear babies whose birth weight was too low. Low birth weight had come to be recognized as a major cause of infant mortality.

In 1970 the National Academy of Sciences jumped the desirable average gain to twenty-four pounds, and it kept climbing. The American College of Obstetricians and Gynecologists arrived at twenty-four to twenty-eight as the ideal range. Late in 1990, as Susan was moving through her first trimester, the Institute of Medicine of the National Academy of Sciences issued a report urging a gain of twenty-five to thirty-five pounds. Some doctors even suggested that OBs stop weighing their patients because it might make them self-conscious and likelier to stop eating.

Rod didn't buy that argument. If a patient was on her way to gaining sixty or seventy pounds, it was in her best interest to know it, he believed, because she would have a hard time losing it later and might keep it the rest of her life. It was confusing for a pregnant woman to try to monitor her weight without regular weighing. People ordinarily know they've gained weight when their clothing gets tight, but pregnant women, in their loose garments and their stretch fabrics, have more difficulty detecting it. Not only that; their bodies are undergoing changes they've never experienced before, and they feel very different. It is difficult for them to know where they are, physically. Rod didn't berate his patients, but he did keep them carefully informed about their weight and, when it was called for, suggested countermeasures.

Women dreaded weight gain for the usual cosmetic reasons but also because they assumed that fatter mothers make bigger babies, ones tougher to squeeze through the birth canal. The Institute of Medicine debunked that notion. There was very little relationship, it said, between the mother's weight at the time she gave birth and the size of the baby. The real danger, they said, echoing what others had been saying for some time, wasn't too much weight—though that could be a problem—but too little. Up to a point, the less weight a woman gains, the greater the chances of infant mortality. A case in point is the relatively high death rate among babies of teenage mothers; these very young women are still growing and, typically, storing little fat—which means their babies get less nourishment than they need.

Rod worried about weight a lot less than his patients did. As long as the woman was in the right range for her height, all was well. One thing he did care about, though, was that she gain the weight in synch with the fetus's own natural growth pattern. A baby puts on 90 percent of its weight after the fifth month and 50 percent of it in the last two months, which is to say that its weight increases slowly at first but climbs fast. Its mother's gain, therefore, should start slowly too—three to four pounds during the entire first trimester is fine. Then, during *each month* afterward, she should expect to gain three to four pounds, or a total for the last two trimesters of about fifteen to twenty pounds. Despite the confusion about the MacGregors' scale, the office scale, and Susan's heavy sweater, she seemed to have gained about the right rate for the first trimester. But now the real blossoming would begin.

"The right weight," Rod told Susan, "depends somewhat on your height and frame. You're what, about five-seven? So let's say something like maybe twenty-five to thirty. Plus or minus. Somewhere in there. The rate you gain it, though, and the timing, they're important too, and we'll be watching that closely."

Rod was under no illusions that he'd exhausted the inexhaustible topic of weight for this patient. There were so many things Susan could have asked and didn't and at some point probably would.

Where, for example, would the new weight go? All over, he'd say. The breasts enlarge one or two pounds worth. The uterus enlarges and thickens and eventually weighs several pounds more. The placenta, a brand-new organ, contributes a few more. The amniotic fluid weighs something, and so does the increase in the patient's blood supply. There's also the fluid that collects in various places, particularly the legs, producing swelling. And of course there's the weight of the baby itself. A couple of pounds here, a couple of pounds there—it adds up. Which often leads to a question about waist size: What will, say, a twenty-seven-inch waistline become by the ninth month? Rod's answer: between fifty-four and sixty inches; the mother's skin has to expand until it doubles. No wonder some women get stretch marks.

Another common question was about the belly bands that some women used to support the weight of the baby. Every so often a magazine article somewhere suggested that wearing one would somehow make it easier for a woman to lose weight later, after the birth. Patients would then ask about it, and Rod and Jack would say no. Belly bands and maternity girdles are cosmetic; that is all.

Rod raised the leg support of the examining table and latched it in the horizontal position. Susan, responsive to the signals, swung up her legs and lay back on the table. Rod placed his fingertips on her lower abdomen and pressed, then moved them and pressed again. "Check your tummy here, my dear. You're getting puffy, huh?"

She brought her hands to the spot he indicated. "A little."

"A little, huh? I think you're going to be showing pretty soon." He went around to the other side of table. "Let me sneak over here," he said. He picked up the Doppler, the small black plastic cylinder that measured sounds within the body. A cord extended from it to a small speaker so that the sounds it picked up could be heard in the room. "Let's take a listen," he said. He touched the Doppler to Susan's belly.

While Rod moved the Doppler from point to point, concentrating, as if searching for something, Susan teased Tracy. "They take your blood yet?" She knew Tracy hated needles.

"Bea saw me in the hall and she said, 'You owe me some blood.' But I got away."

Rod overheard. "She'll get you," he said. "Bea always gets her man." He had seen the red flag on the chart warning of a possible Rh incompatibility problem.

"Tell you what you do," he said to Susan, returning to his search. "Hook your thumbs right in there and pull down a little, okay?" He needed to move his Doppler device a little farther down her body, and rather than pushing back her underpants himself, he let her do it. Good obstetricians were skilled at respecting their patients' privacy and had little ways of creating in the patient the sense that, though considerably exposed, she was in control. When the new area was exposed, he moved the Doppler into it. "Let's see what's down here," he said.

Softly at first and then emphatically, a rhythmic pulsing sound came from the speaker. *Boom*-boom-*boom*-boom-*boom*-boom-*boom*-boom. About two beats a second. A thumping, throbbing noise, like something from a sci-fi movie. It filled the little room.

"That's it," Rod said with satisfaction. "That is your baby's heartbeat."

Tracy had been sitting in a chair to one side. He shot to his feet, astonished. Susan's eyes opened wide and her lips formed an O. The MacGregors had just met their first child.

"Wow!" Tracy said.

Susan laughed in glee, and static drowned out the heartbeat.

"Isn't that great?" Rod said. "But don't laugh, if you can help it. The Doppler picks up the noise."

"It's beating so fast," Susan said.

"Supposed to be that fast?" Tracy asked with concern.

"Yeah. Babies in utero, their pulses are about twice as fast as ours."

"What can you tell from that heartbeat?" Tracy asked. "Anything?"

"Well . . ."

"No predictions?"

Rod smiled. "Oh, I see what you mean. Boy or girl. No predictions. Those theories about females having faster heartbeats, they aren't reliable anyway."

Rod put down the Doppler and the sound had stopped. "Can we hear it again?" Tracy asked.

"Sure you can," Rod said. "We'll just find out where the baby's lying now." He moved the Doppler until it found the spot and the urgent cadence resumed.

"That is neat!" Susan said.

"So there you have it," said Rod, to whom the fetal heartbeat was a very old tune. "You're not just missing your period. This is for real."

Tracy, moved, took off his glasses and wiped his eyes with his handkerchief.

"The sound is stronger this time," Susan said, listening hard.

"Yeah, it's really a strong one," Rod said.

"He's real big?" Tracy asked.

"No, it's real little. We hear it so loud because of the way the baby's lying now."

He let them listen for another minute. "Okay, little baby," he said, "you're doing great." He moved the Doppler away, and the pounding ceased.

Susan was beaming. "There *is* something in there," she said. Everyone laughed.

"Now we believe you," Tracy said, and everyone laughed again.

Rod was scanning Susan's chart once more, looking for something. "You had your AFP done, Susan?"

AFP stands for alpha-fetoprotein, a chemical that, if present in the mother's blood in unusual amounts, suggests that the fetus has a malformed central nervous system—spina bifida, perhaps, or anencephaly, the condition that afflicted Maria Ramirez's baby.

"She took my blood a couple of minutes ago," Susan said. "Could that have been it?"

"Oh, yes," Rod said, still looking at the chart. "Here it is. She's marked it in." He buttoned his white jacket. "All right, folks," he said. "Any questions otherwise?" It was his routine wrap-up line, delivered in the awareness that there were patients waiting in the other two examining rooms and that he was the only doctor on duty. "All right, so we plan to see you in four weeks. Probably shortly after your next visit you'll start to feel your baby."

"Will you do an ultrasound?" Tracy asked.

"I was thinking about that. It's probably a good idea. A scan really does tell you an awful lot about the baby. Primarily what it would do, it would confirm your dates. We'd measure the baby lots of different ways and see just how far along it is, and that would tell us exactly how old it is and whether your expected date is correct. That might be important later on, if you go well beyond your due date and we begin to wonder if the baby should be induced. Also, you can get a look at the baby's heart. You're fifteen and a half weeks. We'd do the scan in about three weeks."

Tracy turned to Susan. "You want to do it?" It was plain he wanted to.

"Yeah," she replied, with just a shade less enthusiasm. Her fundamental view was the fewer gadgets the better.

"It's a fantastic experience," Rod said, "to see your baby swimming in there."

"I want to do it," Tracy said.

"Ask Eleanore, out at the desk, to give you an appointment."

"Don't you want to do it?" Tracy asked Susan.

"Yes, okay," she said, "I'll do it."

"If you want," Rod said, "you can call me after talking about it. Anything else? Okay. Nice to see you. You're doing beautifully. Happy holidays."

.   .   .

"How about that heartbeat!" Tracy said as soon as they'd left the office and the door shut behind them.

"Wild," Susan said. "So fast. And so strong."

"Must be a boy," Tracy said. He was teasing.

"That does *not* mean anything."

"I'm sure it means something."

"It means there's a baby in there, for sure. We better get our fill now of sleeping in late, because our carefree days are numbered."

.   .   .

A week later the lab report came back on Tracy's blood test. He was Rh positive. Rh incompatibility was no longer just a possibility; it was certain.

9.
Wrap-Up

Rod lived a half dozen miles from his office, in Essex Fells, a village so small and out of the way that its existence was something of a local secret. The O'Driscoll house, a turn-of-the-century place covered with shingles painted gray, had "Family" written all over it—big, with many rooms for many children and wide porches on three sides.

Rod's father was an immigrant. "The only choices open to him back in Ireland," he said, "were the priesthood and teaching. He became a teacher but ran head-on-head with a difficult parish priest, which resolved him on the course of getting out of the country. He went to the United States and spent the rest of his life trying to better himself. He was a great influence on me. He was horrified when I decided to be a priest." Rod had spent his high school years studying Latin and Greek, preparing for the seminary. Before graduation he'd realized he wasn't meant for the priesthood and chose medicine instead. One way or the other, he wanted to care for people.

Rod and his wife, Joan, had both been only children. "When I was a little boy," Rod said, "I'd come down in the morning and my mother would put the red velvet cape around my shoulders and the crown on my head, and I was ready for another day. It made me very independent—it made me feel there was nothing I couldn't do—but all that focus isn't good for a child." The couple had agreed from the start that they'd have a big family.

On one hand, a lot of children; on the other, a father with a job that consumed him—it was a combination that could have meant trouble. What had made it all work, Joan O'Driscoll believed, was a family agreement that to a large extent Rod's work came first. Not first in affection but first in allotment of time. Joan accepted that premise, and the children had been raised to accept it. It was understood that everyone would make a point of being available when Rod was and would help make the most of those occasions.

Once when Rod was a resident—done with med school and going through an intensive four-year training program at a hospital, working round the clock—he came home exhausted. Joan had prepared his favorite meal, and she served it in the dining room with candlelight and all of the children—they had four by that time—on hand. While Joan was speaking to a child she noticed the conversation had lagged. She looked across the table. There was Rod, fast asleep, his face in his plate, right in the mashed potatoes. She was aghast and the children howled with laughter. She led him upstairs, washed his face, and took him into the bedroom, and he dove for the bed.

When Vietnam came along, he became what was called an "obligated volunteer" in the army; he could finish his residency but must then be an army doctor. He served at Fort Knox, delivering the babies of the troops stationed there, and when the war ended he joined a hospital in Newark. The head of its OB-GYN section was James Breen, a distinguished physician who would eventually become a national figure in the specialty. Breen was hired away by St. Barnabas. His assignment was to make it into a top teaching institution in the OB-GYN field. Breen was impressed with Rod and took him with him, and Rod became a "Breen's marine," the staff's name for OB-GYNs trained in Dr. Breen's way of doing things. Over the years, under Breen's guidance, Rod flourished in his specialty and built a strong career at St. Barnabas. And now he was a senior member of his department, and his children were grown, and the most remarkable thing was happening. The obstetrician's daughter was pregnant.

Her name was Margaret O'Driscoll Chapman, and she was Rod's oldest girl. In February, if her dates held, she'd be the first to bear him a grandchild. She'd stopped by today not for an appointment but to pay her dad a fast visit during a Christmas shopping expedition.

They called her Peggy. She was her father's height, and her face was an attractive feminine version of his own. Once someone who'd never met her saw her in a restaurant, a face in the crowd, and identified her as Rod's daughter. She had brown hair, as he had once had, and like him she wore glasses. The spring before, she'd married a young advertising copywriter named David Chapman, and the wedding, presided over by both a priest and a rabbi, was held on the lawn of the O'Driscolls' house in Essex Falls. Rod escorted the bride out of the house and down the front steps, and the two of them together, those two faces, provided a touching double-take.

Peggy's resemblance to her father was more than visual. She was studying to be a doctor, probably an OB-GYN, at the University of Medicine and Dentistry of New Jersey. But Rod was not her obstetrician. Except in rare circumstances—in remote rural areas, for example, where there was only one OB-GYN for many miles—obstetricians' wives and daughters generally went instead to a colleague. The very thought of tending the females in his family professionally gave Rod the shivers. The intimacy of the family connection argued with the detachment that doctors must achieve when treating patients.

Peggy had chosen a female doctor, the young woman Rod and Jack often referred patients to, Sandra Fornwalt. Rod was content with that choice. Several years before, when Dr. Fornwalt had applied for a staff position at St. Barnabas she'd been so impressive that she'd been accepted even though she hadn't gone through its acclaimed residency program—the first non–St.-Barnabas-trained woman it had accepted in ten years.

Like Peggy Chapman, Sandra Fornwalt came from a medical background. Her father, too, was an OB-GYN, and her mother was a physician who worked in family planning. Her grandmother had become an OB-GYN in 1915, a time when such a thing was almost unheard of for a woman: when she made house calls, women would often slam the door in her face, saying, "I wanted a man."

How times had changed. Today many women preferred female OB-GYNs. A fifth of all doctors in the specialty are women; by the end of the twentieth century the figure will be 35 percent, and it's expected that by the time Sandra Fornwalt retires the proportion will be half-and-half. The preference is clear from the statistics on how long it takes new doctors to establish themselves. A male OB-GYN needs five years to build a practice. A female can do it in just one.

Rod, who had suggested Sandra Fornwalt to his daughter, was pleased that so many young women were attracted to the profession, but he disparaged the notion that women made better OB-GYNs.

Patients who selected women simply because they were women, he maintained, were headed for disappointment. "They're obstetricians first," he'd say when the subject came up, "who happen to be women. They're going to do all the suitable things they've been trained to do."

How far would the pendulum swing? A maverick male gynecologist, John Smith, had recently written a book asserting that "men have no business being gynecologists. The role properly belongs to women. They are the only sex truly able to understand, empathize with, and relate to women in the already difficult doctor-patient relationship." A strong subconscious motive for many men who choose gynecology as a specialty, he'd written, was the "need to be in a powerful and controlling relationship with women." Yet even that doctor had admitted that female physicians could be just as domineering and money-grubbing as their male colleagues and that medical training could bleach the sensitivity out of them.

Another male OB wrote that when it came to OB-GYN, males had an advantage: They *weren't* women. True, they couldn't know the pain of childbirth or the misery of menstrual cramps. But that, he argued, made them more, not less, sympathetic toward their patients. What a female doctor, using her own experience as a reference point, might dismiss or belittle, a male doctor would treat as a legitimate problem. Sometimes female obstetricians, he observed, had no patience with women's complaints and their need for reassurance. Males could have more compassion for women because they weren't women.

Peggy Chapman's visit didn't last long, just long enough to say hi to her father and kiss the scrape on his forehead. Two days before he'd been trying to get something out of the trunk of his car, and he'd leaned so far forward that he'd lost his footing and tumbled in headfirst. The trunk lid had come down on top of him, and for three or four minutes, caught in the jaws of his big blue Mercedes, he hadn't been able to extract himself. The office had gotten a kick out of that—the thought of Rod's legs sticking out of the trunk, waving. "Not as bad, though," Barbara Valente said when Peggy came out to see the staff, "as the time he was trying to remove a vaginal pessary from a patient and fell off the stool."

"I'll have to say this for him," Bea said. "He never missed a beat. He just knelt there and kept working until he got that pessary removed. I don't think the patient ever knew what had happened."

• • •

The morning's other special visitor was Maria Ramirez. Her awful ordeal—four months of carrying twin babies knowing all the while that one was anencephalic and would die—had ended three weeks before.

When her labor began, she and her husband had no one nearby they could ask to take care of three-year-old Peter, so they had to bring him to the hospital. Maria's husband had to watch over him instead of being with Maria. Rod O'Driscoll delivered the babies by cesarean section. Both were girls. The anencephalic baby was stillborn, which was perhaps a mercy; the Ramirezes had been spared the additional pain of watching a doomed child cling to life for days or weeks. The other little girl was fine, a perfect baby.

Father Leo Farley, the Roman Catholic chaplain at St. Barnabas, was called. He was a tall man in his early sixties, with salt-and-pepper hair and rimless glasses. In his five years at the hospital he had been summoned to many such situations, and it was his practice, in dealing with the parents, to avoid all the time-worn comforts such as "It was God's will." Meaningless palliatives, he called them.

He was there to provide a sympathetic presence and, as he put it, "to honor the reality of the grief." Each loss was unique. The grief was real. He baptized the stillborn baby with the name the Ramirezes had given her, Danielle.

Late that evening, as Maria lay in the recovery ward, a nurse brought her little Catherine to feed and afterward asked if she would like to have the stillborn child, Danielle, brought to her. She said yes, and in a few minutes the nurse came back wheeling a bassinet with a tiny, motionless, swaddled figure in it. For two hours, tears streaming down her cheeks, sometimes quietly sobbing, Maria held Danielle in her arms and told her again and again that she loved her, while from here and there around her, elsewhere in the darkened ward, came the sounds of other new babies sucking or fretting. At midnight the nurse came again; her shift was over, she said, and she would have to take the baby back. Maria handed up her little lost child.

Two days later, Father Farley celebrated mass for Danielle in the hospital chapel. The next day was the funeral. In a final anguishing touch, Maria could not go. Her stitches had become infected. She stayed home with Catherine. It was her thirtieth birthday.

A week after the birth, Maria came to the office so Jack could see how the resewn incision had healed and to show him and Bea and the rest of the staff her daughter Catherine. Small and peaceful and pink, Catherine had fine black hair an inch long sticking straight out all over her scalp. She looked at everyone calmly, her lips moving to indicate that as far as she was concerned, it was lunch time.

Maria's demeanor had changed since her last office visit. The sadness was there, but her expression was clearer, the blurred appearance gone. In the examining room, waiting for Jack, she talked with Bea. "I think sometimes it would have been better not to know," she said. "I've had to go through such a long period . . . four months. Still, if we'd spent all that time preparing for twins, preparing two of everything, and then the sudden shock. . . . There's no answer, no way to solve it."

"I just feel so bad for her," Bea said after Maria left. "Everybody is saying how cute the baby is, and this and that, and nobody talks about the baby that isn't there. But she needs to talk about it, because that's a part of this whole thing. You know, people come into our lives all the time who have just such quiet strength. You don't know the burdens they carry. Maria Ramirez has that strength."

•   •   •

That afternoon, office hours ended early. It was the day of the annual Christmas office party, which Jack and Suzanne Bonamo were hosting this year. Last winter they'd bought a place thirty minutes west of the office, in a rural area. The Bonamos' house, large and new and done in the English half-timbered style, was high up one side of a valley, with an unobstructed fifteen-mile view across the national forest called the Great Swamp.

Suzanne Bonamo wore a black silk pants suit with black lace over the shoulders—a dignified version of the lingerie look. Twelve-year-old Sara, tall and slim like her mother, with a dimple in one cheek, and ten-year-old Nick, with his surfer haircut, passed hors d'oeuvres to the guests; counting husbands and wives and children, there were about forty of them. Alex, five, kept close check on the two fireplaces, eager to tell his father when another log was needed. The party was thrown in an atmosphere of prosperity and accomplishment. It had been a good year. The practice, in fact, had just set a record for new obstetrical patients signed up in one week—eighteen. "It's going to be a busy July and August," Barbara said.

Presents were handed out. The staff gave Jack a special bag for his skis. Rod got golfing lessons; it was a sly comment on his game. Rod and Jack had given personal presents to each member of the staff earlier that week; now Jack gave everyone T-shirts with sassy messages printed on them. For those in the know, each message referred indirectly to a trait or specific incident and was full of hilarious meaning. There were screams of laughter when each was displayed.

The first went to Jane Rissland, a nurse who worked mainly during GYN hours. Her sisterly, solicitous personality was ideal for GYN, whose procedures included some that were upsetting. Jane was a widow with an active social life, and Jack gave her a T-shirt saying: I GAVE UP DRINKING, SMOKING, AND SEX. IT WAS THE WORST 15 MINUTES OF MY LIFE. To his wife Suzanne: I SAY IF THE KIDS ARE STILL ALIVE AT 5 PM, I'VE DONE MY JOB. To Barbara, who was always concerned about her weight and always thinking about food: INSIDE THIS BODY IS A THIN PERSON SCREAMING TO GET OUT. I ATE HER. In the elation of the moment, they all seemed brilliantly appropriate. But the one that caused the loudest shrieks was the one Jack gave Bea.

Jack and Bea respected each other professionally. Both were excellent at what they did, and each recognized the gifts of the other. They also possessed the two sharpest, quickest tongues on the staff, and they enjoyed each other's wit—most of the time. But in the five years Jack had been with the practice, a certain strain had grown between them.

For twelve years Bea, as Rod's right-hand person, had been accustomed to doing things a certain way—her way. Rod, a casual fellow who ran a taut office, but casually, had given her considerable authority. She was first-class, and she got the job done. Jack, whose public manner was also casual, was in fact intense. Highly organized and systematic, he came from a generation of medical school students different from Rod's; they placed more emphasis on the profession as a business. For Jack there was a great deal more to obstetrics than mere dollars, but he did have his convictions about how an office should be run. Rod was grateful; thanks in no small measure to Jack, the practice was humming.

Bea, however, did not like change in general and Jack's changes in particular. She was not humming but rather, it sometimes seemed, rumbling. Jack rumbled too. "I love Bea," he once said in a moment of exasperated candor. "She's a terrific nurse, she's a lot of fun. But sometimes she drives me crazy." Bea, it had to be said, liked a certain amount of encounter in her life. She was a master of the fast comeback, and when she had something to say, she did not blush daintily behind her fan—she said it.

For the rest of the staff, confined in a small space with two sizable and contending personalities, things sometimes got a little claustrophobic. At tense moments they'd exchange glances, look to the ceiling, then bend their heads over their work. All this was out of sight of the patients and never interfered with performance. Bea and Jack worked together every day, laughed together, knew what was going on in each other's life, and cared. But the tension was there.

And so, as Jack unwrapped his T-shirt for Bea, those in the know held their breath wondering how pointed the message would be and how Bea would receive it. Jack held up the shirt. IF YOU DON'T LIKE MY ATTITUDE, it said, CALL 1-800-WHO-CARES.

When Bea saw the T-shirt Jack had bought for her, she roared with laughter. Then everyone else laughed too, partly in relief: Bea had taken it well. The T-shirt, however, wasn't accurate. Bea cared, a lot. During her years with Rod when he was in solo practice she had enjoyed her work as much as a job could be enjoyed. When things changed and the practice took on a new character, it was difficult for her. The truth was that Bea's attitude wasn't 1-800-WHO-CARES. It was closer to 911.

• • •

On Friday, December twenty-eighth, Rod and Jack had their annual year-end review lunch. They chose Spectators, a mile west of their offices on Northfield Avenue, conveniently near the hospital if a beeper should summon. Spectators was a theme restaurant, an all-out elaboration of the sports motif. The handles on the plate-glass doors were baseball bats, and as the diners walked in they passed through turnstiles as at a stadium. The bar was done up like a hockey rink, with blue and red lines on the floor and enclosed by original Plexiglas hockey boards from the Meadowlands, home arena of the New Jersey Devils. The dining area was a boxing ring, with ropes on stanchions. Spectators was mainly and deliberately a male preserve, maybe just the change of scene that two male obstetricians needed after yet another year of deep immersion in the world of women.

They entered the boxing ring and sat down. Rod ordered a scotch and a Pro-Burger, and Jack, in reluctant obedience to his diet, asked for seltzer and the Spectators salad.

Rod pulled out a piece of paper with some numbers scrawled on it. "Well," he said, "as of this morning, and assuming that nobody goes into labor over the weekend, we'll have had 278 births for the year."

"Not bad," Jack said. "In fact, it's a record." Two hundred and seventy-eight usherings of squalling newborns into the state of New Jersey, many of them involving, for the doctors, anxious, last-minute telephone calls from contracting mothers and dashes to the hospital at unappealing hours. Mary Jo had said she'd actually been able to see the increase: The stacks of patients' folders for her to file had been steadily growing all year long.

"One hundred fifty-two boys," Rod went on, "and 126 girls."

"Sounds about right." More boys were born, usually, but the girls, over the years, would outlast them.

"Three sets of twins. Two vaginal, one cesarean. All uneventful."

"They all did well," Jack agreed.

Over their lunches they went on to discuss the other statistics that bore on the success of the practice: the numbers of referrals—new patients sent to them by other patients or by doctors or nurses; the number of gynecological visits and procedures they'd performed; and so on. They talked about costs, including staff wages, and whether or not their own fees were adequately covering those costs.

Jack raised his favorite subject: new offices. Rod owned the entire, two-story building that housed the practice. The idea was to move up to the second floor, taking it over entirely, bumping its present tenants to other space, and rebuilding it into the most modern and convenient and attractive OB-GYN facility in the county. Rod was willing—he could see the need; the practice was growing—and Jack was avid.

Toward the end of the meal they fell into reminiscence. What they recalled was not the several hundred routine, stressless births, the stream of beautiful babies and delirious parents. Those births supplied the doctors with a steady flow of satisfaction, but it was the background music of their craft and didn't need to be talked about. Like ballplayers reflecting upon the season, they spoke of the exceptional cases, the tough ones that went up against the odds.

Rod remembered a patient named Marie. Sixteen weeks into her pregnancy, he had discovered that she had an ovarian mass the size of a soccer ball. He operated, removing the mass, which was benign, and Marie went on to have a nice normal baby. And then there was Kathleen Krueger. The fact that she'd had a baby was a particular satisfaction. As a girl she had been stricken with Crohn's disease and had undergone removal of her large intestine. Her doctors told her she could never become pregnant. She got married and for ten years tried to conceive, without success. Giving up, she and her husband adopted a baby. This year, when that child turned two, Kathleen became pregnant, and Jack helped her deliver a healthy baby boy.

One young patient, a college student, had come home on spring break and told her parents she was pregnant. Her mother wanted her to have an abortion, but she refused and went on to have a nice baby and to marry the baby's father. Those stories didn't always work out that well.

Several sets of parents had been in great suspense before the birth of their babies, anxious to see if the children had inherited family diseases. Deborah Dunleavy's first child had a rare form of muscular dystrophy, one that couldn't be tested for. The Dunleavys' second child had been fine, and during the spring and summer she had carried her third, wondering all the while. In September, in an atmosphere of fierce suspense, she delivered an eight-pound, nine-ounce girl, Caitlin. She did not have muscular dystrophy.

Another woman's previous baby had had spina bifida. This time her baby was perfect.

Donna Gabelman had had bleeding and other complications, and in February, at twenty-four weeks, she was hospitalized for premature labor. Her baby, born by cesarean, was almost unthinkably tiny, a mere one pound, five ounces, scarcely more than a grapefruit. Named Jessica, the baby suffered from a number of medical problems but, as of her first Christmas, was doing fine.

Among the most vivid memories for both doctors were women who, while pregnant, had undergone dreadful experiences that had nothing to do with the pregnancies themselves. One patient's father was murdered. The husband of another patient, during her pregnancy, came to her and confessed he was a sex addict. He had a high-profile New York job but picked up hookers on Forty-second Street. He had confessed because of fears for the baby. Both parents were tested for AIDS, and they were negative. The husband got therapy, and it all turned out pretty well.

Still another patient, a school principal, had gone through an agony several years before that persisted throughout her new pregnancy. She and her husband had gone to a convention. During the sessions they put their toddler in the convention's day-care facility, from which it wandered and died in a fall down some stairs. It was the most annihilating kind of shock. Only recently had the two parents been able to bring themselves to begin a new child. The pregnancy had been tense; so much was riding on it. Jack saw them through.

In those three cases, though all hell raged outside the womb, the pregnancies proceeded serenely within and the outcomes were happy. But sometimes the hell invaded the womb and smote the baby. One patient was brought to her obstetrical visits by her father because her husband, a vicious drunk, beat her, and she'd had to have him thrown out of the house. A week before her due date, she failed to feel the fetus move, and she gave birth to a stillborn baby.

One day Jack got a phone call from a woman who, a week before, had given birth to her second child. She was in a closet, she said, hiding there. Her husband wasn't home. She wouldn't come out of the closet, she said, because if she did she'd kill herself; she couldn't handle her two kids. Jack stayed on the phone with her an hour and a half, until her husband came home. Eventually, she was persuaded to go into therapy.

Among Jack's greatest challenges that year had been the pregnancy of JoAnn Cuccolo. At just seventeen weeks her membranes ruptured; membranes sometimes give way due to a weak spot in the amniotic sac. The rupture drained her of amniotic fluid. Without enough fluid the risk of problems shoots up—lung trouble, cerebral palsy, learning disability, birth defects. One particularly bizarre result of early membrane rupture is an affliction called amnionic band syndrome, in which small fragments of the torn membrane form tight, tourniquetlike bands around the fetus's finger or toe or arm or leg, pinching it sometimes to the point of amputation. When bands form around the umbilical cord, the result can be death.

Jack was obliged to warn JoAnn of these dangers and at the same time to tell her that because she was still producing amniotic fluid, there was a chance the baby might escape them and she could go on to bear a healthy baby.

For further counsel he sent her to David Hollander, the St. Barnabas perinatologist, its specialist in high-risk births. Hollander painted a very bleak picture. He repeated everything Jack had said about complications and told her there was an 85 to 90 percent chance of a "less than optimal outcome." He suggested that she consider terminating the pregnancy. JoAnn could not accept the suggestion. She told the doctors she was resolved to do her best to have a healthy baby.

With that, once JoAnn had made an informed decision, both doctors shifted from extreme caution to full emotional and medical support. For the rest of the pregnancy, they told her, in order to retain the most fluid she possibly could, she would have to stay home in bed. Not easy, they knew, for the mother of three small children.

When JoAnn was in her twenty-sixth week, she felt contractions and began to bleed. Jack found that her cervix had opened slightly more than halfway. He sent her to the hospital. The baby was monitored on ultrasound; it was fine.

The labor didn't progress. The bleeding subsided. For one, two, three, four weeks JoAnn was kept in the hospital and closely watched. Each week was a precious gain. In mid-August, in her thirtieth week, the bleeding began again; it was not severe, but it threw her into labor. Rod, who was on duty when the emergency occurred, decided not to use drugs to prolong the pregnancy further; the uterus was determinedly trying to empty itself. He performed a cesarean and delivered a three-pound, one-ounce boy, whom the Cuccolos named Vincent. His scores in the physical examination given at birth were high, and he did well in the Intensive Care Nursery.

"A wing and a prayer," said Rod over lunch in Spectators four months later, recalling the Cuccolo birth.

"Sometimes you just get lucky," Jack said. "A higher power was obviously involved."

The waitress, who in keeping with the sports theme was dressed as a referee, asked them if they'd like dessert. Rod ordered apple pie, and Jack, stoic, had a second bottle of seltzer. A huge TV on one wall was showing highlights of the New York Giants games from the year before, and there on the screen was the Giants' huge, powerful defensive end, Mark Bavaro, mashing one ball carrier after another. That, of course, made both doctors think of the third of May, when, with Jack's help, Susan Bavaro had presented her 245-pound husband with a six-pound, fourteen-ounce son.

The other notable sports birth of the year was to a patient of Jack's who was a nurse in the St. Barnabas emergency room. Her first baby had been born in the hospital elevator, and she was determined that with this baby she would get to the hospital in plenty of time.

This time, her wheelchair racing through the hospital halls, she made it up the elevator and into a bed in Labor and Delivery, where Jack immediately delivered her of a baby girl.

"Wow," Jack said to the parents when it was all over. "Another close one. Why did you wait so long to come to the hospital?"

The wife looked at the husband, who lowered his head. "Tell him," she said to her husband.

"My fault," he said sheepishly. "I was watching the World Series. The score was tied and they were into extra innings. I just had to see who won."

10.
Showings

Three days after Christmas, Tracy got home from work first. He'd just begun setting the table when he heard Susan's car in the driveway. As soon as she came in he sensed something was wrong. Her face was flushed, and she was slightly hunched over.

"I think I'm going to die," she groaned. When she saw the concern in his face, she managed a smile. "Oh, don't worry. I'm all right. It's just that these pantyhose are killing me. They don't fit anymore. I've been in agony all day. Nothing fits any more."

It had happened so suddenly. At Christmas parties friends kept saying Susan didn't even look pregnant. But that night as she dressed for bed, Tracy studied her belly and he could see the difference. Susan had begun to show. Soon, for all the world to see, she would be unmistakably, undeniably, a Pregnant Woman. She would cast a new shadow.

Ten days later, on the first Monday in January, came another surprise. Tracy was up early—he had an early meeting—but Susan was still asleep. He tiptoed through the dark house, not wanting to wake her. He was packing his briefcase when he heard her call from upstairs. "Tracy, Tracy, Tracy! Come here! *Fast!*"

Susan was in bed, lying on her back, her hands on her belly. She was agog. "I just felt the baby move!" she gasped.

Tracy put his hand on her abdomen.

"There it is!" she said. "Can you feel it?"

"I can feel it!" he cried. "I can really feel it! That's wild!"

The two of them fell silent, huddled over her belly, their four hands spread out on it as if it were a crystal ball. The pregnancy books talked about the "quickening," but these movements they were feeling were not the feathery little butterfly brushings the books described. With no diffidence or subtlety, this baby was knocking to announce its presence. Sometimes they could even see the flesh rise in response to the impacts.

Tracy was late for work that day and every day for the rest of the week, enjoying the baby's morning workout. As soon as he woke up, he'd ask, "Any activity?" and Susan would take his hand and place it on the spot. They'd linger under the covers, communing with their child. The seven A.M. show, they called it.

As she lay there, Susan was enveloped in an emotion new to her but instantly recognizable: strong, distinctive maternal feeling. *I have a baby inside me. This is something I have to take care of.* No more running around as though she weren't pregnant, working too hard, carrying heavy things. She was receiving a highly specific instruction to conserve herself, to take things seriously. *You and me, baby.*

The baby was always active in the morning and sometimes in the afternoon when she was at work. Wherever she was, she would sit down and put her hands on her belly and try not to think about anything else. *My baby.* No distractions. If somebody wanted to speak to her, she'd say, if she could, "Let's talk about that later." Sometimes it would happen when she was talking to people, and if she could she'd let herself zone out for a minute and be in her own little world.

One day a week and a half later, the first thing in the morning, Eleanore Steel filled a pitcher with water and placed it on the reception counter, along with paper cups. That meant it was Wednesday, the day for ultrasound scans. The water was for patients who hadn't yet managed to drink the thirty-two ounces they'd been ordered to drink before the scan, to achieve the full bladder essential to a good result.

"Are you uncomfortable?" Eleanore said to Susan.

"Well, I drank the amount you told me to," Susan said.

"Can you fit in another cupful?"

"I guess I can."

"All right, drink another one. If you're not really uncomfortable, you didn't drink enough." Obstetrical staffers could tell whether a patient's bladder was right just by looking at her. If it was fully distended, the woman shifted from one foot to the other as she stood, and when she sat down she lowered herself tentatively.

Susan was scheduled for the second scan of the day, but the first patient had failed to drink her quota; she was sitting in the reception room with a pitcher of her own, forcing down cup after cup. So Susan was moved ahead of her. Bea led her down the hall to the center examining room, where the ultrasound scanner was, and Tracy followed.

The routine Wednesday-morning scans were done not by Bea Perez, who had to take care of the nonscan patients being fed into the other two examining rooms. They were performed by a freelance technician named Frank Conte, a tall, thin, thirty-seven-year-old with reddish brown hair receding from his forehead. Frank was softspoken and serious. His first job out of high school was in construction, but he lost it and became an X-ray technician. In a hospital he saw a demonstration of ultrasound, then still a new technology, and was intrigued.

Ultrasound, or sonography, was a spinoff of sonar, the World War II device that located enemy submarines by sending sound waves down through the water and measuring the echoes returning to the surface. By the 1970s the principle had been applied to many other uses including, in medicine, locating those hidden submersibles called babies. Frank trained in ultrasound. Now he had his own business as a freelance technician, travelling to obstetrical offices all over northern New Jersey to do their ultrasound work. He had scanned his own wife during her pregnancies, including her most recent; the baby, their third, named Adam, was born at twenty-six weeks, not much further along than Susan's baby now was, and he weighed a bit less than two pounds. From years of scanning Frank knew all too well how much nurture in the womb is missed by a baby born that early, and as it turned out Adam had a tough time well into infancy.

Susan had no idea what to expect from the ultrasound experience. At a previous job she'd known two women who'd had ultrasounds, and she'd meant to phone them and find out what it was like. But she didn't get around to it, and all of a sudden the day had arrived. One thing she did know—something not many patients were aware of— was that the ultrasound machine was capable of making a videotape of what it saw, so she'd brought a blank tape with her. Frank took it and slipped it into a slot.

The ultrasound machine was the size of a portable computer, which was partly what it was. It rode on a stand supported by tubular chrome legs on casters. There was a typewriter keyboard on which Frank could type the notations he wanted to appear on the images he took. On top was a video monitor that could be swiveled so that the patient could see what was going on inside her uterus.

Susan lay back on the examining table, and Frank spread electrolytic gel on her stomach. The probe was a small, smooth, rounded steel container, like a bar of soap at the end of a cable. It would send sound waves into Susan's body and pick up the echoes. The computer would measure those echoes, change them into moving pictures, and display them.

No sooner had the probe touched Susan than an image filled the vacant screen. It was like the negative of a black-and-white photograph. The background—the amniotic fluid—was black. Wherever the sound waves struck flesh, the echoes registered in gray. Bones were white. To some parents the depiction is alarmingly spectral at first; every ultrasound technician is used to nervous Spiderman jokes. But once they are helped to identify what they are seeing, unease changes to fascination.

"Here's the wall of the uterus," Frank said, pointing to a double line of white running across the bottom of the screen. "We're looking at a profile of the baby. Side view. You can see the legs down here. Here's the abdomen. You can see the heart motion. We can see the spine over here."

Susan and Tracy stared at the little screen, spellbound, trying to understand what they saw.

"What's the baby doing?" Tracy asked.

"It's lying on its back, lying on the mother's spine, feet toward the exit. The mother and baby are spine to spine. We're getting a side view."

The baby's entire spine was visible. Frank's practiced eye examined the row of ghostly white knobs, the vertebrae of the spinal column. He was looking for openings between them. If there was a gap—spina bifida—the spinal cord could squeeze through it, forming a meningocele, a hernia of the nerve endings. What Frank saw pleased him. "That's a beautiful spinal column," he said. "Nice curvature." He inspected the lower back carefully. On a scan two weeks before he'd seen an omphalocele, a sac full of intestines that had bulged through a defective abdominal wall. The baby had died soon after birth.

"We just saw the stomach bubble there," Frank said. "See it? That dark hole right there?" He moved the probe, examining the baby section by section.

"We just had a four-chamber heart there," Frank said with the hushed excitement of a birdwatcher who'd spied a rare species. "I just saw it. There it is again. Four chambers: two ventricles, two atria. The chambers you see pumping away, they're the ventricles." The ventricles looked like tiny gray fists, ceaselessly clenching. The motion was not clipped and mechanical but fluid. Susan and Tracy gazed at the tiny apparatus, in every sense of the word the heart of their baby. No bigger than a marble, it was already pushing volumes of blood throughout the body. To look at it was to wonder. What, for example, had flicked the switch that turned that little engine on? How many decades would it throb before something else turned it off?

Every mother, Frank knew, wanted to make sure that the brave little heart was beating. That was one of the main concerns. So Frank always made a point of confirming that it was fine. "Well, here's the heart beating," he'd say as soon as he could so they'd know the fetus was viable.

Susan and Tracy could have watched the heart for hours. But Frank, knowing that by now there were two or three women in the reception room with very full bladders, and others now starting to drink water for appointments after lunch at another doctor's office ten miles away, shifted the probe. When the image of the heart disappeared, Susan sighed and Tracy said, "Oh, gee . . ." The show, however, was not over.

He traveled now to a glowing white ring at the top of the spinal column. "The head," he said. "Here's the skull; here's the brain. This is all brain tissue in here." He changed the angle of the probe so that it aimed directly down onto the top of the baby's head. The image became a cross-section of the cranium, ear to ear. It was as if he'd placed the probe on the crust of a loaf of bread and photographed just one slice; the sound waves went in until they hit something, then bounced back up to the probe. The computer received the bounced signals, analyzed their intensities, and displayed them as a moving picture. In the course of this process the computer did something flashy: It took the vertical slice and turned it ninety degrees, so that what Frank saw on the screen was not an end view of the slice but the slice resting flat, as if on a plate. That way he could study it.

A small white arrow appeared on the screen, and with the machine's controls he moved it until it touched one side of the skull's image. Then he moved an arrow to the opposite side. He pressed a button and there was a click. He was measuring the distance from the outside of the skull on one side to the inside of the skull on the other. The distance, called the biparietal diameter, was one of the key dimensions he'd check to calculate the age of the baby. It was 5.5 centimeters—a little over two inches.

The probe moved again, and for a moment the image was streaked and confused. Then it cleared, resolving into a gray oval—the placenta, the temporary organ through which Susan and the baby exchanged blood. One of the main objects of a scan is to examine the location of the placenta. If it is low in the uterus, too near the exit, that is not good. Toward the end of the pregnancy, during labor, a low-riding placenta, or placenta previa, might block the fetus's path and be forced out ahead of it, causing severe bleeding and other complications. Susan's placenta was in the ideal spot, back against her spine, not near the cervix, well up in the uterus. It could never present an obstruction. At the moment the baby's head was lying on it as if lolling on a pillow.

"Here again we're looking at the spinal column," Frank said. "You can see all the vertebrae coming up and around." A white halo rose from each bright vertebral knob, and together they created a delicate architecture of ribs. Once more, this time from another perspective, Frank checked the spinal column for defects.

The baby turned, and Frank followed the motion with his probe; keeping up with the baby's shifts was one of the challenges of his job. Then the baby came to rest on its stomach. The probe was looking straight down at the spine. Frank concentrated on the lower back, the lumbar and sacral areas. If any place was disconnected, it was usually there.

Frank moved to the legs. "Here's the femur," he said. Along with the dimensions of the skull, the length of the femur—the long leg bone between the knee and the pelvis—is a crucial indication of the baby's age. The femurs of virtually all babies, whether destined to become jockeys or Boston Celtics, are almost exactly the same length at each stage of fetal development. "Basically all babies grow at the same rate. Every baby at, say, twenty weeks should have the same femur length." Frank measured off 3.1 centimeters. The thigh bone was an inch and a quarter long.

The third age-determining measurement was the circumference

of the abdomen. The probe took a slice through the baby's midsection and turned it flat. Frank marked off two diameters—front to back and side to side—and clicked them into the computer, which would use them to figure the circumference. From Frank's various measurements it would be determined that Susan's estimated date of confinement would be the tenth of June instead of the seventh.

Next Frank examined the structures of the brain. The left and right hemispheres showed clearly as dark spaces on either side of a white line. Frank checked to see that the ventricles of the brain were not enlarged. A swollen ventricle might indicate hydrocephalus, a pool of spinal fluid that as it grew would put pressure on the brain and force the skull to expand. The oversized skull might impede labor and delivery. One baby in two thousand has hydrocephalus; it accounts for 12 percent of serious malformations found at birth. Again, the MacGregor baby passed inspection.

"You did a good job of drinking your liquid," Frank told Susan. "The bladder is pretty well distended. It has to be full, because a full bladder pushes the bowel and other things out of my way. But that's just part of it. The bladder acts like a window into the lower part of your body. Sound travels better through liquid than it does through air. If your bladder wasn't full, I couldn't see the vaginal canal."

He moved the probe back up Susan's abdomen. "Now I'm just generally searching for things. There's a hand. See the arm coming up and the hands curled? We can see the hand moving up and down. You can see how active the baby is."

The baby turned. "There's the baby's bottom," Frank said. "If I see its sex, do you want to know?"

"No!" Susan said.

"No," Tracy said, much less emphatically. "We want to wait and be surprised."

It was so interesting to Frank, the strange discipline young couples imposed on themselves. They would absolutely refuse to learn the sex of their baby, put a lot of effort into not knowing and making sure that people didn't tell them, and then spend months desperately trying to guess what the sex would turn out to be.

"There's the umbilical vein," Frank continued. The umbilical cord looked like twisted rope, spiralling out of the placenta.

Until now the ultrasound portrait had been fragmentary: a glimpse of this, a hint of that. To the amateur eye the images weren't immediately recognizable as a baby. Now, however, the baby assumed the perfect position for a full-length portrait. Frank got a good angle on it, and a bright, crisp picture of a human infant popped onto the screen. There it was, unmistakable, a well-formed fetus. It was lying on its back, moving its arms and legs.

"There's the face!" Susan cried. "I can see the nose and the mouth; I can see the lips."

The baby raised its hand to its mouth, and the jaw began to move.

"Look at that!" Tracy said. "It's sucking its thumb!"

Frank was busy with what he was doing, which was counting fingers and toes. To oblige, the baby spread both hands. One, two, three, four, and the thumb's over there. And the other hand. All present and accounted for.

Some babies, like this one, really cooperated. Some didn't. The baby would refuse to get into position, and Frank would tear his hair out trying to get a decent shot. He felt it important that the parents saw a good picture of their baby, because for many, he believed, this might be where bonding began. Watching their baby, most were too moved to speak. This was their child. *Here's my baby. It's alive. My little baby's leading a life in there.*

When Frank had started doing ultrasounds, fourteen years before, the husbands seldom came along. Over the years, that had changed, and now nearly every woman was accompanied by a man. And no matter what attitude or lack of it the men brought to the scanning room, they left it genuinely moved, if Frank was any judge. They stood there stunned, often with tears slipping down their cheeks.

It had to be a good thing, Frank felt, for a man to identify strongly and personally with his child at this point in pregnancy, half way through, not just on the day of delivery. Fathers who'd fallen in love with their babies via Frank's ultrasound screen had to be more involved with the pregnancy, he reasoned, better companions and helpmates to their wives during the last five months, which could be such heavy going, and later on maybe even better fathers. That, at any rate, was how Frank liked to view his vocation. People criticized ultrasound as being too technological, unnatural, another medical rip-off. The criticism couldn't have conflicted more drastically with the everyday truth that Frank experienced.

Having counted everything he was supposed to count, measured everything he meant to measure, and checked everything he could check, Frank prepared to take the baby's first portrait. He directed his computer to send an image of the baby to a Sony printer. As the printout emerged, he saw that the picture was particularly good, one of the sharpest and best composed he'd ever done. "Here," he said to Susan, "the first photo for the baby book."

"Wow, look at this!" Tracy said. "This is great!"

"Oh, it's beautiful!" Susan said.

"We really can't thank you enough," Tracy said.

Frank blushed. He never knew how to handle all the emotion that parents showered on him. The picture had a practical use: It caused so much excitement that parents hardly noticed he'd turned off the machine, the screen had gone blank, and their precious visit with their child was over—as if he had summoned a loved one's spirit from another world and now must let it return. "And don't forget this," he said, reaching down and extracting the video tape. "You'll have fun watching this on its twenty-first birthday."

• • •

When it was time for lunch, the staff always turned off the telephones and let the answering service take the calls. It was a special answering service, accustomed to dealing with doctors' offices, and when they got a call from a patient who was distressed they knew to contact the office on the private line. On this day, they were having tuna salad and discussing with pleasure the birth of a baby boy to Karen and Michael McDonough the day before. The brain tumor that had stricken Michael early in Karen's pregnancy, causing her such fear, had never returned, and Michael was growing heartier with every passing week. When lunch was half over, the service forwarded a call from Anne Marie Lipper, who was nearly six months pregnant with her first child. Anne Marie had been at work and had just received a call from her husband Steve, who with his father ran a service in Manhattan that evaluated mutual funds. Steve had told her of the death of one of his grandmothers, a dear old woman whom Anne Marie had come to love very much. The death still on her mind, she'd decided to go down to the next floor to get some fruit juice. As she stepped from the first of the carpeted steps she caught her heel and started falling forward, knees first.

Her first thought, she told Steve later, was of the dramatic plunge that Scarlett O'Hara took in *Gone with the Wind*. Her second thought was more typical of the strong-minded, practical person she was. *No!* she commanded herself. *This is not going to happen. You're going to reach over and grab the rail and you're not going to fall.*

Down she went, taking the impacts on her knees and shins. But she had managed to seize the rail, and after four or five steps she managed to check her plunge. She lay across the steps, shaking and crying, partly because of pain and partly in suddenly released grief for Steve's grandmother.

Other workers rushed over to help. They comforted her and dabbed at her bleeding knees and urged her to visit the medical department. Instead, after sitting down for a little bit, she drove herself home. At home she'd begun to worry about the baby. She called Dr. Bonamo.

When the answering service put the call through, Bea Perez picked up the receiver and talked with Anne Marie. "I'm sure you're fine," she said comfortingly. "In all my years in nursing I've never once seen a baby in utero injured by a fall. But you should talk to Dr. Bonamo. He's at the hospital now, but I'll have him paged, and he should be calling you very soon."

Ten minutes later Jack phoned. He listened to her account of the fall and asked a half dozen questions. "I honestly don't think you have anything to worry about," he said. "You took all the punishment on your legs. Anyway, babies are beautifully protected. It would take a pretty strong blow to the stomach to cause any trouble. Patients in their eighth and ninth months often call and tell us they've fallen on the stairs. Some fall down the stairs, but some fall up because the weight of the baby tips them forward. Either way, in virtually every case they're fine."

Much reassured, Anne Marie took a nap, and when she woke she felt better. A week later Frank Conte performed an ultrasound examination. All was well.

•   •   •

The young-married life Susan and Tracy had been leading had involved a couple of ski weekends each winter. This year it wasn't happening. Everything in Susan was telling her to be careful, to watch her footing, to avoid a fall that could hurt the baby. She knew rationally that the uterine walls and amniotic fluid protected babies against blows, but her instincts were commanding her to act as if the baby were as fragile as a teacup. If she saw a patch of ice on the sidewalk, she walked around it. She wore a seat belt. She took no chances. She loved to ski, but this year it was out of the question.

"Dr. Bonamo said you could go on the bunny hill," Tracy said at dinner.

"I know," Susan said, "but what's the point? Why spend all that time to get there and all that money on a lift ticket unless you're really going to have fun? Anyway, it's solved itself. At this point I couldn't possibly get my ski pants on."

•   •   •

Susan had an OB visit the week after ultrasound, and Jack reviewed Frank's ultrasound photos with her. "I have to say, you're doing fine," he said at the end of the session. "Your weight is right and you're carrying it well. You look wonderful." And she did. She was lovely—lustrous hair, ivory complexion with soft pink blush, her expression the ethereal-madonna look that made some who saw her think of Renaissance paintings. She was just slightly, attractively fuller in the face, not to mention the bosom. For the moment, at least, she was the idealized pregnant woman. She had entered her fourth month, and this was the famous second-trimester glow.

For many women, the second trimester is the golden time of pregnancy. The nausea generally vanishes, and sexual desire proves it hasn't. Whatever mischief the hormones are causing, they also pump up the vitality. Skin, if it isn't blemished by the hormones, is perfected by them. Hair and nails are never better. The belly is big enough to bring the attention that is a pregnant woman's due but not big enough yet to be unwieldy.

And the mother can get to know her unborn baby. Its movements are now not random twitches but so well defined that they immediately call to mind the specific body parts that seem to make them— the bottom; the hard, round little head; the foot; the knee; the elbow. Now the baby develops its own cycle of sleep and waking, which its mother can learn and have the fun of anticipating. All of it gives her the feeling she is coming to know her child, that she is its companion, not just its ride.

The second trimester is the peaceful interlude between difficulties past and difficulties perhaps to come. Ahead lies the third trimester, which can be another kind of experience altogether: an exhausting crawl, encumbered by an ever-increasing weight, toward a climax full of unknowns.

11.
Detour

It was February at last. Judy Lombardy, the forty-three-year-old psychologist, was in her ninth month now and nearing her time of delivery. Although she'd be glad when it was over, she had loved her pregnancy. "It's like having a companion with you all the time," she told a friend. "You're never lonely; you always have someone to talk to." But it had been going on for a long time, and she was ready for it to end. "I'm tired of having the baby on the *inside*. I want to *have* it, carry it, see it, be with it. There's this connection between us already. It's in me; it moves; I feel it and touch it. I know its schedule, when it's frisky, when it's sleepy. It's as if I know a little bit about its personality, just from carrying it. I think it's going to be a mellow little baby."

Rod had been after her for months to cut down her practice; he was worried about her blood pressure. She'd tried, and two weeks earlier she'd begun her full-time maternity leave. "For the first time in thirty years," she told Michael, her husband, "I have nothing to do."

"If only you were doing nothing," he said. True, she wasn't seeing patients anymore, but she'd switched into full-time housework, cleaning drawers, vacuuming, scrubbing floors. She'd chosen some wallpaper for the baby's room and, stomach holding her away from the wall, was in the process of hanging it.

Ten days earlier, she had called the O'Driscoll-Bonamo office full of anxiety; her baby didn't seem to be moving very much. She was instructed to come right in. "I'm a little frightened," she told Bea. "The baby's usually very active in the morning, but today I've barely felt it. I mean, I have confidence in the tests and so on, but I still get scared."

Bea did an ultrasound scan. Rod came in to take a look at it. Then he examined her. "The baby looks fine to me," he said. "All his signs are swell. He's not moving much this morning, but sometimes they do that."

The further along a pregnancy got, the more calls Rod and Jack received about lack of fetal movement. There was usually a simple explanation. As fetuses grow they have less maneuvering room in the uterus and a harder time performing what OBs refer to as "gross movement," the somersaults and other extravagant gymnastics that make mothers say "wow!" There is another aspect to it. Patients at first are enamored of their babies' movement and fascinated by every punch and kick. But eventually they become used to it; it becomes like background noise, something they aren't consciously aware of as long as it continues. This accustoming is especially common among women having their second and third pregnancies. Activity registers on them less vividly than on the new mother—until it seems to stop.

Even though Judy's baby had seemed fine, Rod had sent her up to the hospital to be checked on their more sensitive instruments. The baby's heart had been steady. But Rod had been unsatisfied. He'd decided that in another week or so, as Judy's pregnancy approached term, the birth should be induced; she'd be given medication that would dilate her cervix—make it open up to allow a baby to pass—and start contractions. Judy had hypertension, and if the birth became overdue, she might suffer complications. The job of inducing her would probably fall to Jack. Rod was taking his family to Florida for some tarpon fishing. Jack would have the practice all to himself.

Now it was nine days later, and Judy's impending delivery was on Jack's mind. This morning he had called her, inquired how she felt, and asked her to drop by in the afternoon to repeat the test, just in case. Bea put her on the electronic fetal monitor. While Jack was watching, the baby's heartbeat went way down and stayed down for five or six minutes. He didn't know why.

"Probably the umbilical cord was around the baby's shoulder," he said later, "or maybe it was wrapped around the baby in such a way that when the baby moved in certain directions, it put pressure on the cord. I mean, those are the kind of in utero accidents that you can't predict and that can be tragic. They put pressure on the cord and pinch off the oxygen, without anyone being aware of it. The heartbeat slows, and the baby is injured or dies. Or sometimes, afterward, you find the placenta had separated and was hanging on by just a thread and the baby was in a lot of distress."

He decided to induce her immediately. "Let's get you up to the hospital," he said. Judy was too upset to drive, so Genevieve volunteered. On the way, Judy's anxieties poured out. "I'm forty-three and I'm having my first baby," she said, "and it's not supposed to be like this."

At Jack's direction Genevieve, who had worked in the hospital and knew the ropes, skipped the admissions procedure and took Judy right up to Labor and Delivery. Jack had called the resident on duty, Dr. John Scaffidi, to let him know Judy was coming and to ask that the operating room be set up for a cesarean, just in case it proved necessary. Dr. Scaffidi met her and took her to the recovery room; all the labor-and-delivery rooms were occupied. He immediately put her on the electronic fetal monitor. The heart was normal. He gave her a biophysical profile test, and she scored a perfect ten. What was going on here?

Jack arrived at the hospital, and while he and Scaffidi were talking to Judy, it happened again. The heartbeat went way down, then came back up.

"Let's get that baby out," Jack said to Dr. Scaffidi, "before one of these decelerations happens and the heartbeat doesn't come back. We'll make one try to induce, but if that doesn't work . . ." Judy was given Pitocin, a birth-inducing drug designed to start contractions. With her first contraction, the beat went down again. So they turned off the Pitocin and prepared for cesarean section.

As it happened, two of those unavailable beds in Labor and Delivery, Rooms 2 and 3, were occupied by other O'Driscoll-Bonamo patients, both of whose labors had begun. Jack realized that he could well be delivering three patients at once, a juggler with three balls in the air, a catcher with runners on three bases, an air controller landing a squadron of cherubs. It didn't faze him at all. He loved it when two or three patients were in labor at the same time. It was efficient, and it used his abilities to the maximum.

The patients would not be given short shrift. St. Barnabas was a teaching hospital, and so Jack would be assisted by residents—M.D.s learning obstetrics. These residents were experienced; by this stage in their residency they'd done many deliveries, all of them under the watchful eye of veteran OBs like Jack. However, Jack would fully participate in the births. He was in command. And unlike a solo obstetrician who during a delivery was huddled down at the end of the bed dealing with the emerging baby, hidden from the patient's view, Jack could come up and stand next to her and keep her company. "You're actually closer to the patient," he would say. "They can see you better if you're not lost somewhere down between their legs." What was important to the patient, he knew, was not whose hands were delivering the baby but that someone was in control.

Cesarean section is an ancient procedure. The writers of the Talmud gave rules for operating on a living pregnant woman to rescue her baby. It was commonly thought—because of the procedure's name—that Julius Caesar was born through his mother's belly, but historians have debunked that notion. For one thing, his mother survived the birth, which was then unknown in cesareans. The name probably came from the fact that the Romans codified their regulations on the operation in their *lex cesaria.*

In the old days the purpose was simply to save the baby and to get it baptized; it was assumed the mother, if not already dead, soon would be. In the Renaissance, however, accounts of successful cesareans began to appear. In 1500 a Swiss who castrated hogs for a living performed one on his wife. Both mother and child survived, and the wife went on to have six more children, all of them normally. The first successful cesarean reliably reported in the United States was performed in Nassau, New York, in 1822 by a fourteen-year-old girl upon herself as she lay in a snowbank; her wound was dressed by her employer, a doctor, and she lived. The first American doctor to perform a mother-sparing section was John Lambert Richmond of Newtown, Ohio, in a log cabin. Throughout the 1800s more and more doctors tried the procedure, though debate raged. In 1882 a doctor in Prague developed a technique for sewing the uterus, and from then on cesareans became ever safer and more popular. Since then, the lives of many millions of women and babies have been saved and many cases of cerebral palsy and birth injuries to the newborn avoided.

Jack explained to Judy the need for the cesarean and what would be involved. "Dr. Scaffidi and the nurses will get you all ready," he said, "and Dr. Fox will give you an anesthetic. You'll be completely awake throughout the whole thing, but you won't feel any pain. I'll be right across the hall while they're getting you ready. If you need me or if you have a question, I'll be right back in while they're preparing you. I'll be ready for you as soon as all the preparations are done and you have your anesthesia."

With Judy busy with the preparations for the cesarean, and now that the fetal heartbeat was back up, at least for the present, Jack switched his attention to the other two patients. First stop was Room 3, where Marsha Phelps was just starting to deliver. Her situation was now the most urgent.

A shy young woman with rich brown skin and a gentle expression, Marsha had come in the night before. This was her first baby, so she'd brought her mother with her for support. She was two weeks overdue, with no signs of labor, and Jack had decided to induce her. During the night, to encourage her to dilate, a resident had inserted into her cervix a Foley catheter, thin plastic tube with an inflatable bulb, and slowly expanded it, "ripening" the cervix. When that process had reached a certain point she'd been given Pitocin, which had brought on contractions. All had worked as planned, or better. The labor had moved rapidly, and she was now in the throes of delivery, her feet in stirrups, her legs held up and back. Her mother, Edith Phelps, dressed in a yellow hospital smock, held her hand.

Jack had seen Marsha twice during her labor, in the morning and the early afternoon, and the resident, Dr. Jerry Ciciola, and the nurse, Dana Fedroff, had been there throughout. Now, much sooner than expected, she was in active labor, and Jack joined in. "That's it, Marsha," he said. "Push down on your bottom. Push down real hard. On your bottom. Good for you. Come on. Come on. Good! Chin on your chest. Come on, come on, come on. Good, good, good."

To the side, Dana Fedroff readied a small platform the baby would be examined on. Then she came back to help Marsha. "Okay, deep breath," she said. "Hold it. Hold it there just a sec. Hold it on your bottom. Five . . . six . . . seven . . . eight . . . nine . . . ten. Let it out." Marsha let loose a mighty exhalation.

"On your bottom," Jack said. "Get it out of your face. All on your bottom. As if you're constipated. Real hard. Push down on your rectum. Good. Good."

In the background the television, set to the station Marsha had been listening to before all the action started, jabbered away—a noisy game show. And over all came the steady, sonorous thump of the electronic fetal monitor as it unflaggingly reproduced the beat of the baby's heart.

Dr. Ciciola probed the vagina with his gloved fingers. "Good! Good!" he said. "The baby is right there! Lift up. Lift up once more.

A little more. It's almost there. Come on. Beautiful. Give it to me. It's almost there."

Pale yellow water gushed out, which told Jack that the baby's head was moving down. The membranes had ruptured earlier, but not all the amniotic fluid had come down. The head was like a cork in the birth canal, holding it in. When the cork moved, more fluid slipped through. "Good, Marsha," he said. "After this push, we're going to ask you to move down the bed a little bit, okay?"

She pushed, and Jack said, "Marsha, scoot all the way down to Dr. Ciciola, okay?" With help from Dana and Jack she moved down the bed until her bottom was at the very end.

"Come on," Jack said. "Give us a good push. You've only got a couple left, I think."

"Chin to chest," Dana cried. "Chin to chest."

"Marsha, I see dark hair," Jack said. "No resting now."

The baby's matted wet head was visible. Dr. Ciciola and Jack, standing on either side of Marsha's right leg, were moving gloved fingers between the head and the vaginal opening, thinning out the bottom of the vagina, easing the way. "Hold it. Hold that breath."

The TV game show host was shouting that he had a winner.

"It's 120 now," Dana said, referring to the baby's heart beat.

Dr. Ciciola performed an episiotomy, snipping the skin at the bottom of the vaginal opening with surgical scissors to ease the baby's way. Marsha felt it through her anesthetic and winced. But she was almost smiling now.

"Dana, will you fix the light for me, huh?" Dr. Ciciola asked. Dana adjusted the bright surgical lamp so that it bore directly on the vaginal opening.

Marsha's face, glowing with sweat, grew tense as she felt the baby moving rapidly through the birth canal now. A contestant on the game show was singing, "Way down upon the Swanee River . . ."

"Here comes the head," Dr. Ciciola said.

"Mama, put my glasses on me," Marsha said.

Dr. Ciciola held his finger in the baby's mouth, and Jack suctioned the mucus out of the mouth and nostrils. Jack pushed the head down. "Don't push now," he told Marsha. "Don't push. We don't want your bottom to rip." Water poured out as the baby's lower body emerged.

"A girl?" Marsha asked.

"Yup. Yup," Jack said. "Looks like a girl."

"Oh."

"What do you mean, 'Oh'?"

"I mean Oh."

"I'll take her," Jack said. "I'd love to have another little girl."

Dr. Ciciola put a plastic clip on the umbilical cord near the baby and a clamp on the end near Marsha.

"She's cute!" Jack said. "She's cute!"

Marsha, now adoring, gazed at her child.

"Dr. Fox," he said to Marsha, referring to the anesthesiologist, "is going to get her warmed up and straightened out. Congratulations."

"What's her name?" Dana asked.

"Marissa."

"Very pretty."

Dr. Ciciola cut the umbilical cord, and Jack rolled it up onto the clamp and began to pull gently, massaging Marsha's belly, bringing down the placenta. The placenta came out and plopped in the up-held plastic pan.

"What's that?" Mrs. Phelps asked.

"That's the afterbirth. Kind of messy."

"I've never seen all that before."

"Well, we didn't use to show you what we show you nowadays."

Mrs. Phelps sat back in her chair.

"Grandma, you okay?" Jack asked. "That's a beautiful baby you've got there."

The new grandmother smiled. "I'm getting old and tired," she said, fanning herself with her hand.

"You should be fanning *me*," Marsha said.

Jack was happy, enjoying this swift, uncomplicated birth and the healthy new baby. "We made a very tiny cut in your bottom," he told Marsha, "and now we're sewing it back up. You won't feel it much, if at all."

As Dr. Ciciola worked, nimbly moving a curved needle, Jack chatted—the kind of light, inconsequential chat that keeps patients from focusing on needles and stitches. "They say the women have to have the babies," he said to get a reaction, "because the men never could do it."

"They never could," Mrs. Phelps agreed.

"How many have you had, Grandma?"

"Six."

"Wow. No wonder you're sitting down."

Dana handed Marsha her baby. A nurse came in and whispered something to Jack. In the hall he spoke to the nurses of his other patients and learned that Judy Lombardy was prepped and anesthetized and calm but that Barbara Betz's baby was beginning to move fast. He went in to see Barbara; it was clear she was nearly ready for him. Then he visited Judy and explained to her and to Michael that another patient was on the fast track and would deliver quickly, since it was her third child, and that Judy was to rest and be peaceful and he'd come as soon as he could. She said she understood. Then he crossed back to Marsha's room. "You wanna keep her?" he asked Marsha. "Or shall we throw her back?"

"No, I think she's beautiful."

Dana retrieved the baby and took her footprints. Dr. Ciciola was still suturing the episiotomy, making tiny, precise stitches. Marsha kept craning to see her baby, which was swaddled now in a white blanket with an overpattern of pink and blue ducklings. Dana had given her a little stocking cap to keep her head warm. "Here, let me give her back to you," she said to Marsha.

"Who does she look like?" Jack asked.

"Looks like Grandma," Marsha said.

"I think so too," Jack said. He turned to Dr. Ciciola. "You take over here," he said. "I've got to go deliver my other patient." He turned back to Marsha. "You didn't have to push long at all."

"About ten minutes."

"That's wonderful. Usually it's a couple of hours for a first baby." Dr. Ciciola was sewing up the outermost layer of the perineal skin. "I've ordered pain pills for you, if you want them. You going to nurse the baby?"

"I'm going to try."

"You can do it. You can do it. All the medication we give you is compatible with nursing, so don't worry about that."

"Okay."

"All right?"

"You're going to stay in the hospital a few days. You'll go home Sunday, okay? And they'll bring you the baby at 10 P.M., 2 A.M., and 6 A.M. I'd suggest you don't take the sleeping pill until after you feed her. But do get some sleep. When you go home, you're going to be busy. You'd better sleep while you can."

Dr. Ciciola finished the episiotomy, and Jack examined the site. "I'll see you in a little bit, okay?" he said to Marsha.

"Okay."

"Gonna take care of another patient. Everything here looks great."

He went to the phone at the nurse's station and called his wife.

"I'm not sure when I'll be home," he said. "Maybe eight-thirty or nine."

Judy Lombardy's husband, Michael, had been called to the hospital by someone in the doctors' office. He stood in the hall, barred from the delivery room until the anesthesiologist had finished installing the epidural catheter in her back. He was wearing a pale blue hospital gown and throwaway shower cap. Framed by all that pastel blandness his black beard, still uncovered, stood out starkly. Judy had pinned to his chest a snippet of the black cloth she'd had blessed in the name of St. Jude, the patron saint of hopeless cases. Judy had put herself in Jude's hands when it seemed she would never get pregnant. As Michael stood there, feeling out of place, worrying about his wife, the continuing tumult of labor and delivery raged around him.

Jack was in Room 2, delivering Barbara Betz. On his way out of Marsha Phelps's room he'd been intercepted by Barbara's husband. "My wife needs you," he said. "She's sort of straining."

Barbara was almost two weeks overdue, and Jack had planned to induce her next Monday. But this morning he'd seen her in the office and found that she was four to five centimeters dilated. This was her third baby, and third babies usually come easily, like plums falling from a tree. He sent her right up to the hospital, the second in the stack-up of O'Driscoll-Bonamo patients.

Michael Lombardy saw Jack's head suddenly appear from behind the door of Room 2. "Where's the nurse for this room?" Jack said to no one in particular.

A blond young woman in gray appeared, Dawn Ammirata. "Here I am," she said, rushing by Jack. "I can't be in five places at once." In less than a minute she was out again and moving fast down the hall, swinging her arms.

Through the slightly open door, Michael heard Barbara Betz call out, "Oh, I can't move!"

Dawn, the nurse, was back. "Room 2 is delivering," she said to a nurse at the desk. "I need a cart in there." She went into Room 1, which now was vacant, took a cart, and wheeled it pell-mell into Room 2.

"Oh, oh!" Barbara Betz's screams were thoroughly audible where Michael stood.

Dawn poked her head out the door and called to the desk. "Can you bring me a water container please in Room 2? I'm delivering my patient here." Galvanized, two nurses in pink pajamalike costumes ran this way and that, one of them fetching the container, the other a portable incubator.

"Oh! Oh!"

". . . Five . . . six . . . seven . . ."

Jack's voice was heard now, rising above the screaming. "Listen to me! Listen to me!"

Dawn came out again. She yanked a stool out from under a resident who was sitting at the desk and raced it into Room 2.

"Come on, you're doing it!" Michael heard Jack shout. Barbara Betz screamed.

"Okay," Jack said with excitement, "move down. Good. Good. That's what I want."

"Open your legs and push!" Dawn entreated.

"Beautiful," Jack cried. "You're doing it!"

A big scream came out, so anguished that Michael wanted to cover his ears.

"It's right there, Barbara!" Dawn said.

A howling scream, and then an improbable moment of silence.

"Don't push, don't push!" Jack commanded. *"Don't push!* You've got a baby boy." It was 4:39 P.M. Michael could hear young Betz making his first sputtering attempt at complaint.

"Look at this guy!" Jack cried gleefully. "Is this *okay?*"

A nurse in pink came out of Judy Lombardy's room. Michael recognized her and took a step in her direction. "She's okay," the nurse said in a motherly way. "She's comfortable. The epidural's in. You can come in now."

He was greeted by the anesthesiologist. "She's epiduralized," he said. "She's stable. We're waiting for Dr. Bonamo. He's just delivering another baby."

Is he ever, Michael thought, and went to Judy's bedside.

A small black St. Jude's swatch was pinned to Judy's blue gown, and around her neck was her gold St. Jude's medallion. The electronic fetal monitor was pinging out the baby's heartbeat; 160, said the red digital readout. Her arm was taped to a support board extending straight out to the side, parallel to the floor, and inserted in the arm was an IV connector and a tube. Michael looked around him. This was a full-scale operating room, very large, three times the size of the labor-and-delivery rooms. Off to the side was a big, elaborate electronic fetal monitor. Everywhere was gleaming medical equipment.

The anesthesiologist examined Judy to see how the anesthetic was taking. He rubbed her with a Velcro pad, first on the breast, then the thigh, then the belly. "Can you feel that? Can you feel that? Not at all? Can you feel that?" He put away the pad. "You're having a very nice response to the epidural," he said.

"How long will it be before Dr. Bonamo comes?" Judy asked.

"Well, by the time your epidural really takes effect, he'll be here."

Several nurses were laying out the equipment for the cesarean, moving automatically through the ritual they had performed countless times before. "Did you hear about the new radio station?" one asked. "Its call letters are WPMS. One week rag, three weeks blues." The other nurses laughed.

The main nurse was Patty Peña. She was small and round, with cropped dark hair and a warm manner. "Well, Judy," she said. "It's the moment of truth. Everybody's washing their hands." Jack, who had finished with Barbara Betz and had donned a fresh hospital garment, was scrubbing up in an alcove off the hall.

"What does that mean?" Judy asked, slightly apprehensive.

"That means," Patty said, "that it must be time to start." She looked carefully at Michael. "Are you nervous?"

"No," Michael said, a little too lightly to be convincing.

"Michael wanted the baby born on Thanksgiving," Judy said, needing to talk, "but I didn't. I wanted to be home from the hospital by then, feeling well, being a princess."

"Judy," Patty said, "I hate to tell you this, but you're no longer going to be the center of attention."

"You mean the baby?"

"I mean the baby."

Jack came in, his wet hands raised. "Hello," he said, as if he'd just happened by. "I was temporarily waylaid. One and one—a boy and a girl. The boy is huge. He must be about nine pounds."

"How much is my baby going to weigh?"

"Oh, I just guessed a baby's weight right on the nose. I don't know if I can do it twice." He examined Judy's belly thoughtfully. "I'd say . . . seven-five."

"Eight-five," Patty said.

"Will I lose all my weight now?"

"You'll go home a size three," Jack kidded.

"I started a size six."

A nurse pulled rubber gloves down over Jack's hands. "How much did you gain overall?" he asked Judy.

"Thirty pounds."

"You'll lose twenty in the next three weeks. Baby, water, placenta, body fluids . . ."

"Now that the moment is here, I hope he's okay."

Jack waved his rubberized index finger. "Don't worry. He'll be fine."

Patty slid Judy's gown up, revealing the dome of her belly. She painted the whole thing with a bright brown-red liquid—Betadine, an antiseptic—then continued down the body, covering the thighs and upper legs. Finally she lowered a sterile green cloth onto the belly with a hole cut out where the incision would be—low, at the base of the globe, two fingers' width above Judy's pubic bone.

Michael, the mechanic, laughed. "They're putting a drop cloth on you," he said.

"No," Jack said, "these things are no good for that. I tried it once. They don't absorb. The paint runs all over the place."

Patty mounted a half circle of metal tubing to the bed so that it arched over Judy's chest. She covered it with a blue sheet, forming a shield that prevented Judy and Michael from seeing the operation directly. Without the shield, too many patients panicked and too many husbands passed out.

There were three doctors in the room now, including Craig Fox, the anesthesiologist, and the resident, John Scaffidi. Michael stood at Judy's left shoulder, caressing her cheek with his finger.

"Just talk to me," Judy said, fear in her voice.

Jack looked away from his preparations. "Judy," he said comfortingly, "you should be excited. You're having a baby!"

With a small shining steel scalpel, Dr. Scaffidi made a horizontal incision across Judy's lower abdomen.

"Done yet?" Judy joked.

"Come on," Jack said lightly, now extending the incision in his direction. "Too fast is no good. You don't get the full experience."

Standing on opposite sides of the table and cutting away, the two doctors began a collaboration that would take them deep into Judy's body and back out again. They worked in concert, like two musicians playing a duet, sharing the melody, each yielding to the other at just the right moment, knowing when to fall back and let the other take the lead, resuming on cue. They knew all the steps, shared an unspoken language. "When two people who can do a procedure by themselves do it together," Jack said later, "it's done more elegantly. It's a neater, faster, classier operation."

A tray bearing a heap of Kelly clamps—small, blunt, scissorlike instruments that would pinch off the blood vessels flowing into the wound—rested on a tray set across Judy's legs. As the incision deepened, Jack and the resident applied clamps to the severed vessels so promptly that there was almost no blood. Steadily growing piles of clamps accumulated around the cavity's perimeter.

"Is everything copacetic?" Jack asked Dr. Fox, the anesthesiologist, without looking up, inquiring about Judy's condition. He was assured it was.

"Can I have another Kelly, please?" Dr. Scaffidi said to a nurse.

"May I have the Deaver?" Jack asked, referring to the retractor used to hold the incision open so the doctors could see what they were doing. One doctor held the Deaver as the other cut, and then the situation reversed.

The opening was eight inches side to side and eight inches deep. Looking in, one could see most of the seven layers of Judy's body. They were clearly apparent, as distinct from each other as layers of rock at Grand Canyon. The fat at the surface was brilliant yellow; the muscle was rich, dark red. The peritoneal layer was a glistening whitish pink. The walls, virtually free of blood, looked as tidy and schematic as an illustration in a home medical guide. If one repressed all associations with battlefield carnage and the sci-fi weirdness of looking deep into the body of a woman who, at the other end of the table, was whispering softly with her husband, the spectacle was fascinating.

"What are they doing now?" Judy asked Michael.

Jack, his hands entirely within the incision, heard. "We're having lunch," he said jovially, then corrected his tone. "We're right down to the uterus, dear."

He began to cut the uterus across its base. When a woman has gone through a lot of labor before her cesarean, thinning the lower uterus, the uterine wall can be sheer. In Judy's case it was unthinned and nearly an inch thick. The baby's head was jammed against the muscular uterine wall, and the surgeon had to cut right down to it without cutting the head itself.

Jack moved very slowly, his scalpel delicate. "Go in fast and get out fast," went the cesarean maxim, "but take your time while you're in there." He studied the tissue fibers as he went; their patterns told him how deep he was. He could feel the baby's head through the tissue, more and more palpably the deeper he went. He was almost there. The uterine muscle fibers were separating now, almost of their own accord. He turned the scalpel around, using the handle in place of the blade to go through the last millimeter. Jack had never cut a baby's scalp, though once when he was a resident he had cut one's bottom. Sometimes the finest of doctors cut the baby, not because they were careless but because the tissue yielded so unpredictably. The wounds were minor and seldom needed stitches.

Jack gently rubbed away the last filaments of amniotic membrane still wrapping the hairy little skull. "We're through, Judy!" he said. "I see your baby!"

Four minutes had passed since the scalpels had first touched Judy's skin. It was time to remove the baby.

Patty bustled around the room, preparing the baby's identification bands, checking to see that the infant warmer was working, putting out suture for the doctors to use when closing the incision, and picking up the bloody cloths they'd discarded and counting them to make sure none were left in the incision. She served as a sort of traffic director and facilitator for everyone who had scrubbed.

Jack and the resident began removing Kelly clamps to clear the exit for the forthcoming baby, handing them off to nurses.

The resident placed his hands on Judy's belly, ready to nudge the baby along toward the incision. Jack slipped his hand into the uterus and cradled the baby's head. "A little pressure," he instructed the resident. "A little pressure." As Jack lifted the head just a fraction of an inch, he broke the vacuum that had locked it in its pelvic fastness, and up from out of the cavity came a loud, wet sucking noise. Jack loved that noise. He could hear it and feel it, and it meant something. It made birth's relinquishment audible. It also told him that the baby's head would come out without trouble.

"Ah, here comes the baby," he said, doing a play-by-play for the Lombardys. "Very fast. Tiny baby. Beautiful round head."

Once the head was out, the nose was suctioned free of mucus. Then up came the torso, slick with fluid and traces of blood. "Waah," the baby cried without prelude. "Waah, waah, waah."

"Oooh, listen to him!" Michael said.

Jack took the baby and raised it above the shield that kept Judy and Michael from seeing the incision. "Oh my God," Judy said in awe.

From the ultrasound test, the Lombardys had known their baby was a boy, but they weren't prepared for this much maleness. His testicles were as big as walnuts—large walnuts. Michael opened his mouth to comment, but Jack anticipated him. "The husbands," he said, "always look at the testicles and they say, 'Hey look at my kid!'

But don't feel too good about it. It comes from the mother's hormone." Judy laughed.

Michael handed Judy her blue-and-black plastic horn-rimmed glasses. She put them on and studied her child. "He's a beautiful baby," she said feelingly.

"Is he all right?" Michael asked.

"He looks great," Jack said, "he sounds great, and he's pink as could be. Look at him! Look at him!"

Patty took the baby over to the little table and handed him to the neonatologist, then waved to Michael. "Come on over, Michael." Fathers these days were invited to witness the physical examination. The baby's scores were perfect. Absolutely no indication of what could have caused the heart decelerations.

Dr. Scaffidi was reaching down into the incision, groping for the placenta. He found it and with a smooth motion lifted it out.

Jack looked across the room to the baby. "God, he's beautiful!" he said. The baby was crying again, good punchy howls.

"What are you doing to me now?" Judy asked.

"We're cleaning out your uterus. We wipe it out with a sponge. We want to get any tissues that might stick to the uterine wall." Judy, who by now had become accustomed to drastic happenings in her innards, wasn't distressed. Jack was pleased that the uterus was tightly gripping his hand, which meant it was contracting nicely.

The tip of a small hose was placed in the incision, and the machine the hose was attached to began to suck.

"Do I have a flat stomach now?"

"Yes, you do," Patty said.

Michael had the baby in his arms. "What's his name?" Jack called over.

"His name is Michael," Michael said. He brought the baby over to Judy and held it down so she could see, stroking him gently, saying, "Oh, oh, oh. Want Mommy?"

"Who does he look like?"

"I don't know."

"Me."

"Got your nose, I think."

"I think he looks a little like the obstetrician," Jack said. "He saw so much of me."

Spread out on the floor was a large blue sheet, and on it, as the doctors used them, six bright-red blood-soaked rags had piled.

Patty took Judy's wrist. "I'm giving you a bracelet to match the one on the baby's ankle. Bracelet number 4878." She took the baby from Michael and gave him to Judy, placing him on her chest. Judy stretched and tried to kiss his hand. After scarcely a minute, Patty took the baby back again. "Take your son," she said to Michael.

Now began the ascent back to the surface. Positioned across from each other, Jack and Dr. Scaffidi began sewing. They began with the large uterine incision Jack had cut and clamped as he had gone in. Once the uterus was closed and dry and there was no further bleeding from the suture line—often there was more bleeding, requiring extra stitches—the rest of the sewing up would be a piece of cake. As they worked, they kept removing clamps and handing them off to a nurse.

"Start your count," Patty said to the other two nurses. "One, two, three, four . . ." The nurses had counted the clamps and sponges before the cesarean began and were counting them again now that the peritoneal layer was closed. They would make a final count when the skin was being sewn. It was an earnest effort to keep track, to keep from leaving hardware or gauze inside the body.

"What do you feel, Judy?" Dr. Fox, the anesthesiologist, asked. "Hard breathing, or dizzy, or nauseous?"

"I feel a little pain. Oh, I just feel a little funny."

"In what way?" Jack asked. "Light-headed? Do you feel light-headed?"

"A little."

"You're great," Jack said, "and the baby's fine, so there's nothing to worry about. We're almost out of the interior part of your abdomen."

"Ow. It hurts when you press."

"Judy," Jack said as he worked, trying to distract her, "you gonna want the baby circumcised?"

"Yes."

"Well, then, I'll take care of that, okay? I'll try to do him on Sunday. I think Sunday's a nice day for a circumcision."

"Now Michael," Patty said, "it's time to find out what your baby weighs. Would you go with the baby, please." A nurse led Michael out the door of the operating room, his baby in his arms.

"Judy, how are you?" Jack asked.

"It hurts," she replied, sounding like a little girl with a skinned knee.

"Okay, the hurting will stop in thirty seconds. No more. You have a beautiful little bikini cut."

Michael's head appeared at the door. "I just wanted to say thank you," he said to Jack.

"Oh, you're welcome, Michael. See you outside." He spoke to Judy: "Now it shouldn't hurt anymore. The layers that hurt are done." The suturing level was above the peritoneal layer.

Jack and Dr. Scaffidi were relaxed now, enjoying themselves doing beautiful stitching jobs that no one else would ever see. Every layer was closed with a different suture material using a different stitch. They looped the little curved needles round and round, over and over again, gabbing as they stitched. "This morning," Dr. Scaffidi said, "we had a woman who began to deliver in Admissions. By the time we got to the elevator, the baby's foot and some of the umbilical cord were coming out of the vagina."

"Yeah," Jack said. "I heard. That elevator has seen some incredible moments."

The scrub nurse began counting the needles, calling out the numbers, and the circulating nurse watched intently, as if the needles were the most amazing things she'd ever seen.

"Judy," Jack said, "we've only got one more layer."

"One, two, three, four, five, six, seven, eight Kellys," said a nurse.

"And I have twelve," said another.

"I'm gonna want a plain," Jack said, referring to plain catgut suture.

"The baby's weight is six-twelve," Patty reported.

"Oops," Jack said. "My guess was a little high. But this is a good weight."

"Thank God it's a good weight," Judy said.

"A good weight," Patty said, "doing fine."

"Ouch!" Judy cried. "That hurts a lot."

"Judy, we are really done . . . almost done." The doctors' fingers were moving swiftly.

"Our counts are correct, Dr. Bonamo," said a nurse.

For the skin they used the subcuticular stitch; it went through the base of the skin layer. It was made with a single strand of very strong and flexible suture that ran back and forth from one side of the incision to the other. It was sewn so that, once it was done, you could hold both ends of it and slide it to and fro. Four days after the cesarean, when the wound was healed, the physician could simply pull on one end and the entire suture would slip right out. Cosmetically, it is the most successful of all the possible stitches, leaving just a thin pencil line—no puckering of the wound, no old-fashioned railroad-track type scars. In most instances, no one would ever guess surgery had been performed.

And then they were finished. Jack stripped off his blue gown. "Thank you, ladies," he said to the nurses.

"You've done a real Hollywood production," he said to Dr. Scaffidi, examining the incision. "Judy, you've got a beautiful baby."

"Thank you," Judy said, groggy but happy. "Thank you."

"You've made it." Jack chuckled. "You did it."

"I'm so tired."

"That's a combination of things. It'll pass." He said to Patty, "I'll be back in the office at six o'clock. I thought I was going to get the night off, but no such luck.

"Judy, I'll see you tomorrow, okay? Don't try to move until they get you all cleaned up. They'll get you all washed up and put you in a nice clean bed. I'll see you in the morning, and I'll do the circumcision, probably on Sunday." He waved to the nurses. "Thank you all again."

He went down to the doctors' parking lot, found his black Mercedes sportscar, and sped off. The waiting room at 95 Northfield Avenue, he knew, was full of patients.

There were, in fact, sixteen people jammed into the waiting room, patients and children and spouses. Avoiding them, Jack entered the office through the back door.

"I know, I know," he said to the staff in the defensive manner of the perpetually tardy. "Rod would have been back by six o'clock sharp. I'm five minutes late."

"No," Bea said emphatically, leaving no room for dispute. "It's six-fourteen on the digital clock."

"Okay, Rod would have been back an hour ago."

"But you're not Rod," Bea snapped, plainly exasperated by the wait. The other staffers, Eleanore and Mary Jo, exchanged a pained glance. At last Bea had given voice to her implicit, imperishable indictment of Jack: he wasn't Rod.

Jack pretended not to have heard the crack. "I just delivered three babies," he said.

"Three babies!" Bea said. She had regained control of her tongue and was making nice. Jack told them all about it, then plunged into the evening's work, seeing patients and, in between, returning calls.

12.
Natural

Susan MacGregor wanted to see Jack alone for a few minutes this visit. She'd brought a series of questions written on an index card, and in the waiting room she'd reviewed them with Tracy. These were matters they'd discussed a lot together. But it wasn't Tracy's answers she needed; it was Jack's.

She went through the usual preliminaries. Bea announced a gratifyingly small weight gain; Susan had put on just a quarter of a pound, which brought her to 134. ("I think I've gained more weight than you have," Tracy had said that morning.) Then Jack came in. "Tell me what's on your mind," he said. He'd been through this many times before, he'd been confronted with many lists.

Susan paused, not sure how to begin, not wanting to seem insulting or antagonistic. Other women had been telling her about doctors who were dictatorial and ignored the mother's wishes, doctors who imposed a high-tech childbirth on women who yearned for natural delivery. She'd developed faith in Jack, but it was all by inference. She'd suddenly realized the birth was just five months away and she really hadn't worked anything out with him on some of the most important matters.

"I think the main thing is cesarean," she said with emphasis. "That's something I definitely do not want." She had dressed to look earnest, in a dark green jumpsuit with a subdued paisley print. She wore a gold necklace and fingered it absently.

"I hear you," Jack said. "And I agree with you. In this practice, we think of cesarean as pretty much a last resort."

"I just don't want a cesarean to be an easy way out," Susan said. "I realize things come up. Two of our friends recently had babies, and both had emergency C-sections, and oddly enough both for kind of the same reason. They're both relatively small women and apparently had big babies, and while they were in labor the cord was behind the head, and the pelvis was pinching, or something, and the baby was in distress."

"Well, in cases like those, the only alternative might be a cesarean," Jack said. "But we wouldn't just go ahead and do it. We'd come to you and say, this is the situation and this is what we recommend."

"I know women who felt they'd been hustled into a cesarean. The next thing they knew they were in the operating room being cut open. I don't want that to happen to me."

"It won't, I can promise you that. The only way you'll have a cesarean is after you fully understand why it's the way to go. But if it does happen that a cesarean is called for and you decide to go ahead, you shouldn't be afraid. It's not a nightmare kind of thing. It's a real operation and it has some risks, but it's a fairly routine procedure."

Susan consulted her list. "Another thing is anesthesia," she said. "I'd really like to avoid it if I can. I don't want to be out cold when my baby is born. I want the birth to be as natural as possible."

· · ·

There it was, the word "natural." Many patients, especially younger and educated women, ask for what they call a natural birth. But what, exactly, does a natural birth consist of? To some it means delivery at home assisted by a midwife or perhaps just a friend; these patients use an OB-GYN practice only for gynecological care. To others it means a hospital delivery with a minimum of medical manipulation. One thing it always implies to some degree is defiance, some measure of opposition to what they see as a trend in twentieth-century obstetrics, the overuse of technology in childbirth.

It was inevitable that science would try to improve childbirth; the demand for it had been building for so long. In most of humanity's time on earth there was pathetically little anyone could do for mothers and babies in births that went wrong, so much pain and innocent death. Those who stood by helplessly as tragedy struck could only pray that mankind would someday find remedies. The new profession of obstetrics was a response to that prayer. Nature in that sense became the enemy, and subduing it through innovation became a holy mission.

To an amazing extent the mission succeeded. In modern times, there was an explosion in obstetrical technology, another in pharmacology, and still another in knowledge of the female body. In the spirit of William Smellie, the eighteenth-century London physician who helped found the obstetrical profession, his successors closely observed and learned from what they saw, exchanged their new knowledge with one another, and built up a tremendous store of obstetrical information and technique. It was the age of salvation through science, and with the new equipment and procedures available to them, obstetricians came to feel mightily empowered. There was so much they could do now, and their instinct was to do it. They expected women to be grateful, or at least to lie there and cooperate.

The one thing they did not expect was that women would rebel. In the 1960s, however, more and more patients and even some doctors began complaining that childbearing, one of the most personal and fundamental experiences of a woman's life, was being dehumanized. In the big, modern, elaborately equipped hospitals, women said, they felt like production units, not mothers-to-be. They claimed that the doctors behind the machines had become mechanical, too—cold, stiff technicians and efficiency experts, who had no time to waste explaining their complex procedures to mere patients, no time to wait patiently while a woman had a real try at delivering her baby the old way. Cesarean rates boomed; it was almost as if the cesarean, which the doctor could completely control, was becoming the preferred method of delivery and the vaginal method was coming to be scorned as primitive. Doctors replied that the ever-growing threat of malpractice suits was forcing them to do more cesareans.

Some critics charged that since the machines had cost a great deal of money, doctors felt they had to recoup that investment and make it pay—which meant marching the patients through. Whatever recognized procedure took the doctor the least time, it was said, or made the most money, was the right one. Often it seemed that in perfectly normal labors, the slightest tendency to "fail to progress" resulted in drastic expedients. As if to substantiate these charges, Dr. Saul Lerner, past president of the Massachusetts section of the American College of Obstetricians and Gynecologists, laid his cards on the table. "We now have a very aggressive approach to pregnancy," he told the *Boston Globe* in 1977. "There's a whole new concept plotted out by computers, how long each stage of labor should be. We will not allow a woman to labor for more than four hours without making any progress. We do cesarean sections freely."

Their feelings hurt, obstetricians denounced their ungrateful critics, not realizing that for all their life-saving, pain-sparing accomplishments, they had blundered. They had mistaken their young patients for their patients' mothers. From the OB's end of the examining table the two generations may have seemed the same, but up at the other end they often were a lot different. Great numbers of younger women had grown up to think of themselves as independent. They were not to be patronized or dominated. Just because the person telling them what to do—their obstetrician, for example—was a man, that didn't mean that they would obey and do it unquestioningly. They strongly felt that the vaginal delivery, which many regarded as a sacrament of their womanhood, was not to be despised.

Feminism encouraged women to seek each other out for strength, and the most obvious occasion for this was childbirth. Women in childbirth had always turned to other women—that is, until the men pushed their way into it (so the argument went), the way they always pushed their way into things and took them over.

Men and women had battled for centuries for exclusive sovereignty over the female reproductive system. At first the women were the victors. For most of history and in nearly all cultures, women had been tended solely by other women, and midwives had a strictly enforced monopoly. In 1522 in Hamburg, Germany, a doctor named von Wert was burned at the stake for attending a patient in labor. But as medicine became a profession, more and more physicians, moved by scientific curiosity or concern over the cruel and superstition-based practices of some midwives, became "male midwives."

The word obstetrician comes from the Latin word *obstetrix,* meaning midwife or, more literally, "the woman who protects" or "the woman who stands by the woman giving birth." The first man known to practice obstetrics in America was a seventeenth-century Massachusetts veterinarian, William Avery. The first educated Colonial physician to take up obstetrics was John Moultrie of Charleston, South Carolina, who died just before the Revolution. A number of male physicians studied in London under Smellie and his colleague William Hunter and came to America. Some of these doctors and their disciples introduced obstetrics into medical school curricula; some also tried to educate female midwives to help them improve their skills. But not many. In 1820 a professor at the Harvard Medical School, writing anonymously, argued that midwives should not be allowed to deliver babies without proper training but that such training was out of the question: "We cannot instruct women as we do men in the science of medicine" because the nasty work of dissection would endanger their character.

As an obstetrical establishment began to coalesce, it did what the midwives had done: tried to monopolize the business. In many states obstetricians had midwives outlawed as incompetent and dangerous. Some probably were, but many who were driven out were the hard-working, attentive, motherly care-givers with great practical experience and devotion who had always been the mainstay of women. In 1934 the New York Obstetrical Society called lay midwives "a menace to the health of women." The number of midwives began to decline sharply. In the running battle between the sexes for control of birthing, the men at last prevailed: Childbearing was largely moved out of the home and into the hospitals. Despite all pressures, however, midwives never vanished, especially in remote and impoverished places where few obstetricians cared to practice.

The bossiness of many physicians, so out of synch with the times, affronted post–World War II women and left them wide open to other approaches. First published in the 1940s, Dr. Grantly Dick-Read's book *Childbirth Without Fear* introduced large numbers of ordinary readers to the principles of natural childbirth. He believed that much of the pain of childbirth came from tension and fear, and he suggested techniques for lessening or eliminating those emotions. In the late 1950s, in her book *Thank You, Dr. Lamaze,* Marjorie Karmel popularized the theories of a French physician, Ferdinand Lamaze. Lamaze complained that "women in birth are cared for in the same way as ill patients." Childbirth, he said, should be a shared event for both mother and father, and he described breathing and relaxation techniques they could do together. In *Birth Without Violence* another French obstetrician, Frederick Leboyer, argued that babies at the moment of birth were extremely sensitive to noise, bright lights, rough handling, and bad vibes from those around them. He urged that the delivery room be darkened and hushed and that the infant be laid immediately upon its mother and given a gentle massage, then placed in water at body heat to ease the shock of transition from the 98.6-degree womb to its 30-degree colder new surroundings.

To many women these approaches had great appeal. The natural childbirth philosophy promised them a restored womanhood, a replacement of something male and mechanical with something mystically female. Natural childbirth became a cause, a creed, a passion. A counterrevolution was underway.

Many women, when their offended obstetricians scoffed and refused to go along with the natural birth approach, turned to midwives. The modern-day "lay midwife," as they were called, was an updated version of the ancient midwife figure whose training had come from other midwives and whose main credential was her experience. Lay midwives delivered mostly at the patient's home, and "home birth" became a hot issue in the OB-midwife controversy.

"Home birth," said one of the more than two hundred midwives who attended the First International Conference of Practicing Midwives in 1977, "is a civil rights issue. It's a woman's civil right to give birth where she chooses to give birth."

"Home birth," said the president of the American College of Obstetricians and Gynecologists in the late 1970s in a remark that was greeted by natural-birth advocates as gasoline is greeted by flame, "is the earliest form of child abuse."

More and more city and suburban women were turning to midwives and finding comfort in their sisterly gentleness, their simple, unintimidating techniques. In 1990 there were about two thousand lay midwives performing home births despite a skeptical, often hostile medical profession.

An alternative developed. In the 1920s the federal government had sent registered nurses with advanced training in obstetrics and gynecology—they were called the Frontier Nursing Service—into the hills of eastern Kentucky to help poor doctorless women. The idea spread. In due course nurse-midwives were practicing legally in every state. Some delivered babies at "birth centers," some of which had backup doctors on call, but most delivered in hospitals. By 1991 there were more than four thousand nurse-midwives, a doubling in ten years. Some were men.

They were good—even some doctors had to admit it—and their results with uncomplicated, low-risk births matched the OBs' own. Furthermore, they were getting a noticeable share of the business. During the 1980s the number of babies they delivered yearly quintupled, to about 100,000.

Telling obstetricians they were being inconsiderate merely made them grumpy, but taking 100,000 delivery fees out of their investment portfolios every year made them sit up and take notice. Some hospitals and obstetrical practices responded by co-opting the enemy: hiring nurse-midwives. Nearly all of them, showing more adaptability than they were given credit for, quietly adopted many of the principles of the natural birth pioneers in some form, humanizing themselves as best they could. They created attractive birthing suites that let a patient stay in one place, without shuttling, throughout her entire childbirth, if there were no difficulties. They introduced flexible birthing beds that let a laboring woman assume almost any position she wanted. Instead of giving babies warm baths, nurses put them in electrically heated, thermostatically regulated Plexiglas bassinets until they were used to their chilly new world—technology's approximation of the little bath that Leboyer had in mind.

Even the mentality began to change, or at least the manner. Younger doctors, like Jack Bonamo, came out of med school saying what the best older doctors, like Rod O'Driscoll, had always said, "You're not sick, you're pregnant"—music, no doubt, to the aging ears of Dr. Grantly Dick-Read. Most OBs stopped ridiculing the relaxation techniques, and hospitals started offering Lamaze classes.

One of the most welcome and refreshing capitulations involved fathers. In the old days they'd been exiled to smoky waiting rooms while their wives went through the parturitional cataclysms. Now they were allowed to stay with the mothers throughout the whole process and, what was more, encouraged to perform many helpful tasks as partners in the birth. To everyone, even doctors, that simple change brought rich benefits. "At times now," said Dr. John T. Queenan, chairman of the department of OB-GYN at Georgetown University School of Medicine, "I catch myself wondering: How did we get along without them!"

One mother, Malie Bruton Heider, of Columbia, South Carolina, had three babies during the five years of greatest change in obstetrical attitudes, 1977 through 1982. "For the first birth," she recalled, "we asked about having my husband in the delivery room. We'd heard they'd started permitting it in Charlottesville. But the hospital said no, there was a firm policy against it. The doctor said, 'Fathers can't stand blood. They pass out cold. I've got to take care of *you;* I can't take care of your husband too.'

"The physicians' attitude back then was: 'We'll take care of everything, now lie down and put on your gas mask.' The doctors hated the Lamaze people for giving away all the secrets.

"By 1982, when we had our third, at the same hospital with the same doctor, there was no problem. By then it was routine for the father and mother to be there together, experienced, with knowledge."

The professional magazines and organizations started urging OBs to talk with their patients, and busy doctors, even when communication was against their principles, paid it lip service. But putting flowered curtains into a birthing suite was a great deal easier than thrashing out dozens of controversial labor-and-delivery matters with somewhat informed patients. Despite all the efforts the profession had made to adjust to the new world of childbearing, there was plenty left to interrogate a doctor about. There was a whole series of events in an ordinary childbearing that could be done this way or, if the doctor was of another mind, that.

The episiotomy, for example. Since the early part of this century obstetricians had almost routinely made room for the baby's head as it exited the tight vagina by making a small incision—an episiotomy—in the perineum, the area between the vagina and the anus. Better to make a nice, neat cut that could be sewn up precisely, they argued, than to allow the perineum to shred. Ripped perinea were hard to sew well. In the United States it was the fifth most common surgical procedure, and some 80 percent of first-time mothers delivering vaginally got one. At St. Barnabas the rate was 95 percent.

The natural-birth people said that doctors, as usual, were just trying to make things easier on themselves. It was much better for the mother, they said, to let the perineum tear. Usually the tearing affected only a couple of layers of the flesh there, while an episiotomy cut all the way through all the layers. Anyway, they said, any decent midwife could generally avoid a lot of the tearing, perhaps all of it, by patiently massaging and stretching the vagina as the head came through—"ironing the perineum."

The doctors bristled. They massaged the vagina too, they declared. But you could do it only so much or the patient's vaginal muscles would be lax the rest of her life—not a good thing. And then the argument would shift to comparative infection rates, and stress on the fetus, and on and on.

And there were other thorny matters.

When, if ever, should the drug Pitocin be used to start contractions or to regularize them? Doctors and natural-birth advocates could spend a year together on a desert island without exhausting that one.

The world of obstetrics was a very different place before Pitocin came along. For most of the existence of the human race, when labor went on and on but failed to move the baby through the pelvis, the pregnancy would founder like a ship on a rock, unable to advance or retreat, and death would follow. Faced with the dread prospect of prolonged labor, ancient peoples resorted to remedies handed down from generation to generation. Sanskrit texts written three thousand years ago advised Hindu midwives to burn the skin of a black snake and direct the smoke at the vagina. The Romans prayed to the goddess Opigena, the divine midwife; more practically, a Roman physician named Soranus advised creating spasms by making the patient sneeze. In the Middle Ages, the power of amulets—"eagle stones," "birthing stones," "women's stones," and, in some parts of France, fossilized shark teeth—was widely believed in; women lent them to other women, and midwives arranged them ceremoniously around the birthing chamber. If the amulets failed to bring on labor, many midwives shook the woman or pummeled her belly.

Midwives in many places, until modern times, thought vomiting useful in childbearing. Tending women in long, drawn-out labor, they often fed them nauseating concoctions in the hope that the violent act of vomiting would move the birth along. In the south of France, rhubarb mixed with cinnamon water was the emetic of choice. Afterward, to make a woman expel the placenta, midwives would bring on more vomiting by putting threads or hairs down their patients' throats. Some favored potions made of animal afterbirths.

None of these techniques had much effect. One substance, however, used in Europe since the Middle Ages, did work. Called ergot, it was made from a fungus that grew on rotting rye and other grains. People eating food made from diseased grain often died from ergot poisoning, but when administered carefully, in small amounts, ergot could speed labor. American obstetricians in the eighteenth and nineteenth centuries argued violently about ergot. John Stearns, an early president of the New York State Medical Society, declared in 1807 that he had used it "with the most complete success. It expedites labor," he said, adding, as a tip to the pennywise physician: "It also saves [the obstetrician] a considerable portion of time." Thanks largely to Stearns, many American doctors began to use ergot. Others maintained that it was too potent and caused countless accidents.

Wherever ergot was given, they pointed out, there was a great increase in the number of stillborn infants. By the end of the nineteenth century, the use of ergot in labor was almost universally damned.

Out of the ergot controversy and the toll of new lives lost to the drug came the resolve to find out what in ergot made it work and to produce that essence in a synthetic form. What was needed was a gentler, more reliable substance that could be administered in a highly controlled manner. This breakthrough was achieved in the early 1950s by a Chicago-born biochemist, Vincent du Vigneaud, and it brought him a Nobel Prize.

The commercial name of the substance was Pitocin. It was an exact chemical copy of oxytocin, the hormone produced by a woman's pituitary gland to make the uterus contract. Like many medications it had some questionable uses along with the good ones. Pitocin made it possible to deliver babies on schedule—a human schedule. Obstetricians acting in the spirit of Dr. Stearns' advice in 1807 about saving the doctor's time no longer had to wait on the vagaries of female physiology but, like a dentist, could book their extractions. It was efficient and convenient. No more lost time hanging around the hospital waiting for something to happen. No more missed golf games or dinner parties because labor dragged on too long. A shot of Pitocin would jump-start the uterus and the doctor would be on the first tee by the time the baby got to the nursery. Some women collaborated in the mechanization. They loved the idea of picking a date and having their baby on that date, and farewell to the stressful wait.

During the 1970s there was a strong reaction among advocates of natural childbirth against what they considered the chemical blitzkrieging of childbirth. It seemed to them just one more aspect of the brave new world of obstetrics, a factory environment of ever higher tech in which a woman's body was manipulated for the convenience of the doctors and the hospitals. Not that the profession officially disagreed. Early on, the American College of Obstetricians and Gynecologists declared that there must be "strong medical or obstetrical reasons to induce labor artificially." When mothers developed high blood pressure or diabetes, for example, or if the amniotic sac enclosing the baby burst too early, or if there were Rh blood problems that might require transfusions, or if the fetus was in trouble—these, said the College, were sound reasons for inducing labor.

Some doctors continued to induce labor for their own convenience and profit, and some patients continued to demand inductions for nonmedical reasons, such as exasperation—"patient distress," it was called—but that sort of thing came to be considered bad form, and efforts were made to discourage it. More and more, Pitocin came to be used responsibly, to help women whose labors were truly in need.

•   •   •

Another controversial matter was the use of the electronic fetal monitor (EFM), the band wrapped around a patient's lower body to send fetal heartbeat data to a video monitor. Did it provide an unbeatably sensitive and continuous picture of the baby's condition as the contractions throttled it? Or, as the natural birth advocates said, did the doctors and nurses tend to rely too much on their EFMs, which according to studies were not that reliable anyway and no better than regular checks with the good old-fashioned stethoscope? Some opponents claimed that misleading EFM readings were one of the main causes of unnecessary cesareans. Some insisted that since EFMs required patients to be hooked up to monitors, they inhibited the walking around and the position-shifting that allowed laboring mothers to make use of gravity in bringing down the baby; monitored mothers pretty much had to lie there.

Unshaken, doctors stuck with their electronic fetal monitors, crediting them with saving innumerable babies. And anyway, they said, until labor was quite far along a woman could get herself unplugged from the monitor whenever she liked and go for a ramble.

How was a patient with no special medical knowledge but who nevertheless wanted to make intelligent choices and have the best possible birthing experience supposed to work out puzzlers like these over the course of a handful of brief meetings with a doctor who, though he might want to explain everything fully, was still tired from a pair of deliveries the night before and who knew that ten patients were perched in the waiting room coddling their urine samples and feeling peculiar?

At St. Barnabas, no patient had to have an EFM if she didn't want one, but nearly everyone ended up electronically monitored. For most women, the answer was not to say the hell with it and take their business over to the midwife. Most of the women in prosperous, middle-class, suburban, northern New Jersey wanted a great obstetrician and a well-appointed hospital. Far from being leery of technology, they were avid for it. They wanted all the high-tech wizardry and highly educated obstetrical skill they could get if it could boost their chances of having a perfect baby.

Susan MacGregor, for example. Just by stepping across the threshold of 95 Northfield Avenue when she became pregnant, she had made her decision on the key question: to tech or not to tech. She was teching. But she wanted to be sure that the brilliant new devices and medications and procedures would be used with real restraint. For the sake of the baby she wanted the advantages of science-assisted birth. She didn't, however, want it to interfere with something she also fervently wanted, the primordial birthing experience, which she instinctively knew contained psychic nourishments essential to her motherhood.

• • •

Susan had asked Jack about anesthetics, and with special reason. She explained she was the daughter of a woman whose experiences with obstetrical painkillers had been bad. Thirty years before, when Betty Sprague had had her first child, Susan's brother Larry, she received an injection directly into her spinal cord—a spinal. As so often happened with spinals in those days, before the development of very fine, specially shaped needles, it gave her a long, ferocious headache; it also damaged a nerve to her leg, giving her a lasting twinge in her left foot. When she had her next baby, Gordon, she refused to have another spinal. Instead, she was given a shot of anesthetic in her arm (she wasn't told what kind), which sent her into a high-flying state of euphoria. The birth of Susan brought another numbing shot. Susan knew that her mother had always felt the anesthetics had cheated her of the real experience of giving birth.

"Anesthetics have come a long way since your mother had her babies," Jack said. "These days the usual thing is an epidural, which numbs you from the waist down. During your labor you don't feel the contractions at all. From the waist up, you're alert and calm." He went on to describe the epidural technique, how a tube was inserted part way into the spine—near the cord, but not into it—and connected to a pump that sent finely controlled doses to the patient. He told how, in a vaginal delivery, the dose was reduced as delivery drew near so that the patient regained enough sensation to do a good job of pushing out her baby.

"But don't some women at least make a try at delivering without an epidural," Susan asked, "without any anesthetic at all?"

"They do," Jack said, "and you certainly can too. As long as you can hold off and are happy about it, we're happy too."

Susan again checked her list. "I wanted to ask about birthing chairs," she said.

"Birthing chairs," Jack said.

"Yes, I read something in *U.S. News & World Report* about them, how being in a more upright position speeds up labor and delivery by something like 15 to 20 percent. I thought, 'Wow, that kind of makes sense.' It sent me back to when I was taking art history and we were studying a lot of Pre-Columbian art. They used to plant little statues of fertility goddesses in their fields to make the soil rich, and the goddesses would be squatting, giving birth. I imagined myself squatting like one of those figurines, delivering the baby. I thought gravity might help."

"It's not a new thing," Jack said. "It's like an eighteenth-century device. Women used to sit in chairs with holes in the seats to have babies. We gave it a try and found it just doesn't work well. It would be great if it did; anything to bring that baby down. But it didn't seem to make a difference." In the thousands of births he'd witnessed, Jack said, he'd never yet seen a woman want to stand up to get rid of the baby. The old gravity theory—it wasn't that simple.

"If babies just fell out," he said, "we'd make people just walk around; we wouldn't have all that other stuff. They don't just fall out, they have to be pushed out, with an incredible amount of strength, and you need to hold onto something with your hands and brace against things with your feet, and push the baby out. And if you're standing up, there's just no way to do that, nothing to push against but the sky.

"So we don't have birthing chairs," he said. "We have birthing beds. They let you do almost anything. You can squat. You can sit up. You can lie flat. You can get into just any position that might be comfortable."

"Great," Susan said, smiling. "Save the chair."

Going down the list, they touched on other topics: electronic fetal monitoring, episiotomy, and so on. "These are good questions," Jack said at the end, "and we shouldn't knock them off too quickly, like items on a grocery list. It takes time to absorb the answers and even to find out exactly what question you want to ask. The way it usually works is that you and Rod and I will keep talking about these things over the coming months. We'll talk about some things several times."

"I'm looking forward to the pregnancy classes," Susan said.

"They're good," Jack said. "The instructors have all been labor-and-delivery nurses, so they know their stuff. Once you get into your classes, you'll find it all will begin to make sense to you."

Tracy was summoned from the waiting room. "You talked about cesarean?" he asked.

Jack went over the main points on cesarean. "But in Susan's case," he said, "there's no reason whatever to think that a cesarean is in the cards. From every indication I'd say you're headed for a very normal vaginal delivery."

"These two women I told you about who had emergency cesareans," Susan said, "they were both fairly small and their babies were enormous."

"Well, you're not really small, and I don't see anything to suggest that the baby is going to be huge."

"In my family," Susan said, "we have big heads. All the Spragues have big heads."

"Mine too," Tracy said.

"I don't think you need to worry," Jack said reassuringly. "Babies' skulls are ingeniously constructed so that they collapse a little as the baby goes through the pelvis. The plates of bone ride up over each other, and once they're through, they slide back. You've be surprised how big a head can fit nicely through the average birth canal." The MacGregors' concern about the head passing through, he sensed, had been quietly building and building. It was a common fear among first-time parents.

"By looking at me, then," Susan said, "the way I'm built and whatever you can tell about the baby, you're saying the chances are good that I'll be able to deliver normally?"

"They're excellent," Jack said, knowing the question would come up again.

• • •

What Susan was really asking, without realizing it, was not how Jack stood on individual matters like cesareans or birthing chairs but what kind of doctor he was. When it came to labor and delivery, obstetricians ranged from the interventionists, at one end of the spectrum, to the noninterventionists, at the other. The interventionist OBs favored Dr. Lerner's "very aggressive approach to pregnancy." They liked to *run* the birth, not just stand by and let the mothers have it their way. Their focus was not on the patient but on the process.

In contrast to the interventionists were the obstetricians who generally gave nature the benefit of the doubt. They didn't just go along with vaginal delivery; they urged it upon patients who didn't need a cesarean but thought that having one might be more peaceful and convenient. They took time with their patients not because it had become good form but because they really cared about them and wanted them to know what was going on. Whatever the fads and trends, there always had been many obstetricians like that, and finding them involved the same old skills that finding a good spouse or employer or babysitter had always required—effort, intelligence, and a sharp eye for phonies.

Even the most restrained of OBs, however, was likely to feel that the natural-birth thing had been somewhat overdone. "Everybody talks about the natural way and how great that is," said Dr. William Dillon, head of the department of maternal-fetal medicine at Children's Hospital in Buffalo, New York, "but Mother Nature is a bitch. If you look at nature, it's survival of the fittest. Years ago, prior to any of our interventions, we lost many, many mothers in labor— from infection, from uterine rupture, from bleeding. They were horrible deaths. We've seen those days go by. They are gone."

Many obstetricians who, like Rod O'Driscoll and Jack Bonamo, combine mastery of the advanced gadgets and procedures with attentiveness and respect feel that their profession has gotten a bum rap. Jack, for example, usually unflappable, was nevertheless really burned about the midwives who built up their trade by misrepresenting his.

"I have no trouble with the idea of midwives doing uncomplicated vaginal deliveries," he had said one day several months before in a cubbyhole office at St. Barnabas, near Labor and Delivery. "I'm sure many of them have a great deal of skill. And for people who mistrust doctors or are put off by doctors' reputation for coldness, I know midwives provide comfort. But they perplex me.

"I recently talked to a woman who'd been going to a birthing center and was being seen by a midwife. She was telling me all the things the midwife could do for her. If the baby wasn't coming down in the pelvis, she told me, the midwife had maneuvers that could help her have a vaginal delivery, certain positions the patient could assume, and so on. She told me the midwife could spare her an episiotomy by stretching her vaginal muscles and that the midwife had a special oil that would help the baby's head slide out.

"I really had to laugh. I told the woman, 'It's incredible. You talk as if obstetricians don't want you to have a vaginal delivery. A safe, healthy vaginal delivery is exactly what the vast, vast majority of obstetricians *do* want—for your sake and because a simple natural delivery is easy money for an obstetrician. The patient's very happy, the baby's almost invariably healthy, and you walk away with a sense of accomplishment, with a sense that all is well and that you've done some good; you've done what you've been trained for. But midwives love to plant in the minds of parents the notion that this is not what the doctor wants.'

"From what I can tell, midwives never, ever let on that not only can I do everything they do; I can do thousands of things they're not trained to do. I can do surgery, if the need should arise; I can handle all the obstetrical emergencies. And *that* is why you go to an obstetrician. The postman can do an uncomplicated delivery. But, unfortunately, you never know when a birth that was supposed to be simple is going to get very complicated."

He listed the stages of an OB-GYN's twelve-year training—the four years of undergraduate premedical work, the four years of medical school, the four-year obstetrical-gynecological residency. A person doesn't go through all that training, he said, without picking up a great deal of important knowledge and skill. And the surgery that OB-GYNs do gives them an understanding of the female reproductive system that no midwife can faintly approach.

"Midwives don't respect that. They very rarely talk about that distinction between us. They don't let on that I can do all the things they do—can provide a patient with the nicest environment and great labor coaching and a lot of support. They let women believe they know tricks I don't—but they don't. They insinuate that there is some mythical, magical wonder they can provide that I can't. And that is my problem with midwives."

He fell silent, then returned for an addendum. "For a long while at St. Barnabas," he said, "we've had big, beautiful rooms where a woman both labors and gives birth. We have birthing beds where the person can be in stirrups or can use a roll bar to push in an upright position if that's more comfortable. The patient has a nurse with her at all times, and very often a resident, too. During the pushing, her physician's with her constantly. She can have her husband or significant other person with her, and often a mother or a sister shows up for part or all of the time. She can have as many or as few people as she wants. It's the best of all worlds. She can have as natural a delivery as humanly possible, but if an emergency comes up she can immediately, without waiting, have the most high-tech medicine performed on her.

"If her baby's placenta suddenly starts separating, for example, or if its cord prolapses, or if her uterus ruptures, or if she has some type of embolus or catastrophic event during the labor or delivery, or if her baby is in dire distress—her baby can be saved, where it probably wouldn't be saved if she was in another kind of place.

"Granted, these emergencies and others just as serious don't happen very often. But they happen, and the precious minutes that occur during delivery or episodes of fetal distress aren't something that you can recoup or make up for. It's a one shot only."

Jack was now speaking as if he were saying something he'd wanted to say to misguided parents many times in the past but hadn't been able to. "The birth of your child is one of the most important things that will happen in your life. To risk something like that on the hunch that all will go well—how can you do it? This isn't scheduling a wedding in the back yard and if it rains, you had a rainy day on your wedding. You can take your chances on something like that. But if your baby's cord falls and the baby's deprived of oxygen for fifteen or twenty minutes while you're being rushed through traffic to a hospital to have your baby delivered, it isn't just rain on a wedding day. Your baby's retarded for the rest of its life."

Jack sometimes worked with nurse-midwives. "Some of them are wonderful," he said. "Some really understand the patients, they understand what's going on, and they know their limitations. If a high-risk situation develops, they turn to the doctor. I enjoy practicing with midwives who respect what I know if I respect what they know.

"But it has to be in the right situation, where a physician is not just available but readily available—a hospital setting, or a birthing center within a hospital, not a free-standing birthing center. The appropriate backup has to be there, because, again, you only have those precious minutes."

Years of exposure have given obstetricians a pragmatic understanding of what for others is just a statistic: that about 20 percent of women with no known medical problem and no previous trouble with pregnancy develop some kind of problem during labor, and about 2 percent have severe problems that must be dealt with immediately. Rod knew it vividly. An older physician, he had a harder time with what he called "this naturalist thing" than Jack did. It often conflicted with his deep-dyed sense of his profession's purpose—to bring patients the best possible treatment. He'd been brought as close to angry as he ever got by what he considered the purists' careless attacks on obstetrical technology, especially on the epidural anesthetic. In the span of his career, he said, he'd seen a heaven-sent improvement in the management of pain, and he didn't want to go back.

"The epidural has revolutionized this whole business," he said. "I mean, now we can give women pain relief early in labor and not interfere with their labor or their delivery. It's marvelous! But the other night I heard a woman really complaining about the epidural and all this technology.

"I understand, but you know what? It's masochistic. Jack delivered a patient this morning. She had a rough labor and was in a lot of pain. They offered her an epidural and she said, 'No, I don't want anything.' It's crazy. Someone's in pain, and I have something that can take that pain away, and they say, 'No, I don't want any.' Is there any psychological value to pain? I mean, is it important to go through pain to give birth?

"We get a patient who's 4 centimeters dilated. She gets an epidural, and the next thing we know she's fully dilated. She won't believe you. 'I didn't feel anything!' She's gotten to the second stage of labor and she's felt no pain. So now it's time for her to push. So we reduce the dose, and soon she can push as effectively as if she'd never had anesthetic at all.

"Believe me. For someone who's spent twenty-five years or more seeing women in pain, or seeing them numbed out by other kinds of anesthetics, the epidural is a dream come true."

•   •   •

"You're coming along beautifully," Jack told Susan at the end of the session. "Soon you'll *really* be showing. The top of your uterus is right at your belly button—which, no matter how tall or short someone is, is just where it belongs at twenty weeks. Your belly button is going to pop out. It's going to be a total outie."

In the parking lot, Susan and Tracy gave each other a high-five in delight about Susan's small weight gain.

"It was good to run through all those questions with him," she said in the car.

"He took a lot of time with you," Tracy said.

"One thing I have my doubts about," Susan said, "is the epidural. All those tubes and pumps and so forth. I'd really like to try and avoid that if I can."

13.
Special Delivery

Sandra Fornwalt couldn't help but feel under pressure. Every one of her patients mattered to her, but Peggy Chapman was Rod O'Driscoll's daughter, and Rod O'Driscoll was a large star in her particular constellation. He was the chief of the medical staff at her hospital and one of its most eminent OB-GYNs. She had to remind herself that Peggy was a patient first, not somebody's daughter.

She confessed to Peggy, doctor to doctor-to-be. "When it's somebody you really don't know," she said, "you can maintain your objectivity. But I know your father, and I know you. So I have extra, personal reasons for not wanting anything to go wrong."

"My dad wouldn't have recommended you," Peggy said, "unless he thought you were a good doctor."

Rod had done everything he could to take the pressure off the younger physician. He never meddled. He wasn't a hoverer, not the kind who constantly questioned juniors about what they were doing. He was trusting, and Dr. Fornwalt appreciated that. Once, when a medical question arose about the pregnancy, she asked Peggy, "What does your father say about it?" Peggy replied, "I don't know. He won't tell me a thing unless I ask him."

One evening when Peggy was in her thirty-fifth week, about a month before her due date, she went to Dr. Fornwalt for a check-up. The doctor examined Peggy's swollen belly, gently taking the high hard mound of uterus between her hands, first along one dimension and then others. The procedure, called the Leopold maneuvers, was designed to determine how the baby was lying in the womb. Developed near the end of the nineteenth century, the maneuvers had been supplanted by ultrasound, which could absolutely verify the baby's position, but every obstetrician still felt the patient's belly in the systematic way taught by Dr. Leopold for a preliminary sense of what was going on.

Dr. Fornwalt repeated the procedure thoughtfully and then said, "Peggy, I think that's a head I'm feeling up here. I think we've got a breech."

As an OB's daughter and as a medical student with a special interest in obstetrics, Peggy knew what breech meant. If the baby was in a breech position, it was badly placed for delivery. The normal posture for the baby at this point was upside down in the womb, with head low and bottom high. This baby, it appeared, was right side up, sitting in the uterus. Right side up was wrong.

Many babies rode out their second trimester and much of their third in breech position, upright, cruising along on their tail. During that period, it was nothing much to worry about. Sooner or later a good number of those babies somersaulted into the desired headstand. After the thirty-seventh week, however, "version" became less and less likely. By then the baby had grown so large that it almost filled the uterus and was tightly wrapped by it. And there was much less amniotic fluid to move in. The swimming pool had almost dried up and the water ballet was just about over. Some babies turned at the very end, but it was rare. At full term, 3 or 4 percent of babies remained in breech.

•   •   •

The next day Peggy had an ultrasound test. Afterward she phoned her father. "Guess what, Dad," she said. "I just had my scan. It looks like section city."

Most obstetricians at St. Barnabas delivered all or nearly all their breech babies by cesarean section. Sometimes the breech birth was so far along when the patient arrived at the hospital, or when the breech was discovered, that there was no stopping it and no choice but to carry through vaginally. Sometimes when a mother of twins delivered the first normally and vaginally, the second, if it was breech, was allowed to follow; the first had stretched the cervix and opened the way for its sibling, and breech birth became feasible.

Doctors elsewhere made attempts to deliver vaginally, and they claimed reasonable success. But the St. Barnabas obstetricians generally felt the risks were too great. Breech babies delivered vaginally were three to four times likelier to die and much likelier to suffer from congenital anomalies and birth trauma—among them fractures, dislocation and nerve injuries. There was also a slight increase in maternal mortality—not too alarming when one took into account how few mothers died during delivery for any reason. Cesarean section, an operation with its own risks, was thought by most to reduce the risks associated with breech. In any case, cesarean section didn't eliminate them; breech babies were harder to deliver even by cesarean than headfirst babies were.

What made breech a problem was that it reversed nature's own delivery system. In the normal, or vertex, position, the head led the way through the birth canal, and for good reason. The head was the hardest and biggest part of the body and did the best job of battering a path through the tight, muscular exit, the cervix. But if, instead of the head, the bottom came first—a so-called frank breech, the most common kind—that could be trouble.

The bottom was the softest part, a bad battering ram. It did a poor job of thinning and dilating the cervix. Even after letting the torso pass through, the unvanquished cervix still had a lot of elasticity. It could close around the neck, choking off the head and preventing its passage—"entrapment of the aftercoming head," it was called. The baby would be stuck, its body born but its head still locked on the wrong side of the cervix. Extracting it was difficult. The doctor couldn't safely pull on the baby's body to bring the head through; that could injure the baby. He often had to use special forceps—surgical tongs designed to guide the baby through the birth canal—to seize the baby's head. It was doable but by no means ideal. Babies were hurt that way too, and it was hard on the mothers.

If the baby came out feet (or, more likely, foot) first—a footling breech—there was an additional threat. In footling breeches, there was a good chance—thirty times higher than for normal births—that the umbilical cord would come out too early. As the upper body and the head came down, they'd press the cord and cut off the baby's oxygen supply, creating an "acute obstetrical emergency." One in fifteen babies delivered in the footling position died.

According to the ultrasound, Peggy's baby was a footling breech, standing with one foot in the birth canal. When Peggy told her father of the ultrasound finding, Rod, who had seen hundreds of breeches and didn't take them lightly, stayed calm on the phone, but as soon as she hung up he found Jack and told him. "She asked the big question," Rod said. "She said, 'What do you think, Dad? What are its chances of turning spontaneously? Give me a number?'"

"So what did you tell her?"

"I told her fifty-fifty."

"You did?" Jack asked. He was looking at Rod wide-eyed.

"Yeah."

"That's the first time, in all these years, that I've ever seen you not objective."

"You mean . . ."

"I mean the chances of that baby turning are very poor and getting worse every day. Less than 10 percent. At the end, maybe 3 percent. You know it's not fifty-fifty."

"Yeah, I guess I do. You're right."

"It's the first time I've ever seen you kid yourself."

"You know why?"

"I know why. Because she's your daughter. You don't want to believe she's going to have a breech."

"Well, that, of course. But also, she asked me, 'What are the circumstances under which it can turn?' and I said, 'If it's not a big baby, it can turn.' I said, 'I don't get the sense you have a great big baby. But you don't have a tiny baby.'"

"I saw her just a couple of weeks ago. She didn't look huge. But . . ."

"You're right," Rod said, caving in. "I'm not objective."

The day after the ultrasound, Dr. Fornwalt met with Peggy and her husband, David, and talked with them about their options. "We could schedule you for a cesarean," she said. "At the last minute, we'd do another ultrasound, and if the baby had converted and was in good position, we wouldn't do it."

"What's the other option?" David asked.

"The other way is nonsurgical: external version. The doctor places his hands at certain key points on your lower abdomen and gently pushes the baby into the head-down position. Actually, two doctors do it; I'd do it with a perinatologist. First you find out where the baby is, with ultrasound, and then you choose between a 'back flip' and a 'forward roll.' One doctor moves the bottom and the other moves the top. It works more than half the time, though not quite as well on first-time mothers as on mothers who've had a child before. I have to say, though, it can be really uncomfortable."

It was also risky. The baby's neck could be dislocated. The uterus could rupture, or the membranes could rupture. The placenta could separate from the uterus early. The whole procedure would be monitored by ultrasound, however, and the placenta probably could be avoided. If something went wrong, Peggy could immediately be prepared for a cesarean.

"One more thing," Dr. Fornwalt said. "Even if we do turn the baby over, it could turn back and go breech again. It might fail. You have to accept that possibility."

When there were no more questions, Dr. Fornwalt smiled. "Speaking from personal experience," she said, "I've had two cesareans myself, and hey, it's not too bad."

Peggy and David spent a few days considering version. The more Peggy thought about it, the more skeptical she got. She phoned Dr. Fornwalt. "It's cesarean," she said. "We just decided, why put the baby at any risk if there's a safe alternative? Maybe it's because I'm in that medical mode of thinking, but I don't have a big problem with having a cesarean. The outcome is the only thing that's important to us."

Over the course of the next weeks, suspense mounted. Every time Peggy felt something stir in her womb, she wondered if the baby had turned and breech birth was no longer a danger. Dr. Fornwalt examined her and said the uterus somehow felt different. "Dr. Fornwalt says we ought to do another ultrasound," Peggy told her father. "Her technician comes in on Friday."

"Oh, don't wait for that," Rod blurted out, revealing his own apprehension. "Bea is doing ultrasounds tomorrow. She'd be happy to check you out."

•   •   •

"Come on in, honey," Bea said to Peggy the next day when her turn for ultrasound came up. This wasn't the gruff or tart Bea. This was the affectionate Bea. She'd known Peggy since Peggy was a little girl, and she loved her, and Peggy loved Bea.

As Peggy removed her dark green wool top, Bea studied her belly. It was a mammoth bubble about half a yard in every direction. "From the looks of you," she said, "that baby must be lying side to side, like in a hammock. Have you felt a lot of movement?"

"I can't say I felt anything like the baby just turned around. Not as if I could feel it spinning. But it's been very active for a while."

Peggy lay back on the examining table and tugged down the waistband of her black stretch-pants, exposing the crest of her belly. Bea turned on the machine and darkened the room, and then squirted two lines of transparent blue-green gel onto Peggy, a line across the top of the belly and a line across the bottom. She picked up the transducer and put it directly on the jelly at the base of the abdomen.

"You took the day off today, Peg?" Bea asked.

"I took the day off. I have classes until one today, but . . ."

"Peggy!" Bea cried in delight.

"What?"

"It's a *head!*" A large, ghostly circle had filled the ultrasound's small screen.

Peggy's face filled with expectant wonder. "It *is?*"

"Yes! Yes! Yes! Ah-ha-ha!"

"I can't believe it!"

"There you *go!* Just where it's supposed to be. And it's pretty well engaged. So much for that nice, scheduled cesarean. Now you gotta wait like everyone else."

Jack entered, smiling. "What was all that yelling?"

"Guess what we've got," Bea said. "A vertex!"

"Great!" Jack explained. "You see? The best-laid plans . . ."

"I'm kinda disappointed," Peggy kidded. "I was looking forward to that cesarean. You know, no pain, nothing . . ." She stopped kidding. "No, seriously, this is great."

Bea was still scanning. "Nice pocket of amniotic fluid," she said.

"Bea is so great at this," Jack said.

"Baby's heart," Bea continued. "What a heart!"

Bea was now scanning at the top of the abdomen.

"Don't tell me what sex it is," Peggy said.

"I wouldn't do that. Just arms and legs." She moved the transducer and stopped. "Lots of movement here," she said. "Shifting kinds of movement."

Peggy was dismayed. "Oh, please, little baby," she beseeched. "Please . . . don't . . . turn . . . back."

•   •   •

Susan and Tracy were thinking about splurging on a Valentine's Day dinner at Maplewood's most expensive restaurant. Instead, they stayed home and ordered a takeout meal and served it on their best china. The evening seemed an omen. The days of spontaneous, carefree, romantic adventures, with no thought for the cost, seemed to be ending.

Tracy's mother had sent them a baby-name book, and after dinner they once again got it out and started through it. For girls they liked the old-fashioned names. But when they tried them on their friends, the reception was poor. Betty Sprague had to give them the first rule of baby-naming. "Never discuss names with your friends," she said. "They always say, 'Oh, you're not going to name him *that!*' "

Sarah and Hannah were the early favorites. But they learned Sarah was now one of the most popular girl's names, which meant the poor child would constantly be running into other Sarahs. And Hannah had no sooner popped into possibility than they began to bump into Hannahs everywhere.

For a boy's name, they were tending toward the ethnic, with Scottish names high on the list. They considered Ethan and Ian, then switched to Alexander, then decided that "Alexander MacGregor" was a seven-syllable mouthful. So they turned to Alistair, the Scottish version of Alexander.

"If it was Alistair," Susan said, "what would the nickname be?"

"Al?" Tracy suggested unenthusiastically.

"Or Alan."

"Or Ali, I hope not."

"Alistair is hard to shorten."

"Maybe we could name him Alistair but call him Alex," Tracy said. Susan looked dubious. "But," he continued, teasing her, "since it's not going to be a boy, it doesn't matter. We don't have to worry."

"I am not seriously considering the possibility that it will be a boy," Susan kidded.

"You remember the night we told my father you were pregnant," Tracy said. "He thrives on being different on purpose, but he got very close to me and looked me square in the eye—square in the eye—and he said, 'I think very strongly that it's a boy.' He's never said a word about it since then."

"You wait and see."

"We'd better start coming up with some boy's names," Tracy said, "or we'll end up with a boy named Sarah."

14.
Standards

Two steep hills, the Orange Mountains, rise just to the west of the O'Driscoll-Bonamo offices, and from their tops, in the distance, the upper halves of the World Trade Center towers in Manhattan are visible. From West Orange and neighboring towns, New York is just a short drive over or under the Hudson. Many residents work in the city, and many others go over now and then for the shopping or the theater or the night life. But the nearness is only physical.

People in northern New Jersey do not identify with New York. In mind-set they have more in common with Midwesterners than with Manhattanites. They tend to view the city with the mix of suspicion, resentment, and grudging fascination that people in Fort Wayne and Paducah do. When they hear of the latest bit of Manhattan mayhem, another calamity in Gomorrah, they shake their heads as if to say, Well, what do you expect?

With Rod O'Driscoll, a cosmopolitan man who enjoyed much about the city, the attitude showed in his view of its medical establishment. Once, to set him off, someone asked him whether OBs at New York Hospital and Columbia Presbyterian were really justified in charging twice as much for a delivery as he and Jack charged just twenty miles away. He sputtered and said, "Well, I'll tell you . . ." That was all he said, though his expression—popped eyes, raised eyebrows—spoke volumes. Nothing could have pleased him more than when *American Health* magazine, naming the nine best OB-GYN centers in the country, included St. Barnabas—along with Brigham and Women's in Boston and Johns Hopkins in Baltimore—and left out most of the glossy Manhattan institutions.

His courteous skepticism about big-city superiority was not eased by several instances of patients who, before they had come to him and Jack, had gone to "one of those New York specialists" and gotten inferior treatment. One such patient was Grace Findley.

Grace was a New York career woman and, seated in the waiting room that March afternoon, among suburban women in their informal clothes and running shoes, looked it—a pregnant career woman. Her manner, though warm, was businesslike. Her hair, brightly blond, was carefully controlled. She wore an expensive scarf across one shoulder and heavy gold jewelry. She was a fashion director for Lord & Taylor.

But though she was chic, Grace wasn't self-centered. She listened when other people talked, and she liked to laugh. There was a home-town-girl quality about her. Her husband, Dave, was a tall, good-looking commercial pilot.

Rod was her OB-GYN and had delivered the Findleys' first child, Carlyle. The little girl had cystic fibrosis, a congenital disease of the mucous glands that made breathing difficult, but after two years she was doing well and they wanted another child. Grace became pregnant again. She went through a long, difficult series of tests with a geneticist, which yielded the stunning news that this new baby would have cystic fibrosis too.

The Findleys adored their first child. "She's a blessed child," Grace said. "She's beautiful and smart. And she's a positive little unit. She doesn't let the cystic fibrosis interfere with her life." But they knew the impact cystic fibrosis could have on a family. Two CF children seemed more than they could handle. Their little Carlyle had escaped the disease's worst effects, but next time could be drastically different. After a great deal of thought and prayer they decided to terminate.

"The geneticist recommended two doctors in New York who were specialists in genetic termination," Grace said. "She said they were tops; they had all this experience in cases like ours. We checked them out and found out they had excellent credentials. They had offices on Park Avenue; they'd written books. I mean, they sounded like the very best. We knew Dr. O'Driscoll didn't perform terminations, and in my mind I wanted to keep St. Barnabas as the place I'd go when I had my babies."

They made an appointment in New York. The procedure, called a D&E, for dilation and evacuation, was supposed to be fairly routine, the Findleys were told. It was performed in the doctor's offices late one afternoon. When it was finished, Grace was told to go home and was assured she'd feel fine in a few hours. She didn't feel fine. During the late evening she became ever more uncomfortable. The skin in the vicinity of her vagina was inflamed, and she began to bleed.

Dave called the New York doctor's office. The answering service said he'd call back. He didn't, and the Findleys called again. When they got the doctor he was dismissive: everything was all right; she should go to sleep. Her condition grew worse. The bleeding became alarming. After two hours they phoned again. They got the doctor. Grace was on the phone, and as she talked with him she got the distinct feeling he was drunk. She and Dave were appalled and frightened.

At three A.M., Dave became enraged. He called the doctor and shouted, "My wife's losing consciousness. She's been bleeding for five hours!"

"You're overreacting," the doctor said. "Go back to bed."

Grace, seeing her husband turning red, gasped, "Hang up the phone. We're not listening to that guy anymore." She had lost all respect for the doctor's judgment.

She called the O'Driscoll-Bonamo offices and got Jack, who was on call that night. "We wouldn't have called you at this hour," she said, "but we're really scared and don't know what to do." Jack told her please not to worry about that, just tell him what was wrong. The next day he said to Rod: "Grace Findley is the only patient I know who'd be able to describe this entire thing in perfect detail and then faint dead away."

Dave grabbed the phone. Jack said, "Get her to the emergency room immediately. I'll meet you there."

When Jack arrived he found Grace in extreme shock and hemorrhaging. She'd lost more than half her blood volume. It seemed clear to Jack that if the Findleys had listened to the New York doctor and waited until morning, she might have died. The emergency room team rushed her into the operating room and, while Jack cleaned out her uterus to remove clots from the hemorrhaging, she received extensive blood transfusions.

Three years before, there had been a similar case in Alabama. A woman had gone to her gynecologist for a routine biopsy of the cervix. Soon there were burns over almost her entire vagina and crotch and buttocks area. She also suffered a massive hemorrhage. She was rushed to the hospital, where emergency surgery was performed to save her life. It was discovered that instead of the normal 3 or 4 percent solution of acetic acid to clean the area around the vagina, her doctor had used a 95 percent solution—nearly full strength.

Jack and Rod imagined that something comparable had happened to Grace. The New York doctors had used some kind of solution while prepping her for the procedure. The solution had been too concentrated and had severely burned her. "And when she went into shock," Jack explained to her husband, "it got even worse. Burns get worse when you're in shock because there's no blood supply getting to the skin, so a second-degree burn becomes a third-degree burn."

"Throughout the days that followed," Grace now remembered, "Dr. O'Driscoll had my bed positioned right next to the nurses' station so they could check on me every five minutes. He and Dr. Bonamo called the hospital regularly, all through those nights." Fortunately, St. Barnabas has one of the most advanced burn centers in the region, and so the care was skilled. Even so, Grace had to be in bandages for five months, the first three and a half of which she was kept in bed.

"It seemed so unfair," Grace said. "When I went to that doctor I was healthy, and when he was done I had a serious injury, almost lost my life. To think that this man, with his enormous fees and his Park Avenue address, never even called or followed up."

The Alabama woman had sued her doctor for negligence and been awarded $45,000. The Findleys went to a malpractice attorney but were told they probably could not win a suit. She had complications and a possible allergic reaction to the solution, that was all; there was no proof the doctor was at fault. And Grace's education and prosperity weren't likely to win her much sympathy from a jury. "The really awful thing," Grace said, "is that there's just no good way to find out about a doctor, no record on him, what he's done in the past, how many malpractice suits he's been involved in. Do you think that a woman who's in this guy's office at this moment knows anything about my story? Of course not."

•　　•　　•

In 1990 a team of researchers from Harvard University studied the records of over 30,000 hospital admissions in New York State. Taking those New York findings and projecting them nationally, they suggested that each year as many as 300,000 Americans were injured or died in hospitals as the result of medical negligence and carelessness. As startling as they were, those figures, which were just for malpractice in hospitals, ignored mischance in the doctor's office.

According to the main OB-GYN professional organization, some 80 percent of OBs have been sued at least once for malpractice. The average OB-GYN has been sued twice or more, and 10 percent have been sued over half a dozen times. Doctors protest they're sued far too often; trial lawyers insist they're not sued nearly often enough. The Harvard study of the records of over 30,000 New Yorkers reported that one in twenty-five patients (not just OB-GYN but all patients) going into a hospital came out with a disabling injury directly as a result of medical treatment. Of those cases, Harvard said, one in four were due to negligence—but among the victims of negligence, only one in eight ever filed a suit, and only half of those who did sue ever got any damages at all. The lawyers say that taking doctors to court is the only available way to discourage carelessness, because the medical profession generally does a pretty poor job of policing itself.

In most places sloppy doctors can go along year after year, eluding censure or loss of license, concealing their records from public view. Lee J. Dunn Jr., a Boston lawyer who defends doctors against malpractice, reviewed a large number of malpractice cases looking for patterns in which there had been a big judgment against an OB-GYN. He found that many of those doctors had been trained in foreign medical schools. Many overused Pitocin, the drug that can bring on or speed up labor. Many worked in community hospitals. Many kept poor medical records. And, perhaps most important, many delivered more than three hundred babies a year. Juries in malpractice cases, said Mr. Dunn, take a dim view of hyperactive OBs, feeling that doctors who deliver more than 175 babies a year can't give patients adequate attention.

The vast numbers of doctors are conscientious. They grind their teeth in frustration, knowing that the malpractitioners make all doctors look bad. Many doctors serve on boards and committees created to blow the whistle on bad doctors, but their efforts rarely pay off. The system protects the guilty. From time to time there were physicians at St. Barnabas known to be practicing bad medicine; the good doctors tried to get rid of them, but their hands were all but tied. Rod and Jack, both of whom were active in efforts to keep standards up, had known this futility firsthand. "As soon as we get embroiled in one of these ugly situations," Jack said, "and they are always ugly, we are immediately talking to the doctor's attorneys. They charge that we and the hospital are defaming him, depriving him of his livelihood, curtailing his source of income, and so on, and they threaten immense law suits. Which doesn't mean we cave in, just that it's daunting. We know that a tremendous, unproductive expenditure of time and spirit lies ahead."

It's a crazy system all the way around. A few victims get enormous judgments, but most get nothing at all. Because of those gigantic judgments, careful and compassionate obstetricians, along with the rogues, are charged immense fees for their malpractice insurance. Rod and Jack each paid $38,000 a year for the minimum coverage—about 20 percent of their gross income and a tenth of the obstetrical fee each patient paid; as high as those figures seem, they're only a half or a third of what obstetricians pay in some other areas. As long as twenty-three years after the delivery, OBs can be hit with frivolous suits by patients out to make a buck. The psychological and economic wear and tear on the profession is enormous. Fear of malpractice suits, along with the other stresses of the specialty—such as two A.M. summonses from patients in labor—has made many OBs cut down on the number of deliveries they do, or number of high-risk patients they take on. One out of eight OBs have quit obstetrics altogether. And women in more and more places have had to go without any obstetrician at all.

• • •

Jack had been sued twice. The cases filled him with a disillusionment that still made his face darken when he spoke of them.

The first involved a young woman who'd had a one-night stand. Her partner, a bartender, not only made her pregnant but gave her syphilis. She went to a clinic for prenatal care and received the regular tests, including a blood test for syphilis. The syphilis test failed to detect the disease, as happens in 5 to 10 percent of early cases. At four months she came to Jack. He asked the clinic to send him her records, and when they didn't arrive promptly, he did the tests all over again. Again the syphilis test showed negative. A month later she appeared at Emergency at St. Barnabas with a urinary tract infection. The resident noticed she had a rash and told Jack about it, and Jack suggested still another syphilis test. This time it was positive.

The fetus was at risk, but Jack could do nothing except try to comfort the patient. The baby died of congenital syphilis. The uterus had to be emptied, so Jack set out to deliver the fetus. Early or late in a pregnancy, it's relatively easy to deliver a dead fetus; in the first few months it's a D&C, essentially, and at full term it's a normal labor, but at six months the uterus is just not ready for labor. The fetus is a large, formed object wrapped in a tight, resistant, muscular organ. The patient is given suppositories that encourage the uterus to contract. It usually takes twelve to fourteen hours, at the end of which ordeal the fetus can be wrested out vaginally. Hard work for both mother and doctor, but worth it to avoid a cesarean.

The day Jack was removing the fetus, his mother was dying. She was in the same hospital, in a coma in the intensive care unit, barely awake. "I had to decide which bed I was going to sit beside," Jack said, "to sit with this girl or to sit with my mother. I decided to sit with the girl, because she was awake. My mother probably wouldn't have known the difference." Left unsaid was a poignant fact that anyone who knew Jack understood: that Jack's mother meant the world to him, and the forces drawing him toward her bedside must have been almost irresistible.

One day six months later Jack took a call from a lawyer for the company that insured him for malpractice. "You won't believe this," the lawyer said. "She's suing you because her baby died of syphilis."

The woman's attorneys had worked up a deluge of accusations that went on for pages, designed to overwhelm a jury and create the impression that Jack was the world's worst doctor. "Gross negligence and incompetence . . ." "Failure to perform proper testing . . ."—even though Jack had done three syphilis tests where the standard was one. "Failure to properly diagnose . . ." The idea seemed to be to tarnish him in the minds of the jury and make them think that surely *some* of the charges had to be true.

It became the hospital joke that Dr. Bonamo got sued for giving his patient syphilis. To Jack it was no joke. The lawyer told Jack he was sure the woman's lawyers would settle for about $50,000. Many doctors would have thought "The hell with it; the insurance company's going to pay" and settled. That sort of cynicism ran against Jack's grain. He refused to let the insurer pursue a settlement. When the case went to court he was there for every minute of the jury selection and the trial, on hand for weeks.

During the trial, the patient's attorney showed the jury some greeting cards he said his client had given to the baby on its birthday—even though that baby was only a five-month-old fetus. He displayed photos of the room she had decorated for the baby. Jack had an excellent attorney and a distinguished expert witness who testified about the medical science involved. It didn't matter. The jury found for the patient. Jack Bonamo, the embodiment of the careful, caring doctor, was pronounced guilty of malpractice.

When the verdict was announced, one of the jurors stood up and said to the judge, "Your honor, this verdict was not arrived at according to your charge to the jury. We did not apply the law to the case as you told us. That's not how we came up with this verdict."

"All I can do now," the judge said to the juror, "is to poll the jury." She polled the jurors, and they all said they found for the patient, except for that one juror, who said Jack was not responsible.

Jack was crushed. "I felt sorry for the girl for what she'd been through," he said. "I'd feel sorry for anybody who lost a child. But it was of her own doing. She became pregnant and she contracted the disease. I saw her afterward. She told me she'd wanted to sue the guy who had given her syphilis but he didn't have any money, so she sued me!"

The court gave her $100,000: $80,000 for her "lack of society"—not having the baby's company—and $20,000 for her physical suffering.

After she won, the malpractice insurance company decided to make a major issue out of the case. They called it a "shocking" verdict and said it was crucial not to lose cases like this one because losing them encouraged still more rip-off lawsuits. The company wanted to make it a test case and take it to the appellate division. Jack signed consent forms, and over the next five years he and the lawyers prepared the appeal and waited for a court date; five years was how long it took to get a case through the system. During that time the patient was accumulating 15 percent interest on the $100,000 the lower court had awarded her. And during that time Jack was suffering—stewing over the injustice, aching about the unwarranted blemish on his spotless record. He devoted endless hours of his time to helping the lawyers.

As the case was getting ready to go to the appellate division, Jack got a letter from the insurance company saying that the patient's attorney had made an offer: If Jack would give up the appeal, the patient would accept the $100,000 without the interest, and that would be that.

"All of a sudden," Jack said, "the insurance company changed its mind about the importance of turning this case around. Their letter said that this was strictly a business decision. Considering the costs of mounting the appeal, which they expected to win, it would be cheaper to give the patient the $100,000 now and save the $80,000 to $90,000 in interest. They could give her the hundred thousand dollars and 'we all win.' I don't think I've ever been angrier. A negative verdict never counts against the doctor, supposedly. Maybe they'd feel differently if a doctor piled up a series of really large verdicts; I don't know—I've never been there. But it was so disappointing. I thought at least it was going to get turned around. I don't think people should feel they're able to do things like that."

Jack's second malpractice suit, no less punishing, overlapped the first one. The patient was twenty-two, a young woman from a solid working-class family in Newark. "Nice people," Jack called them. He had delivered the woman's sister's baby and then, two weeks later, helped the woman herself have one. The baby was healthy, but an hour and a half later the young woman developed the symptoms of an amniotic fluid embolism.

It is a dangerous condition. Doctors for centuries had been baffled by a mysterious, sudden affliction that killed women who had recently given birth, but it wasn't until 1941 that two researchers discovered its cause. They found that the internal pressure generated during a vigorous labor can force amniotic fluid into the mother's bloodstream, usually through a small tear in the uterus or a place where the placenta has slightly separated from the uterine wall. The bubble of amniotic fluid works its way throughout the mother's circulatory system, bringing on a widespread cataclysm that may include hemorrhaging, breathing failure, and convulsions, among other dreadful complications. In about 85 percent of instances the mother dies. Today, very few American women die in childbirth, but of those who do, about 12 percent are thought to have been lost because of amniotic fluid embolism.

Despite skilled and desperate attempts to save her, Jack's patient died. Shattering for her family, her death was extremely painful for Jack as well. He had never had an obstetrical patient die before. For several years afterward he went into deep depression on the anniversary of her death. This year, in fact, was the first he'd managed to get through the day without sinking.

Several months after the incident the woman's sister came to visit him and told him the family knew the death had been a loss for him as well as for them. She gave him a prayer book.

On the same day that Jack got the devastating verdict in the syphilis case, he was served with fresh legal papers; the dead woman's family was suing him for malpractice. He called her father, a decent, basic man he'd come to know and like. "Just tell me one thing," he said to him. "Do you think I did everything in the world that could have been done for your daughter?"

"Yes," the father said.

"That's all I need to know," Jack said. "That's all I need to know. You can do the rest of this . . . this lawsuit. We'll go through the whole charade. But I needed to hear that from you."

"Doctor," the father said, "I have to do this. Everybody keeps telling me she shouldn't have died. She was twenty-two. She shouldn't have died."

"You're absolutely right," Jack said. "She shouldn't have died. But I was not in charge of that."

Jack felt certain the family had been pressured into the step they had taken. They were good people, and they knew firsthand how hard Jack had worked to save their daughter. They'd been there the whole time, so they knew he'd been there the whole time too. He'd reported to them every hour or so. They had seen the stream of medical specialists who tended their daughter; they saw the effort put forth to save her life.

The insurance company lawyer was frank with Jack. "They've got a very sympathetic case," he said. "A young woman died, and the grandparents are raising her baby. When those nice old grandparents carry that sweet little motherless child into the courtroom, there won't be a dry eye. And the grandparents clearly need the money."

Jack said, "What does that have to do with what I did or didn't do?"

"You didn't do anything wrong," the lawyer said. "That has nothing to do with it. It's how it looks, not how it is."

Once again Jack refused to settle. "I'll probably lose again," he said to his wife. "The grandparents will bring in this little baby, and the jury will see a doctor standing there in a suit and tie, and they'll know he's got an insurance company behind him, and that will be that. But the mother didn't die from a procedure. She had a medical catastrophe, one that's almost always fatal. I did my best, and it bothers me that I'm getting sued for it. But it doesn't bother me anything like as much as the death of that woman. That was the hardest thing that's ever happened to me in my life except maybe the loss of my mother: losing a patient."

The insurance company was also pessimistic. Despite Jack's protests they settled for $300,000. "I realized," Jack said, "that in such a terrible system, you have to expect illogical outcomes. And frankly, having these nice people who had lost their daughter receive money to help raise this little child didn't bother me one hundredth as much as that woman who went out and got syphilis and then used me as her lottery ticket."

Even Rod, loved by his patients, renowned for his sensitivity, known throughout the state for his medical skills, had had his share of malpractice aggravation. He'd been sued four times over his career and was pragmatic in his attitude about that. "We're not fools," he said. "We know we're not perfect. If we've done something wrong, through omission or commission, we settle. The ones that go to trial are the ones in which I firmly believe I didn't do anything wrong. You do your best, and sometimes your best isn't good enough."

One Friday morning Rod was at the hospital delivering a patient whose name, as it happened, was Driscoll. While he was away from the office a call came in from another patient, a stockbroker. She was worried about her eight-month fetus; it hadn't been moving. Bea told her to come in and she'd take a look. A short time later the patient and her mother arrived. Bea placed the sensor of the Doppler device on the patient's belly and listened. She heard the fetal heart.

"There it is," she said to the patient.

"Oh, yes," the patient said.

"But let's have Dr. O'Driscoll take a look. He's on his way back to the office. Why don't you sit out in the waiting room, and as soon as he's here I'll get him to check."

When Rod arrived he listened to the heartbeat with his Doppler. The heart was beating, but slowly. He could be hearing a weak fetal heartbeat or the mother's pulse; it was hard to tell. He decided to look at the fetal heart on ultrasound. What he saw confirmed his fears: this baby's heart was barely beating.

This event was out of the blue. The patient and her baby had been fine, with no "predisposing signs."

"Let's get you to the hospital right away," Rod said. At St. Barnabas he performed an emergency cesarean. The baby was stillborn.

The woman sued. She claimed, among other things, that she had been sent home to lunch and then came back—a fatal delay, an act of obstetrical negligence. Rod knew that this simply was not true; he had sent her directly to the hospital. His lawyer put Bea on the stand and also the secretary, Debbie Kunz, both of whom testified that the woman had never left the office.

Before the trial the insurance company's lawyer said, "I don't like this jury at all. I'm really nervous about this jury. Would you consider settling this case?"

"I really don't want to settle this case," Rod said, "because I didn't do anything wrong. I'd like to have my day in court."

The lawyer's concern proved to be well founded. The woman was good on the witness stand—so good, in fact, that when she started to cry, a juror handed her a handkerchief. The insurance company lawyer asked the judge to excuse that juror for prejudice. The judge refused. To make matters worse, the plaintiff's medical expert turned out to be a physician who had worked at St. Barnabas and with whom Rod had had a number of personal disagreements.The jury found Rod liable. The stockbroker was awarded $250,000. It was the only case he'd lost in his entire twenty-five-year career.

Like most OBs, Rod and Jack talked about malpractice a lot, and when they tried to describe the situation to a nonmedical person they sounded like Vietnam vets describing battles against an invisible enemy that didn't fight fair. To them these three cases weren't malpractice but what they called "maloccurrence." The doctor hadn't done anything wrong. Nevertheless, somewhere along the obstacle course of birth—genetics, conception, pregnancy, delivery—something bad happened and someone was hurt: no one's fault, but a tragedy nonetheless.

"A kid born with heart disease," Rod said. "Who expected that? A limb deformity. Who expected that? People react differently. There are some who were wonderful patients all the way through pregnancy, great rapport, and when something like this happens, they change into malpractice types. The unfortunate outcomes . . . People want a perfect baby for their money."

The quest for the perfect baby places a tremendous burden on the obstetrician. He has to come through; yet he's not in complete control.

"People no longer accept the idea of diverse outcomes," Jack said.

"Today," Rod said, "it's rare for people to have large families. And since they're only going to have one or two babies, by God, they have to be perfect."

The insistence on perfection, and the readiness to sue the doctor if he or she doesn't produce, have led to another craze: a mania for medical tests. Anxious parents want every conceivable test, needed or not, to cut the odds of catastrophe. Anxious doctors, afraid that a malpractice lawyer will someday fault them for not performing this test or that, order test after test, needed or not. Tests tend to cost a lot of money, which partly explains the explosion of health care costs in the 1980s. "Defensive" medicine is thought to cost $30 billion a year.

"A patient of mine," Rod said, "she's twenty-four years old, wants to have an amnio. Well, amnios aren't generally appropriate for women that young. But, if she insists . . ."

Rod and Jack tried not to let the malpractice bogeyman spook them into overtesting. "I have friends who practice OB; they're entirely defensive," Jack said. "They protect themselves all the time. If a patient wants a test, they don't chat with her about whether it's really necessary. They overutilize services like mad. When you ask them about it, though, they point out that in a court of law, somebody who practices defensively will come out better. Nobody sues you for too many tests.

"Except I can't practice that way. I'm not comfortable with it. I feel that people are asking me to be the doctor and make decisions, and so I make those decisions and I have to stand by them. Pregnant people often ask for advice. The advice we give them should be based on our best judgment, not on what somebody *might* say if something went wrong."

"What's happening now," Rod said, "is that doctors don't rely on their judgment. Judgment is going out the window; they just rely on tests. Which is too bad."

"There's a lot of satisfaction in this job that I think many obstetricians lose sight of," Jack said. "You can lose sight of it when you start obsessing about the malpractice thing and let yourself be affected by all the negativity that surrounds it. You could forget why you're here."

"Jack has a great expression: technological insanity," Rod said. "That sums it all up."

In the late 1980s researchers made discoveries that seemed likely to change the obstetrical malpractice picture. The findings revised medicine's understanding of the injury that has been the most common grounds for malpractice suits—brain damage resulting in cerebral palsy. Using a new imaging device that can closely examine the fetal brain before birth, the researchers found that in many palsied children the damaged area in the brain—called white-matter necrosis—was present before birth and so couldn't have been caused by a botched delivery. Dr. John Freeman, head of the Pediatric Epilepsy Center at Johns Hopkins Hospital, declared that only 4 percent of cerebral palsy cases are due to lack of oxygen during labor and delivery. "We do not know the cause of most cases of CP," he said. "Most cases are likely caused by a variety of prenatal developmental insults"—unfortunate events during the pregnancy that affect fetal development. So after tens of thousands of prosecutions, it seemed possible that in most cases involving cerebral palsy the OBs may not have been at fault after all.

No matter what caused the palsy, many babies nevertheless were being born with it—a grave matter. A few of the parents were receiving millions of dollars through malpractice suits, but most were getting nothing. The whole system was focused on what the obstetrician did or didn't do during labor and delivery instead of on the disability itself.

Legislators and doctors in New York State came up with another approach. Rod was enthusiastic. "They're seriously talking about taking 'damaged newborns' out of the court system," he said. "They're neurologically impaired; nobody did anything wrong. Obviously someone has to provide the money to take care of these children, but it shouldn't be charged to a doctor's insurance company. There should be a no-fault system, the workman's compensation sort of thing, a fund into which every physician donates an amount of money—obstetricians a larger amount—to fund it annually. It seems like a better way. Our society recognizes that these infants are going to need a lot of care. Who's gonna pay for the care? So they bring in an actuary to say how long this child will probably live and an economist to say what it's going to cost to maintain him for that time in a state institution. Big bucks. All that money comes out of premiums, and all *that* money comes out of patients."

•　　•　　•

Grace Findley, the patient who'd been badly burned during a D&E, had spent most of the previous hot summer in bandages. They were removed late in August. Three weeks later, without planning to, she and her husband made love. Afterward he said, "You know, we ought to talk seriously about this, before we have another baby. I've seen you in so much pain. I know you've got a will of iron, and I know you're probably ready to do it again, but I just think we should talk to Dr. Bonamo about how long we should wait."

Jack was consulted. "Let's give it six months," he said. "Then we'll talk about it again."

Two days later, while Grace was waiting to have a checkup at the burn unit at St. Barnabas, she started to feel dizzy. "No," she said to herself. "I can't be pregnant. Just that one time!" With the other two pregnancies, it had taken her several months to conceive.

When she went back to see Jack, she felt like a guilty teenager going in to tell her father she was pregnant. She also felt terrified. She dreaded the regimen of genetic testing, the agonizing wait for the test results. But mainly, after her grim experience, she reflexively shrank from the prospect of doctors and hospitals and of once again putting her life in someone's hands.

Jack examined her and picked up his little white calendar wheel. "Well," he said, smiling warmly, "I'd say we're looking at a June second delivery."

The news from the geneticist was wonderful. The fetus was free of cystic fibrosis and entirely healthy.

Now, in March, Grace was six months pregnant and doing well. "That whole business," she said, "it's kind of a chapter in my life that I just want to close and never open again. I concentrate on what happened afterward. I'll never forget the care I got from Dr. O'Driscoll and Dr. Bonamo and at the hospital. If a terrible experience can be made good, that's how I came out feeling. You know, like I know there are decent people, there are good people pulling for you."

15.
Grandpa

Peggy O'Driscoll Chapman, having escaped breech birth and cesarean, had reached her due date. Forty full weeks. The entire O'Driscoll family was on alert. Super-alert. And when, that day at noon, she had light contractions, the word spread fast. Then they all called Rod, one young O'Driscoll after another. "I'm beginning to think I've given up the practice of medicine and become Message Central," Rod told Jack.

Jack had heard these calls coming in all afternoon and was struck by the spectacle of this close-knit family hypercommunicating. "Hey," he said to Barbara, "these people could be Italian!"

A week later the baby was still holding off. The delay had an advantage: Peggy had been able to take her final exams at medical school. But it pushed her into a new problem. The next day Dr. Fornwalt was leaving on vacation. Peggy was losing the obstetrician on whom she'd focused during her entire pregnancy.

She'd been prepared for this possibility. Dr. Fornwalt had said this would happen if the baby was more than a week late, in which case her partner would stand by. But, she said, she realized that Peggy didn't know her partner very well and that coming from a medical family, she might have other alternatives. Peggy was to feel completely free to use any other obstetrician. "Why don't you talk it over with your dad?"

Wearing her husband's down parka, looking concerned and exhausted, Peggy came to the office. She and Rod holed up in his conference room and tried to work it out. The logical answer would have been Jack. Peggy knew Jack well and knew how highly her father regarded him. But Jack was away on a week-long ski vacation—it was the time of year when the slopes of America thronged with obstetricians, those who hadn't gone to Florida or the Yucatan. Peggy could gamble on Jack's returning in time, or . . . The decision that came out of the meeting was to make no decision. She'd wing it.

•   •   •

It was what Rod called a mellow week—a quiet one. The whole month had been mellow: just sixteen deliveries, which was a little bit slow. There hadn't been much to distract Rod from his recurrent thoughts: My daughter is going to have a baby! *When* is she going to have a baby?

Jack returned from vacation early in March, greatly relieved to find that Peggy hadn't yet given birth. He saw her the morning of his first day back and looked her over. The baby's head was hard against the membranes at the bottom of the uterus, but there were no contractions at all. "Enough," he said. "You're almost two weeks late. Let's have us a baby." He was putting her in the hospital that evening. The birth would be induced.

Obstetrical science had come to regard forty-two weeks as an outer limit, beyond which few pregnancies should be allowed to continue. After that point, things got dangerous and the fetal mortality statistics became more and more alarming.

For one thing, Peggy's placenta would begin to age and no longer work as well. That might prompt a whole series of unfortunate developments. An aging placenta would send less blood to the baby, and that meant the baby would urinate less. The baby's urine was an important source of amniotic fluid, and less urine would mean less fluid. Without ample fluid to move in, the crowded baby would be likelier to lean against its umbilical cord, pressing it against the uterine wall, cutting off oxygen and other vital substances and causing "fetal distress." In blunt language, the baby could asphyxiate and die. And that was just one of the dire scenarios. Another was that the fetus would gain so much weight that vaginal birth could become iffy.

Peggy called her husband in New York and had him paged. She told him to come home as soon as he could. Then she and Rod had lunch together, the two of them.

In the early evening, after his office hours, Jack went up to the hospital. Peggy was in a regular hospital room—she wouldn't be moved into Labor and Delivery until her labor got under way—and her husband, David, was with her. Rod had already dropped by— just a social call, he called it—and left.

The induction began. Jack inserted a Foley catheter into Peggy's cervix. By gently squeezing the rubber bulb at the outward end of the catheter, an attendant would gradually pump water into the expandable part of the tube, encouraging the cervix to open. If all went well, its presence would stimulate the release of the acid prostaglandin, which would soften the cervix.

An old method of induction is still often used: seaweed. Lengths of the stems of laminaria, a seaweed found in northern oceans, are gathered, shaped, dried, sterilized, and packaged according to size: small, medium, and large. Inserted into the cervix, they slowly swell and at the same time draw water from the surrounding tissues, causing them to soften and allowing the cervix to dilate. A technique once clearly within the definition of folk medicine—using a weed—has become subsumed into the modern obstetrical armamentarium.

By eleven o'clock Peggy was crampy and uncomfortable. "I'm feeling something," she told her mother on the phone. There was a flurry of mild contractions. In the course of the next hour, the contractions petered out, as they generally did.

"The balloon has been put in and you've experienced a little bit of uterine irritability," Jack said. "Now we have to wait for the balloon to do its job." At midnight Jack went home. He slept, but restlessly. Rod didn't sleep much at all.

During the night the contractions resumed in earnest. The head nurse, Sister Regis Keane, a Roman Catholic nun from the same order as Mary Jo, came in at two A.M. Like Bea, she'd known Peggy since she was a child, and they were friends. At dinner with Peggy and Mary Jo a couple of nights before, Regis had promised to come in and serve as Peggy's private labor nurse when her labor began. It was like having Dr. Spock volunteer to be your family pediatrician.

Hour by hour the contractions intensified. Regis called Michael Schrempf, the resident on duty. He examined Peggy. She was moving along nicely. By five o'clock her cervix was dilated five centimeters—half the way to complete dilation—and her membranes had burst.

Rod appeared on the floor at seven A.M., as was his custom, but this time with special reason. "She's fully dilated," Dr. Schrempf said to him.

"Whoa!" said Rod. "Has anyone called Jack?" No one had.

At that moment Jack called. He wanted to check on Peggy and to direct that she be moved into Labor and Delivery. He didn't want the beds to fill up, leaving no room for Peggy.

"She's already there," the nurse at the desk replied. "We brought her back at three-thirty." That was unusual. When they transferred a doctor's patient, he always got a call. But Jack didn't fume. He knew what had happened. Everyone had been so absorbed in giving Peggy Chapman white-glove service, scurrying all over the place and trying to do everything right, that they forgot to do the elementary thing—keeping her doctor informed.

He jumped in the shower and got dressed, then called the hospital again. "I'm on my way," he said to Dr. Schrempf. "But since she's contracting, go ahead with the epidural."

"We already gave her the epidural," Dr. Schrempf said.

There it was again. It was standard procedure to call the patient's doctor before the epidural anesthetic was administered. "Of all the deliveries in the world I never wanted to miss," he said to his wife as he rushed out the door, "this has got to be number one." Later, at the office, Bea would say, "Oh Jesus, Peggy's the patient and Jack was late?"

Jack arrived at the hospital to find Peggy fully dilated and ready to push out the baby. He also found Rod nervous, unable to stand still, at loose ends. Rod cared very much about this patient and knew all the ropes, but he had no role to play.

Jack was nervous too. He'd done deliveries thousands of times before; he'd just never delivered his partner's daughter. Jack didn't want to have to cope with Rod. He wanted total focus on the task at hand. He wanted to deliver this baby as he would any other baby.

"What shall I do?" Rod asked Jack.

"Go back to the office and see the patients," Jack said. "This is a primigravida. We've got hours of pushing ahead of us." So Rod left, feeling slightly irrelevant but also glad to be going. It would have been harder, he knew, to stay.

Jack went back into Peggy's room, and as she pushed, he and Regis and David coached her along. "She was the best person in the world to coach," Jack said later at the recap in the office. "She's very strong—strong-willed and in good shape—and that's why she pushed that baby out so well. If all patients could push the way she pushed, this would be an easy business. Lots of patients, if they spend three hours pushing, half the time it doesn't do any good, but if they'd pushed effectively for an hour, they'd have a baby."

Jack also admired David. "Sometimes these husbands try to be supportive by playing down the pain," he said. "David didn't do that. He seemed to understand what she was going through.

"And there was another thing he didn't do. A lot of husbands become very concerned with playing their role. They ask a million questions and try to expand their knowledge base. They are into being informed about everything and being part of the process, almost forgetting the fact that their wife is going through one of the most painful things she'll ever go through. Rather than being her support they become the costar. I think the woman has to be the star of the show and the husband very much the supporting player. And that's what David was. Certainly he had his questions; he's a bright, intelligent guy who wanted to understand what was going on. But he didn't let that become the point of it all. He was a totally supportive husband."

Peggy pushed for an hour, as hard as she could push, moving the baby from high in the birth canal right on out, a spontaneous delivery with a small episiotomy. When the baby was born, tears were in everyone's eyes, particularly David's. "It was just a real nice delivery," Jack reported. "Peggy was so goal-oriented; she knew that there was going to be something worth having."

Back at the office, Rod had been seeing patients, not distractedly, but Bea could tell he had something else on his mind. He was controlled but clearly excited. The staff tried to amuse him. Rod loved Mary Jo's stories about the first-grade classes she taught, so she told one. "I was talking the other day with my students," she said, "about physical differences between people and how different we all are. I asked them, 'How many of your fathers have moustaches?' One little boy had his hand half up, and he looked unsure, so I called on him. 'My father doesn't have one,' he said, 'but my mother does.'" Rod, who ordinarily would have loved that story, hardly reacted.

Forty minutes after he'd returned to the office, Regis called and announced the birth. "I wasn't even there!" he said. The phone rang again. It was Peggy telling him he now had a grandson. When he hung up the phone, he sat for a minute. There were another half dozen patients to see, and they'd been waiting awhile. He called his wife and told her she'd better go to the hospital without him. He'd join her soon.

"I feel bad for him," Barbara Valente said. "He should be free to just run up there and look at the baby."

When Rod came into the office the next morning, he pulled a little hospital snapshot out of his pocket and showed it around. "At the risk of sounding obnoxious," he said, "this is really a cute kid. He really is a cutey-pie, gorgeous features, lots of black hair. He's long, twenty-two inches. Seven pounds, thirteen ounces."

He went over to the nearest photo-studded bulletin board and pinned the snapshot to it.

"May we assume," Eleanore said, "that you're happy about being a grandfather?"

Rod smiled. "A friend of mine," he said, "got his first grandchild two months ago. I said to him, 'Franco, what's the best thing about being a grandpa?' He said to me, 'Going to bed with grandma.' "

One of the patients that morning, Susan Conacher, came in for her first postpartum visit and brought her baby, dressed in pink with a pink band attached to her scant wisps of hair. Mary Jo couldn't resist reaching out to take her. "I'll hold you, honey," she said, "as long as I can give you back."

"Isn't she cute?" Barbara said to Rod.

"She's adorable," Rod said. "But my baby's got more hair." He studied the baby. "They're really beautiful, aren't they," he said.

"He's had six children of his own," Bea said to Barbara later, "and he's delivered millions of them. But it's as if he's seeing them for the first time."

·   ·   ·

Something of a ritual for Tracy, a holdover from his bachelor days, was the annual golf weekend. He and his best friends from college would pile in a car and drive all night to a first-class golf course in Myrtle Beach, South Carolina. This year, on his first night there, he was jolted awake by a nightmare. He'd dreamed that Susan was delivering without him. The dream was so real he couldn't shake it.

The next morning, as early as he could, he phoned her. She told him not to worry, to go have a good time. But he couldn't. His golf that day was worse than usual, and that evening he confessed to his friends he was for bagging it and heading for home. His friends were understanding; anyway, it was raining. Susan was astounded to see him two days sooner than expected.

"It was my worst fear," he explained. "I kept saying, 'Oh, God, please don't let her have it without me.' "

"In your dream," Susan asked, "what did we have, a boy or a girl?"

"A girl."

"And how did you feel about that?"

"I was delighted."

16.
Five

At the dot of nine A.M. the phone rang. "Aw, shut up!" Bea called out.

It rang again. "Go call another doctor," Bea said, knowing that Barbara was about to answer it.

Barbara listened for a minute, then said to Bea, "This patient wants to know if she can take some lactate pills."

"Where did she get that crazy idea?" Bea said.

"*Bea!*" Barbara gasped, rushing to cover the phone's mouthpiece with her hand so the patient wouldn't hear. "She said her friends told her that maybe her nausea is caused by allergy to milk."

Bea harrumphed. "Tell her that when she starts paying her friends for medical advice, that's when she should start listening to them."

Barbara gave Genevieve the there-she-goes-again look. "Arla," she said to the patient with strained calm, "lactate pills are a new one on us. Maybe you shouldn't try it until you talk with one of the doctors. You want me to have one of them call you?"

When Barbara hung up, there was a silence, which Bea broke. "I know, I know," she said. "I'm terrible. Sometimes even I can't stand working with me."

"Glad to be back?" Genevieve asked her wryly. It was Bea's first day back from a prematurely terminated vacation, and Genevieve and Barbara and Eleanore knew it had been the vacation from hell. Bea and Oscar and their teenage son, Adam, were driving south through North Carolina, heading for Florida for a March break, when a tire on the truck ahead of them began to shred, flinging big chunks of rubber into their path. Oscar swerved, and their car went off the highway. It rolled over and over down a seventy-foot embankment and came to rest upside down at the bottom, totalled. None of them was hurt. The state trooper who pulled them out said they were lucky; other cars behind them crashed into each other, causing a big pileup in which several people were killed.

"Hah!" Bea said. "I feel like I've never been away."

Susan MacGregor had started the day badly too. An hour before her appointment she had forced down half the bottle of an intensely sweet orange liquid that Rod had given her at her last visit in preparation for a glucose screening test, designed to detect a special affliction in pregnancy called gestational diabetes.

"I had a patient who had to take this test, and she put the bottle in the refrigerator," Rod had told her. "They were moving, and a friend was helping them, and it was hot and he was thirsty. This guy grabbed it and took a big swig and he almost lost his lunch." Now, the cloying taste still making her shudder, Susan knew how that man had felt.

"Up there, Susie," Bea said, indicating the scale and sounding like a jovial top sergeant. "All righty, here you go."

Susan got on the scale and manipulated the measuring weight herself, reluctantly edging it higher. "One-forty-two," Bea said. Susan started to speak, but Bea made the correction before she could. "No, sorry, one-forty-one. How are you feeling after that orange poison?"

"Nauseous."

"Well, you can't complain. You didn't have any morning sickness, so now you're getting yours."

Bea recorded the weight on the chart. "That stuff can give you a sugar high, with nausea and maybe a headache. But in the scheme of things, though, you feel well?"

"Yes. I feel great."

"Well, I can fix that. Come let me take a blood sample."

Bea talked as she worked. "Some of the blood," she said, "is for the glucose tolerance test; we want to see how well your body coped with that big dose of sugar you got from that orange drink. And some of the blood is for an Rh screening test, to see if you've been forming antibodies, which you might have if the baby's blood type is different from yours." Bea carefully set aside the scarlet vials with the color-coded caps. "Now," she said, "you get your Rho-GAM shot."

"Where does that go in?"

"Your ass."

"It does?"

"You bet."

"See?" Tracy said. "I told you. It's like the muscle of your hip, right?"

"Right. An intramuscular injection. Women don't have a big enough muscle in their arm to accommodate an injection. Okay, I'm going to ask you to stand here at the side of the table. Just lean over the table, raise your skirt, lower the waistband of whatever you're wearing. Good. Now lean over the table on your elbows."

"It's going to hurt?"

"Well, it's a needle. I mean, it's not bad. Okay, I'm feeling for your hip bone so I know where I'm going to put this."

"And the Rho-GAM protects me?" Susan asked, trying to distract herself from the shot.

"The Rho-GAM protects your next baby," Bea said and delivered a refresher on the topic. She tapped Susan's bottom. "Okay, kiddo, it's over. You didn't feel a thing, right?"

"Right," Susan said, not meaning it. She straightened up and adjusted her clothes.

Jack came in and after the greetings picked up Susan's chart. "You're eating?" he said.

"Yes."

"You're not dieting, are you?"

"No."

"You seem to be gaining in that nice, slow way, and I want to be sure you're not doing it by heavy dieting just before the visit." Binge dieting before appointments is a fairly common and potentially dangerous practice. Weight control has to be achieved through balanced diet, not by avoiding calories the baby needs.

"I'm not dieting, just being careful. I always have an ice cream cone right after each visit."

"My wife and I were up in Vermont," Jack said, "and we drove by the Ben & Jerry's plant. My wife was practically crawling out the car window. I had to pull her back."

As Susan laughed her whole belly shook. Jack began examining her. "Wow!" he said, lifting his hands. "Even I could feel that one!" The baby had kicked powerfully.

Susan too looked startled. "That was a *big* one," she said.

"It's the sugar from the orange drink. He's full of energy."

Jack was paged: Rod was calling. He excused himself, hurried out to the hall, and picked up the phone. Rod was at the hospital, where two of Jack's patients were in labor, Donnalu Marucci and Virginia Kirschner. "How's it going?" Jack asked. "Oh, I thought they told me she was four." Four centimeters dilated. "How's Virginia doing? Okay, all right, I'm here. Bye." Things were moving slowly for the two women. Plenty of time.

Lots of patients were delivering now, and lots more, apparently, were conceiving. There had been a rush of new OB patients last week, eight or nine of them.

Jack returned to the examining room and resumed talking with Susan. "How about iron?" he asked. "You taking your pills?" Iron is a remedy for the anemia that a fifth of pregnant women experience. Anemia means the blood isn't carrying enough oxygen, a condition that makes for fatigue.

"One in the morning, one in the late afternoon."

"Anything else on your mind?"

"I guess my calf muscles sometimes still get a little bit tight."

"How much milk do you drink?"

"A quart a day, plus."

"You hurt mostly at night?"

"At night."

"Try to drink some of the milk at night. Six o'clock or later. Your muscles cramp up at night because by then your body's used up all the calcium you gave it during the day. The muscles need the calcium. During the day the baby and the mother use up her calcium stores, and during the night the mother gets cramps."

"Sometimes I get these welts all over me. They really itch."

"She got them before she was pregnant," Tracy said. "But now they seem to be recurring more often."

"Any kind of dermatitis or skin problem that you had prior to pregnancy," Jack said, "can be worsened. People who never had any skin problems have a lot of skin problems in pregnancy. The pregnancy hormones affect the skin, which is also why your nipples get darker and you get that dark line down the center of your abdomen. Those are all hormonally related skin changes. Some people get something called 'the mask of pregnancy.' It's a dark area across the eyes that makes them look like raccoons. That's hormonal too.

"If the welts are really bothering you," he went on, "take an Aveeno oatmeal bath. It takes some of the irritation out of the skin and cuts the round robin of scratch and itch. They sell it over the counter at the pharmacy."

"Thank you."

"That's it?"

"That's it."

"See you in four weeks. And then after the next visit we go to twos." OB visits every two weeks.

"Wow!" Susan said. It was a sudden and unexpected signal that she was well down the road.

"I'll see you at thirty-two weeks, then thirty-four and thirty-six. After that, every week. How long are you going to work?"

"As long as I can."

"I hope not too long," Tracy said. "She does a whole lot of driving, and she's on her feet all day long."

"You'll know when the right time comes," Jack said. The remark seemed a veiled suggestion, Susan and Tracy later agreed, that she stop sooner than later.

• • •

Susan found it hard to imagine what her working future would be. Just a few months before, her career had been a given. Her marriage and her job—that had been her life. She'd been looking toward a climb right up the ladder. Now, however, so slowly she'd scarcely been aware of it, the premises had changed. There was a powerful new factor—the baby. The prospect of the baby colored everything.

She still intended to work until late in the pregnancy, but maybe not quite as late. She still wanted to go back to work after the birth, of course, but perhaps not as soon. And she wasn't as sure that her present job, her treasured managership at the Coach shop in Princeton, would be the right one.

"Princeton is beginning to feel a little unrealistic," she said to Tracy one night at the kitchen table. "It's awfully far away, forty-five miles. I wouldn't want to have the baby way up here and me way down there, in case anything happens. And I can't see taking an infant with me in the car for that long."

"It's not as if the shop had day care," Tracy said. "For that matter it's amazing to me that AT&T, the third largest employer in the state, doesn't either."

"Day care," Susan said. "That's something we've really got to look into."

The pregnancy was moving fast. It was hard for the MacGregors to believe Susan was in her seventh month, or that two months from now they'd be parents. "It's happening almost faster than we can absorb it," she told her mother. "You kind of want to pull the reins and slow it down a little bit. The baby's getting bigger and bigger, and every time it kicks I think, 'It's getting closer.' "

·   ·   ·

What was vivid to Susan about the pregnancy, as to any other woman with a seven-month fetus, was its impact on her—the size of her belly, the way she felt, the pregnancy's effect on her marriage, how much longer she had to go, and, in delivery, her relative chances for joy and pain. But events far more important to her were taking place out of her sight and feeling. For this was the month her child would become intelligent.

Just nineteen days after her baby was conceived its central nervous system began to form. Its brain, an empty blob at first, appeared and started extending delicate neural filaments to every part of the body. Now, in the seventh month, the process began its spectacular finale. The front of the brain began to swell, burgeoning to blanket nearly all the rest of the brain. It was evolving into this new human being's main center of thought and feeling.

As the seventh month progressed, the surfaces of this brain mass were developing grooves called fissures. It was a way of creating more functional brain surface, just as alcoves give a room more wall space. In the brain of the MacGregor baby these fissures were appearing in exactly the same places as in the brains of every other normal human being on earth, precisely as deep, and linked to the other fissures identically. Experts on the brain long ago mapped the fissures and from the map could identify the centers for sight, smell, speech, hearing, walking, and so on. This sort of localization of function—each tiny area of the brain being assigned a highly specific duty—was the great work begun in the seventh month.

The hookup was a colossal undertaking: ten trillion connections, by the time it was over, almost infinitely more complex than any artificial system such as a computer. And not just colossal but consequential. To the degree the fissures were properly connected to each other and the rest of the body, the MacGregor child would have that much more potential. There was nothing Susan could do to help the operation along except, some studies indicated, to eat a protein-rich diet during the last trimester.

The baby had had reflexes for a long time, some of which made it grasp at nearby objects, search for a nipple, suck when its lips were touched, or startle at loud sounds. It had also learned some things. For instance, it could recognize Susan's voice, which was why, when it was placed on her chest moments after its birth and heard that voice, it would turn to it. Now, however, with the detailing of its brain, it would be capable of a different order of achievement. It would develop traits and behavioral characteristics that would make it an individual.

The amplified brain made a huge practical difference. Babies born at six months seldom make it; most of their internal organs work, but their brains aren't yet up to running them. But if Susan had her baby tomorrow, it would have a chance of survival—a 20 percent chance, with expert care. Its brain was well enough developed now to control breathing, swallowing, and body temperature. The child wouldn't be able to do those things on its own, but it could with assistance. It could even cry.

• • •

Rod had some news. Two days before, he said, on Easter Sunday afternoon, he'd been called to St. Barnabas to deliver a patient. While he was there a first-time mother-to-be named Karen Bongiorno, a young grade-school teacher from Mount Olive Township, had been admitted to Labor and Delivery. "She's a patient of Hollander's," he said.

That caught the office staff's attention. David Hollander was a perinatologist, an obstetrician who specialized in difficult or unusual births. And Karen Bongiorno's pregnancy was authentically unusual. "She's gonna have quints," Rod said.

The news had quickly spread from Labor and Delivery out through the whole hospital. In the 126 years that St. Barnabas had been in existence there had never been quintuplets. In the whole year of 1990, in fact, in all of the United States, only thirteen sets had been born. A pregnant woman's chances of having quints are one in 300,000.

Having five babies at once, however, is no longer the mind-blowing, media-maddening stunt that it was in 1934, when a woman in northern Ontario named Dionne produced history's first medically and genetically authenticated set of quintuplets, creating an international sensation. Quints are not quite as rare these days because of ovulation induction therapy, the use of drugs to promote fertility. That was the explanation in the case of Karen Bongiorno.

Karen and her husband, Rick, had been married nine years, childless. Finally they went to a fertility clinic, which found that though Karen's ovaries regularly produced eggs, other parts of her reproductive system, most notably her fallopian tubes, had been damaged by endometriosis. After a series of operations to remove scar tissue from the uterus, she was deemed ready for an attempt at in vitro fertilization.

In late October, to increase her chances of conception, she was given Perganol, a drug that made the ovaries release not one but a dozen eggs. Using a needle, the doctor removed them all, and mixed the five or six most promising ones with sperm. He watched them and measured them, and at the time when Karen normally would have ovulated he took the ones that had successfully been fertilized and, bypassing the damaged tubes, placed them into her uterus via a syringe through the cervix.

The fertilized eggs floated free in the uterus. The question was whether at least one of the them would implant itself in the chamber's wall. To increase its chances Karen was sent to her bed for two days. She and Rick and the doctor anxiously waited. On Thanksgiving Day or thereabouts, conception took place, and six weeks later—her cycle was unnatural because of all the drugs she'd been given—as a sort of Christmas present, Karen learned she was pregnant. The Bongiornos were overwhelmed, and soon they were celebrating along with the clinic staff.

A few weeks after Christmas they went to the clinic to see if the gestational sacs, containing the fertilized, implanted eggs, could be seen on the ultrasound screen. The astounding truth was spread out before them. There, as if glued to the uterine wall, were flecks of light—one, two, three, four, *five* of them! Karen later described that sight to a friend. "You know how planes look when they're flying at very high altitudes? You can't see the planes themselves. All you see are little flashes of light as the sun hits them. That's all they were— glimmers of light. We were stunned, Rick and I. And so was the doctor. In all his years in fertility work he'd never had more than triplets. And here were five."

The doctor, who'd become very close to the Bongiornos, was worried about them, concerned about the drastic adjustment they'd have to make: for nine years no children and suddenly five. "We went through the anxiety," Karen said several months afterward, "the how-will-we-this and the how-will-we-that. But we'd been praying for a child so hard and for so long that the fears quickly passed, and we realized we were blessed. They were sent for a reason."

At sixteen weeks of gestation, in late February, it became possible to hear the heartbeats. Five at once. To Karen, listening to them over the amplifier of the Doppler, they sounded like a team of ponies clopping along. At eighteen weeks, in early March, and from then on, the fetuses were regularly examined by ultrasound. It was discovered that each baby occupied its own private amniotic sac—the best possible arrangement. In all, there were four separate placentas, with two of the quints sharing one. That worried the Bongiornos until they were told there was nothing to be distressed about; each baby had its own umbilical cord.

The normal task of the ultrasound technician, which is to get an accurate measurement of the size of the fetuses, is especially important in the case of multiple births. It is vital that the babies' sizes be roughly the same. If four of Karen's babies had been growing well but the fifth had been puny, that would have been alarming. If one of the fetuses was in trouble, it could endanger all the others.

Multiple gestation—being pregnant with more than one baby—is by definition riskier than single pregnancy, the more so with each additional baby. The danger is mainly in the increased chances of premature delivery. The greater the number—especially quadruplets and quintuplets—the larger the chances that some of the babies, at least, will be stillborn and that some or all the surviving babies will suffer from cerebral palsy, mental retardation, lung trouble, or coordination problems.

Faced with the grim facts of the situation—the dreadful odds against the higher multiples—perinatologists have developed a safe but dismaying technique: multifetal pregnancy reduction. To diminish the negative odds, the number of fetuses is reduced. Within the first twelve weeks the doctors decide which fetuses have the worst chance of survival—usually a matter, at that early point, merely of where their sacs are positioned in the womb. Those imperilled fetuses are then terminated in any of a variety of ways. It is a terrible choice to put to parents: Either allow the doctor to end the lives of some so that those spared will be healthy, or spare all the babies and accept the cruel irony that they might well die anyway or be tragically disabled.

The doctors presented the Bongiornos with that choice. It was very unlikely, they said, that all the babies would survive. The wise thing might be to reduce the number to three or two. The Bongiornos refused the option. Through January, February, and March, all five babies continued to grow in Karen's womb. All of them were doing well, falling into the right size range and growing in tandem. There was a reasonable chance that all five would survive in good condition.

On March thirty-first, Easter morning, Karen began to feel pressure in her cervix. She didn't think much of it, but when she went to the bathroom before bed she started to bleed, rather rapidly. She was twenty-one weeks pregnant. It was much too early to be having the babies. They wouldn't have a chance. Rick rushed Karen to St. Barnabas, and the cause of the bleeding was discovered. The fetus they would name Travis, positioned lowest in the uterus, was lying on one of the placentas, perhaps making it separate slightly from the uterine wall. Travis shifted, and everything was all right.

Karen's actual due date, the end of a full forty-week term, was in August, but Dr. Hollander, the St. Barnabas perinatologist, was prepared to settle for a date much earlier. On May twelfth, for example, Mother's Day, Karen would be pregnant twenty-seven weeks. That would take her out of the danger zone. But March thirty-first was six weeks too soon. The quints needed those six weeks in the uterus while their organs developed.

He decided to take no chances. He kept Karen in the hospital, in the antepartum wing, a part of the maternity section reserved for mothers-to-be who, like Karen, were having high-risk pregnancies and had to be observed closely. Karen had joined an exclusive club. The mothers, all of them waiting, endlessly waiting and confined to bed, felt close to each other and exchanged notes and phone calls, but because they were bed-bound they never could meet. The best they could do was to wave through the doors as their wheelchairs were being rolled by on their occasional trips to the shower.

17.
Slide Show

It was mid-April, the day before Susan's twenty-ninth birthday. The crocuses she and Tracy had stuck into the ground along the front path in October were blooming now, purple and cream and yellow.

At thirty-two weeks Susan felt enormous. She had trouble reaching around her belly to pull her socks on, and weighing herself was impossible; she couldn't see the dial on the scales beneath her overhang. She had to ask Tracy to read out her weight to her. Two weeks before, she had paid an Easter visit to Hilda Sprague, her father's mother, who had suffered a stroke and couldn't talk and had trouble connecting. When she saw Susan's abdomen, a sight that transcended language, the old woman came alive. Slowly, her expression full of delight, she extended her hand and put it on the large, high globe that contained her first great-grandchild.

The baby was so active it was unbelievable. Sometimes it got so animated, with every limb going a mile a minute, poking her everywhere, that she felt it was going to pop right out. When she wore one particular dress, a snug jersey, she could see its motions vividly, like a cat in a sack. She wondered if there was something wrong with it, if it was under stress. Tracy said the baby was just athletic; according to the books he'd read, the movements were essential to development.

Its favorite time for aerobics was right after she herself had been exercising. She was doing all the swimming she could, and she often walked around the neighborhood and up into the Reservation, a public woodland along the crest of the hills near the house. When she was moving, the baby was still; when she stopped, it geared up.

Susan was still working, but now, for the first time, she was looking forward to staying home. She kept recalling Jack's advice to get plenty of rest before she delivered. She desperately didn't want to go into labor exhausted. She hoped to gain a certain composure before the whole process began but wasn't at all sure she could. Perhaps the Lamaze classes at the hospital, which were about to begin, would help. If things were ready at home, she thought—the baby's room, the layette, some sewing she had to do—she might be a little more together.

Her good fortune, she felt, was that Tracy got steadier the further along the pregnancy went. She might be all over the place, but he was calm, usually, and loving.

•   •   •

There was a flurry in the staff area of the O'Driscoll-Bonamo office. A celebrity patient had arrived. It wasn't Elsa Howard, who sang with the Metropolitan Opera. It wasn't Susan Bavaro, whose husband Mark played tight end for the New York Giants, or Suzanne Lees, who was special assistant to the governor of New Jersey, or the woman who was an exotic dancer. It was Julie Birchler. Julie was the practice's undisputed champion baby-bearer. She'd had eight of them. Rod had delivered them all.

The staff was fond of Julie and respected her but held her in awe. "Imagine her wash," Eleanore said. "The washing machine has to be going all day."

"How often does she have to go to the supermarket?" Genevieve wondered.

"She never complains," Bea said approvingly. "No fuss, even though all the births have been difficult for her. If you look at her patient's folder: eight babies, tough births, but there's nothing in the folder. Unlike some *other* patients I could name: one perfectly ordinary pregnancy and their folder's an inch thick!" For Bea, the ratio of difficulty of pregnancy to thickness of folder was a gauge of character. Thick folders meant lots of complaints and tests and complications.

"Last pregnancy she was worried," Barbara said. "She's almost forty now, an older mother. But she wouldn't get an amnio to see if the baby had Down's syndrome. It wouldn't matter to Julie if it did. She'd want to have it anyway."

Today, Julie had brought her husband. She was a tall woman with the figure of a mezzo-soprano—a seriously pregnant mezzo-soprano—and her husband, Al, was tall too, with handsome, rough-hewn features. His outdoorsy complexion and broad shoulders and muscular hands, along with his red-and-black checked shirt, made him look just like what he was, a tree surgeon. He had a barter arrangement with Rod: Rod attended Julie's births, and Al tended Rod's trees. "I've got the best-pruned oaks in Essex County," Rod liked to say.

Julie came from a locally prominent Roman Catholic family. She had known since childhood that she would have all the babies she could; it was a matter of conviction and vocation. That was what her life would be about. When she was ready to marry she looked for a man who shared her goal, and she found one in Al Birchler. In many ways they made an improbable couple. He'd gone to high school, she had graduated from college summa cum laude and was just a few credits from a master of science degree in medical and psychological rehabilitation. He was easygoing; she was intense. But when it came to creating a family, they were eye to eye. "They met at the fair," Jack once said about them. "That's what my grandmother's generation used say when two people were perfect for each other: They met at the fair."

"The only difference between Julie and me," Al would say, "is that she uses words this big"—he'd hold his thumb and forefinger widely separated—"and I use words *this* big," he'd add, bringing his fingers close together.

Essential to Julie's quest was finding the right obstetrician, one who'd respect what she was doing. Rod was that doctor. It wasn't so much that he was Catholic and had a big family himself; Rod and Julie were somewhat different varieties of Catholic: the one calm, the other ardent. Rod and Joan had six kids because they'd both been only children and hadn't liked it. Julie, however, was pro-life in the most active sense of the term. She was out to create all the life she could. The thing about Rod that was so important to her was the knowledge that he wouldn't undermine what she was doing, wouldn't treat her with veiled disapproval.

The project had been difficult almost from the start. After the birth of her second child, she soon became pregnant again, but the fertilized egg lodged in her fallopian tube, the duct leading from the ovary to the uterus. Rod had to remove the tube and the ovary.

That left her with only one functioning ovary. With the stroke of a scalpel, her egg-making machinery had been halved. She was anguished, but as it turned out, a single ovary was all she needed.

Months before, when Julie had made her first obstetrical visit for this new baby, Bea greeted her as she emerged from the consultation room. "Pregnant *again?*" she said. Unruffled, Julie smiled and nodded. After all the time she'd spent in these offices, she was used to Bea's megawatt candor.

When she came down the hall to make her next appointment, she paused at one of the five bulletin boards covered with baby photos and found the most recent picture of herself and her children.

"When I first came here," she said, "there was only one bulletin board."

Eleanore Steel, who was just emerging from her office, picked up on that. "Pretty soon," she said, "you're going to need a bulletin board all your own."

•   •   •

Jack and Bea shared a number of qualities—style, intelligence, professional skill, and wit. They also shared a certain irreverence about the patients. Even the nicest patients could be truly silly upon occasion, and the not-so-nice ones could be outrageous. If you didn't acknowledge it somehow—if you simply absorbed it—you could go crazy. Rod's style was to shake his head and roll his eyes. Jack and Bea, both superverbal, were likely to say something.

One morning Barbara was talking to a patient on the phone who thought she was pregnant. "If you're just one day late," Barbara said, "that's really soon. Why don't we see you in about three weeks?" At that point Jack walked in the door. Barbara put the caller on hold and said to him, "She's only one day late and she wants an appointment!"

"Tell her to get out of bed and take a shower," Jack said, "and we'll see her in a week."

One difference between Jack and Bea, in this respect, was that while Jack zapped seldom, Bea zapped often. Another was that while Jack did it entirely out of patients' earshot, Bea often did it to their faces. That was her way. To do otherwise, she felt, would have been hypocritical.

To Jack, rudeness to patients—which was how he saw it—was the unforgivable sin. Where Rod might just shrug and say, "Now

Beasie . . . ," Jack felt he had to say something. He'd speak to Bea, and Bea would do it again. It seemed to Jack that Bea was zapping more and more lately. For several years now the tension between them had been growing, over this and similar issues. The rest of the staff could only stand by and watch and wonder when the inevitable would occur.

"Jack and Bea never bonded," Mary Jo once said to Barbara and Genevieve, using an obstetrical metaphor. Bea, on her part, felt like the child who had come along with the marriage between Rod's and Jack's practices, the older child who feels unloved by the second wife. Jack, on his part, felt like that second wife, who has to endure the constant cold appraisal of the first wife's resentful child.

"It's really unfortunate," Jack once confided. "I love Bea, I really do; she's fabulous at so many things. But I can't watch her do these things to people. It's taking the fun out of it for me. That's why I'm here, this is what I do. I love people, I love to make them feel better, for me that's fun. And I'm not having fun any more."

Recently a first-time mother-to-be had arrived for an appointment. She'd brought her mother and wanted to take her into the examining room with her. Bea, however, had a thing about patients who had to have support people in the examining rooms. She barred the mother. Jack saw the patient's distress and figured out the whole problem instantly. "Didn't I see your mother out in the waiting room?" he asked her. "Why don't we bring her in here with us?" Overridden, Bea steamed.

* * *

A young woman in white leather ankle boots stepped to the front of the room and called the new series of St. Barnabas childbirth education classes to order. Her name was Roseann Toglia, she said, a part-time labor-and-delivery nurse and mother of a two-year-old son. She asked someone from each couple to state why they'd come tonight. "We're here because I'm scared," said one man. A woman said: "We're here to learn to do it without medicine, hopefully." Another woman said: "I'm here to learn as much as I can. And him"— she gestured at her husband with her thumb—"he's here because I dragged him." Susan MacGregor said, "I want to have a fast and painless delivery," a sentiment that brought murmurs of agreement from around the room.

Roseann said, "We want to give you the tools to handle your own experience. Every birth is different. We now call it 'prepared' rather than 'natural' childbirth. There's no success or failure in childbirth, so whether you use medication or you don't or have a cesarean or not, a good experience is one that's pleasing to you.

"I'll be introducing you to the Lamaze approach to childbirth. There are three parts to it. First I'll give you lots of information about the end of your pregnancy, about labor and delivery. Then I'll teach you ways to avoid the fear-tension cycle. When you're afraid of something, such as pain, you become more tense; you feel more pain. That's a conditioned response. You've learned to think that labor equals pain. We'd like to replace that with a new conditioned response: thinking of labor in terms of what it's really composed of—contractions. Labor makes you anxious, but contractions have a purpose, to move the baby out. You'll learn how to relax the rest of your body when the contractions come.

"The third part is learning how to impose rhythmic, patterned breathing on the cycles of contraction, to distract your attention away from the pain. I can't promise you no pain, but I can give you some tools to deal with it." Roseann paused, and the room was silent, not a whisper. Every face was turned toward her.

"An important part of the Lamaze method is the coach. Now we refer to them as the support person. They're real important. Dads, these classes are just as much for you as they are for the moms. When the contractions come, the moms are going to forget a lot of what they've learned, and they're going to be looking to you to help them along. You'll learn all the relaxation and breathing techniques too, so that when the mom says, 'I've forgotten, I don't remember,' the coach says, 'Now look, it's easy; this is how it goes' and helps her reestablish her breathing pattern by counting along with her. A good coach can make all the difference—someone who really knows you and who's prepared with you."

Susan nudged Tracy and smiled.

Roseann darkened the room and showed a film called *Hello, Baby.* It was a soft introduction to the subject—three deliveries, no blood, no screaming, no unfortunate outcomes. "Your baby," the nurse-narrator began, "is getting ready for the big birthday party. . . . You might think the labor is going to last forever, but suddenly the baby is right there in your arms. . . . Don't think of labor as an obstacle to be overcome but a means to a most remarkable end. And it can teach you a great deal about yourself or reveal a new dimension about somebody you love."

One of the three childbearing couples in the film had brought a picture of their cat for the laboring woman to focus on. "Carl did help," she said in the voice-over, referring to her husband, "but sometimes I just didn't want him touching me. But it did help to have him keep me breathing properly." Another mother, shown easing her labor by sitting in the shower while her husband sprayed water on her, said, "If I'd known I was going to like the shower so much, I would have had Leo bring his bathing suit." Leo was singing "She'll Be Comin' Round the Mountain." As her labor wore on into its twelfth hour, a third mother said, "John and I decided we wanted medication to help me relax between contractions."

Throughout the film, Susan was spellbound, and when the first baby finally came, pushing dramatically through the outer vagina like a missile slowly emerging from its silo, she gasped.

And so it began, a gentle, encouraging beginning to five Wednesday nights of concentrated practical information on every aspect of childbearing. In every session the couples spread mats on the floor and practiced the Lamaze techniques of breathing, focusing, reconditioning their conditioned responses, converting fear into purpose. "Take a nice deep breath," Roseann would say, "and blow it out through your mouth. Now tighten up, make a strong facial grimace, tighten your mouth, keep your mouth shut. Raise up your shoulders real hard, real hard, and tense all your chest muscles.

"Now tense your abdominal muscles, bend your arms and flex your biceps, bend your wrists, squeeze your thighs together, tighten your buttocks, lift your feet." Sixteen men and women lying on their mats squeezed their thighs, tightened their buttocks, and raised their feet. "Feel that feeling of incredible tension and how uncomfortable it is and how unnatural.

"Now all at once just let everything release, and take a nice deep breath again in through your nose. Starting with the top of your head, start with a gentle feeling of relaxation, let your eyes close very naturally, let your jaw fall open. . . ."

Then there were breathing exercises, and from all over the room the sound of light panting rose above the thrum of the air conditioner.

Roseann introduced them to a Lamaze relaxation technique called *effleurage,* French for "touching lightly." It was a gentle, grazing massage the coaches gave to the mothers-to-be, using their fingertips to brush the swollen bellies softly. "Try it out," Roseann said, "and see if it's comfortable." At her instruction, each mother lay stretched out on her mat with her coach kneeling behind her, her head in his lap. As Tracy stroked Susan she looked up at him and smiled in amusement and affection.

Most couples took the Lamaze instruction very seriously. One husband grew embarrassed and, with the *effleurage,* finally mutinous; he picked up his pillow and walked out, his wife reluctantly following.

The only mishap was the slide show in the third session. Its aim was to show couples how things worked at St. Barnabas: what the rooms looked like and how the process flowed from stage to stage, from the admissions office and Labor and Delivery to the nursery, the recovery room, and Postpartum. But as the show progressed, it was apparent that something was wrong. "Uh-oh," Roseann said, "these slides are out of order. Somebody must have dropped the carousel and didn't get the pictures back in right."

On went the show with the sequence jumbled, postpartum appearing before Labor and Delivery, the nursery before the admissions office. The photo of the cold, utilitarian delivery room with its operating table and gleaming instruments, where cesareans were done, popped up in the middle of the sequence on normal delivery, which gave the impression that at any point in a routine childbirth a mother could be whisked off to major surgery. In total effect, it was something out of the Marx Brothers.

For the younger parents-to-be, those having their first child, this phantasmagoria only confirmed their worst expectation: chaos. It was Susan's particular dread that she'd be moved from bed to bed, room to room, her meaningful childbearing experience sacrificed to the requirements of a rigid institution. She had heard Roseann say the slide show was askew, but what she saw registered more deeply on her than what she heard. The slide show nourished her nightmare.

Despite all the information Susan and Tracy later picked up in the classes and from the doctors, the impression the slides made would never entirely vanish; the MacGregors would take it right into Labor and Delivery with them. What they wanted was the congenial sort of birthing experiences they'd seen in *Hello, Baby,* and they were afraid they'd committed to another kind of thing altogether, the hurried, high-tech delivery the hospital's presentation seemed to depict.

"There seems to be so much more medicine and equipment at St.

Barnabas," Susan said to Tracy after class, "people hooked up to wires and tubes and everything else."

"It didn't seem organized. Too confusing, like the flow wasn't as easy as it should be."

"So many contraptions," Susan said, "so many things that I didn't feel were necessary. I'm not a doctor, but the whole thing of hooking everybody up to an IV, I mean what's the point of doing that?"

"You can request them not to do it."

"Yeah, you can, but it was kind of overwhelming when Roseann said, 'Everyone gets an IV and 90 percent of the patients get epidurals,' like it's already planned out for you. I feel like I'm going for surgery."

"That movie on TV the other night," Tracy said, "about the babies who were switched at birth . . ."

"That was really bad. Can you imagine? When they brought the baby for feeding, the mother said she didn't think it was hers, but they told her it was."

"That'll be my job," Tracy said. "I'll track the baby as soon as it comes out. I'll make sure he gets the right number."

"Don't lose sight of him," Susan said, "not for one minute."

•   •   •

As if to prove the accuracy of the doctors' assurances that her dreadful morning sickness wouldn't hurt her baby, Linda Cohen, the patient who worked in a travel agency, gave birth to a robust son the third week in April. Rod O'Driscoll did the delivery. Later, at a *brit milah* ceremony at the Cohens' synagogue, the boy was circumcised by a professional called a *mohel* and given the name Daniel. At that moment, throughout the congregation, there were cries of "Mazel tov!"

18.
Floaters

On April twenty-seventh, Anne Marie Lipper, who had fallen down the stairs and worried ever since about her baby, gave birth to a healthy baby girl. And on May third, Beth Keyser, the recovering alcoholic and pill addict, went to St. Barnabas to have her second child.

Beth was frightened, not of delivery but of what might happen afterward. Her first pregnancy she had stayed off pills and liquor and had had a healthy baby but afterward relapsed. Her comeback had been fiercely hard work. Throughout this new pregnancy she'd stayed clean, and there was every reason to believe her baby was fine.

Just before midnight she had a son, David. He weighed eight pounds and was vital and healthy. The day after the delivery, Beth's breasts swelled unbearably. Again she was afraid to breast-feed. She couldn't keep herself from asking for pills.

Jack Bonamo didn't say no. He told her of other ways to reduce the pain. "Put ice packs in your bra," he said. "Sleep with your bra on and wear your bra every minute of the day, or else the weight of your breasts will stimulate letdown of the milk. Keep your husband away from your breasts. And try to stay away from crying babies; crying lets down the milk, too."

This time Beth didn't take the drugs.

•   •   •

Karen Bongiorno was having an emergency. Since her eighteenth week her doctors had been giving her Terbutaline, a drug to suppress labor so she could carry her quintuplets as close to full term as possible. The drug was administered with a special device, a pump that continuously sent small amounts of the drug into her leg. She could control the pump herself. Whenever she felt the contractions beginning again, she could make it supply an extra dose of medication.

The night before, however, at the end of her twenty-fourth week, she had gone into hard labor. Twenty-four weeks was still too early for safety. The babies' bodies were still undergoing important development. Every additional week in the womb now would make a big difference in the health of the newborns. To meet this emergency, the doctors increased the dose and added two other drugs. She got through the night, and by midday the crisis was over.

· · ·

Susan's OB appointment—the first of the biweekly visits—was at five, and Tracy was behind schedule. He raced out of the office and drove for West Orange as fast as he dared. When he got there, he found Susan hadn't arrived.

Five minutes later she appeared. "Well," she said to him, "you have a hot date?"

"What do you mean?" he asked.

"You went flying past me on Route 78. Practically drove me into the ditch."

Tracy looked embarrassed. "I was late," he said, "and I was thinking, 'Boy, am I going to catch it for being late.' Now I'm catching it for being first."

Susan gave him a kiss. She was wearing a new maternity dress—mint green and dusty rose on dark green, with a lace collar, long puffed sleeves, a long skirt, and a loose waist. "Oh, this is really big," she'd thought when she bought it. "Plenty of room." Now she was filling it out.

Jane Rissland, the GYN nurse, was on duty, substituting for Bea. She showed Susan into the examining room at the far end of the narrow, winding hall, the one with the white satin stuffed-stork mobile suspended from the ceiling tiles. Susan laughed when she saw it. It was in this room, back in October, that she'd learned she was pregnant. "Once I saw that stork," she told Tracy, "I knew something significant was happening."

"We've come miles since then," Tracy said. "That was like the dawn of history."

"I don't even feel like the same person," Susan said.

Jane's scales said that Susan had gained fifteen pounds so far.

"Fifteen pounds," Tracy said to Susan, "isn't that great?"

"It's all right."

"You could gain another ten in your last two months and you'd still be fine."

Jack came in and examined her. "The way your belly is now," he said, "there's baby every place."

"Sometimes I feel something here," Susan said, pointing to a spot near the top.

"That's its behind," Jack said. "And there was just a foot or a hand here. Now it's gone."

"This is activity time, I guess," Susan said.

"The baby knows the time's getting close."

"I think it's been getting hiccups," Susan said.

"Yes," Jack said, "and when it does, do you see a little dimpling that's real rhythmic?"

"I see it and I feel it. Why does it dimple?"

"When the baby hiccups, it changes the pressure of the liquid on the outside of the wall."

"And then my stomach periodically just gets tight, like it's going to pop."

"That's a contraction. It gets like a basketball, real tight, then relaxes? You may experience more of that as you get closer and closer. It might start a pattern, every ten minutes. It's not labor, it's just a Braxton Hicks contraction." Braxton Hicks contractions, named after the nineteenth-century British obstetrician who made himself an early expert on the mysterious workings of the uterus, are painless muscular spasms during later pregnancy. Their job is to help the uterus accept and adjust to the expanding fetus.

"And my belly button hurts when I walk."

"Is it pushed out yet?"

"Kind of."

"It'll get pushed out even more. Your belly button's used to being in, and somebody inside there is pushing it out. That's real common. Are you feeling any strange sensations in your groin?"

"Sometimes my ligaments feel like they're being pulled."

"Your whole pelvic floor is starting to relax so the baby can descend. You'll think there's a foot or a hand coming out of your vagina—that's the way people describe it. It's not, it's just relaxation. Everything's just going to move down a little bit. Nothing's coming out."

"Sometimes I feel a little bit of numbing."

"You may feel twinges in your buttocks and down your legs. If you stand up and you feel pain in your leg, try to walk it off."

"Anything exciting you can tell us?" Tracy asked. "Can't you tell how big it is?"

"No. I can tell the baby's size is appropriate to how pregnant Susan is. It's not going to be a huge baby, but that's all I know. It seems to be right on target."

"The kicks are stronger," Susan said.

"It's strong and it's appropriate, but I don't think it's huge."

"Do you ever know for sure?" Tracy asked.

"No, we usually don't. Sometimes we have a tiny woman and we think we have a great big baby, and it turns out to be seven pounds. It just looks big because she's so small. Sometimes we have women who look like they have nothing much there and they wind up with a big baby."

One reason Jack, like most doctors, was seldom willing to say that a healthy woman like Susan was "too small" to give birth vaginally was that the pelvis itself is somewhat elastic. The pelvis isn't one bone but an assembly of them, held together by cartilage and ligament. Over the course of the pregnancy, hormones were making Susan's pelvic joints flexible, so that when the baby came through there would be just a bit more room.

The phenomenon of pelvic expansion was demonstrated a century ago by a Belgian researcher, Theophilus Budin, with the help of an unusually cooperative subject. Budin reported that when he inserted his finger into the vagina of this pregnant woman and then asked her to walk, he could feel the two connected bones that formed the pubis—the bone at the front of the pelvis, which can be felt just above the genitals—moving up and down with each step. How, thus engaged, he managed to keep up with the walking woman, he didn't report.

That flexible juncture of the pubis had attracted the attention of physicians in eighteenth-century Europe. Like all birth attendants since the dawn of history, they were regularly faced with a horrible quandary: what to do for the mother whose baby was too big for her to bear. Since they lacked anesthetics and antiseptics, cesarean section was a dreaded alternative, though it was sometimes attempted. In 1768 a medical student in Paris, Jean René Sigault, suggested an alternative to cesareans: expanding the birth canal by severing the bones of the mother's pubis. At first he was denounced, but nine years later he performed the operation and saved both mother and baby. The Academy of Medicine in Paris awarded him a medal, and he was hailed as a medical pioneer. "Symphysiotomy," the operation was called, after the name of the joint, and throughout Europe, Britain, and America the profession was split between the Symphysians and the Cesareans. But the operation often crippled the mother, and the space it yielded was generally insignificant. So this technique, like so many other grim techniques devised by doctors desperate to help their suffering patients, fell into disuse.

"Everything looks good," Jack said. "Do you have any other questions?"

"I guess that's it," Susan said.

"People tend to run out of questions at about this point," Jack said. "You know what's going on, you've been into it for half a year now, you're getting good at it."

•   •   •

Peggy O'Driscoll Chapman's baby was now two months old. She and David had taken him over to Rod's and Joan's for one of their frequent visits. Rod and Peggy were sitting on the sofa, Peggy with the baby in her arms. "Dad," she said, "I can't believe how much I want to be with this baby. I thought I'd just be able to have it and go right back to med school, and things would be pretty much the way they were before I had the baby, but it's not like that anymore. I just want to be with him all the time."

"Well, even if you were home all the time," Rod said, "you wouldn't be with the baby all the time, you wouldn't be hugging him all the time, you'd be doing other things too."

"I know that rationally," Peggy said, "but that doesn't stop me. I just want to be with him all the time. I think about him all during my classes. I know that my hormones are doing a number on me. But I never could have imagined the strength of the pull, the intensity of the bond between a mother and her child."

•   •   •

The month of May had come at last. It was a fine time to carry a baby. The weather was comfortable—no more heavy coats, but the air was still cool. Strings of cloudless days alternated with occasional spring rain. The lawns of Maplewood were greener than green, and the flowering shrubs—the azaleas, the cherries, the crabapples—were at their showiest.

As they entered the ninth month of pregnancy, the MacGregors saw changes in each other. Tracy was less playful and boyish as responsibility descended upon him, and Susan was less pragmatic, sometimes dreamy. Sometimes reality would break in upon her—when she observed herself in the shower, or when she saw the stacks of baby clothes. Some of the garments, which had seemed so small in the store, now looked so big that she was taken aback, afraid that she'd have to deliver a baby that large. She'd remind herself that the baby, thank God, wouldn't be that big when it was born.

Tracy too had his epiphanies. "It's getting a little scary," he told Susan. "Up until a couple of days ago, I couldn't really imagine life with a baby. And now I can. I can actually see living with this baby, living with something that's completely dependent on you."

"It's different for me," Susan said. "I think it's because I feel the baby pretty much all the time, and because of all the preparation, inside and outside. I already kind of feel that I'm a mother."

A half hour later, still in a philosophical mood, Tracy said, "It's so amazing, because when this child is born I know we'll absolutely love it. I mean totally, unconditionally. I know I'll immediately love this child I've never met."

•   •   •

On a Sunday in May, Susan and Tracy were heading for lunch at the Spragues when Tracy said, "Oh, I forgot. We're supposed to go by the Jonkers and pick up your mother's tickets for the Garden Club house tour." The Jonkers were the parents of Susan's close friend Bronwyn and lived near the MacGregors.

They walked up the Jonkers' front walk, Susan wearing a cotton summer dress. The door opened before they knocked, and Susan was surprised to see Bronwyn, who lived in New York. She wore a silk dress and was holding a glass of wine. "I didn't know you were coming out this weekend," Susan said. "What are you all dolled up for?" From behind Bronwyn came a chorus of female voices calling out "Surprise!"

It was Susan's baby shower. Bronwyn and Mrs. Jonker had arranged it. Susan's friends were there, and so was Betty Sprague with some of her friends as well—about twenty-five women in all. Tracy, in on the secret from the start, had been given the job of getting Susan to the party. The day before, he'd spent two hours with the Jonkers polishing silver.

The presents, a variety of generally practical baby items, were

well coordinated—almost no duplicates, except for two baby bath-
tubs. The prize was the gift from Bronwyn, a carefully crafted patch-
work quilt she'd been working on since January.

The occasion was larger than the presents. The women of Susan's
world were ritually recognizing her motherhood.

•   •   •

Susan came in the back door, her hair still damp from her swim.
She'd always loved swimming. It was the ideal exercise for someone
whose job kept her on her feet most of the time and even better for
someone carrying a baby. When none of her bathing suits fit her new
girth, she'd bought a pregnancy suit, and on her days off and sometimes in the evening she'd drive to the YWCA in Summit and spend
thirty minutes stroking or just lolling, half listening to the music,
half in reverie. "The water supports my stomach," she told Tracy.
"In the pool I don't even feel pregnant. I'm floating, and the baby's
floating inside me. If I put my head under water I can almost imagine what it's like for him—the muffled sounds from the outside, the
sense that you don't know which way is up. We have a great time together."

"Sounds wonderful," Tracy said, slightly envying her intimacy
with the baby. He was dying to see the baby, aching to know what it
looked like and what its sex was—everything about it. He had a
much harder time being patient than Susan did. "Whoever came up
with this nine-month thing?" he said. "I don't think I can stand it."

•   •   •

As they sat in the waiting room that May evening, on hand for the
first of their weekly obstetrical visits, the MacGregors could over-
hear Barbara Valente breaking in a new member of the staff.

Genevieve Collins had left. A year before, she and her husband
had moved to a new house in Pennsylvania, seventy miles away. Ever
since, she'd been driving the immense round trip to and from West
Orange daily, maintaining her perfect attendance record despite
weather and other impediments, but the ordeal had started to wear
her down. So, grieved about separating from Barbara and Bea and
Eleanore and Mary Jo and the doctors, and miserable about leaving
the warm world of her office family, she had quit to take a job closer to home. For the people she left behind, it was like losing a sister. It was an omen of changes to come.

Her replacement was Louise Bacino, who was experienced but

new to the way that phone calls were dealt with at 95 Northfield. "If they catch cold," Barbara was telling her, "we use Robitussin and we force fluids. We tell them to gargle with warm salt water. If in doubt I put them to bed."

"To bed?" Louise asked, slightly surprised.

"Oh, yes. They love to go to bed. People around here tease me because I'm always sending everybody to bed. They call me The Napper. Now, if they have a really bad clogged nose, and they just feel crummy, you know, I kind of try to pamper them. A cup of tea and a cookie. It makes them feel good, which is about all you can do for them. Of course if they have a bad ear or something, they have to talk to the doctor."

• • •

If Jack had really believed the MacGregors had run out of questions, he was mistaken. Not as long as Susan was unsure about the kind of birth experience she'd have at St. Barnabas. Not as long as Tracy was dying to know his baby's sex and when it would arrive.

"Can you tell the size of the baby now?" Susan asked Rod, the doctor on duty.

"About five and a half pounds," he replied. He'd spent twenty-five years making endless guesses about small, hidden creatures. "You're going to have a nice-sized baby, about seven and a half pounds."

"Do you think it's going to be on time?"

"Too soon to tell. Keep in mind that 85 percent of babies are born within five days of their due dates, earlier or later."

"What about traveling at this time?" Tracy asked. "I mean, we were invited to a wedding in Maryland."

"When?"

"May twenty-seventh."

"We tend to discourage travel in the last four weeks," Rod said. "If there's an emergency, okay—a family crisis or something. But probably not for a social occasion. Too close."

"We've been going to the Lamaze classes," Susan said, "and they raised a few questions. I understand you do a routine IV." It was something that she'd asked Jack about earlier but that was still on her mind.

Rod braced for challenge. "Yes," he said.

"What are the pros and cons of that? Is it a matter of keeping a vein open in case of emergency?"

"We're going to assume there won't be an emergency," Rod said.

"The main reason is that when you go into labor, you don't eat anything. We don't want you eating and maybe getting sick. But labor uses up a lot of energy, and the IV lets us give you glucose regularly for nourishment. It'll keep you from getting tired out."

"I was just concerned," Susan said, "because I got the feeling that with all these things hooked up to me, I was going in for an operation or something."

"I don't think you'll find the IV objectionable," Rod said. "You won't feel it's too clinical."

"And you can still walk around, right?" Tracy asked. "You just have to drag the IV stand with you?"

"Well," said Rod, "we like to think that by the time you're in the hospital, you're in good labor, not walking around. The walking-around is when you're home."

"So the IV will be toward the end?" Susan asked.

"Why don't we go back over some of the steps?" Rod said. "We were going to do that next week, but let's do it now. We usually figure first labors will be about ten to twelve hours long. Sounds like an awfully long time, but in the beginning the contractions don't come very often, fifteen to twenty minutes, and they're mild. If you're doing anything, including sleeping, you may not even notice them. But then, over a period of time, they get closer, and you'll say, 'Hey, maybe something's going on here.' And we'll look for a pattern as well. You'll be ten minutes, then they're eight, seven, six, five. And as they get closer together, they'll be lasting longer.

"Now, you live near the hospital, so what we suggest is to give us a call when your contractions are five minutes apart and lasting a minute to a minute and a half. That's when you'll go to the hospital, and in theory you'll hopefully be maybe four centimeters dilated. You're in active labor, and at that point it's appropriate to keep up your energy with some IV fluids."

Susan seemed to be taking it all in without confusion, so Rod proceeded. "There's one chance in eight," he said, "that your membranes will break—an uncontrollable loss of amniotic fluid—in which case, please give us a call. In most cases patients will go into labor six to eight hours after that happens. But if you don't, we ought to give you some help. Once the membranes go, it's important for the baby that labor begins within a reasonable length of time. So, if things don't move along, we'll give you some Pitocin to get things started. And that goes in through the IV connection too."

"The other question," Susan said, touching on another familiar topic, "was the episiotomy, whether that is a routine procedure. What are the chances that I wouldn't need one?"

"The odds are you'll need one."

"You routinely do it?"

"Pretty well routinely for first babies at term. In other words, if someone has a premature baby, the baby is small and . . . I mean, if you went into labor now, you probably wouldn't need episiotomy. I delivered a patient this morning—she didn't need an episiotomy. The baby was almost seven pounds, but it was a second baby. But the right thing is to advise people having their first baby that more than likely they'll need an episiotomy."

"So you make a cut under the vagina so it doesn't tear."

"An episiotomy is a surgical incision that we like to think replaces lacerations. You tear more with first babies."

"How many stitches does it take to sew up an episiotomy?"

"Ten," Rod said, ready to wrap things up. "Enough to do the job correctly."

"And it helps speed up delivery a little bit?" Tracy asked.

"Right."

"Because you don't have to wait for . . ." Tracy groped for the word he wanted.

"That's right, exactly," Rod said, agreeing his way toward the finish line. "Anything else?"

● ● ●

95 Northfield was in turmoil. People were urgently rummaging through cupboards, rifling stacks of papers, looking under dusty piles of medical journals. The halls were knee-deep in anxiety. An important insurance form had been lost.

Jack slammed shut the drawer he'd been searching. "Oh," he called out in profound exasperation. "I can hardly wait until Oscar and Felix have their own spaces."

Felix, which was to say Jack, was finally seeing his dream come true. In a few months the practice would be moving into tidy new quarters upstairs in which both he and Oscar—Rod—would have their own offices. Over the winter Rod, who was enthusiastic about Jack's plans, had given him the go-ahead. The tenants on the second floor of the building were being disposed of one way or another, moved to new space on the first floor or their leases allowed to lapse. Jack, working with an architect, a contractor, and an interior decorator, had created what he considered to be the most logical, efficient, and beautiful new obstetrical offices that anyone had ever seen.

For two months now, the work had been under way. The sound of constant hammering coming down through the ceiling, combined with fear of the new, had done nothing for anyone's tranquility. Tempers were short, particularly Bea's. The old office world may have been worn, but it was cozy and comfortable and familiar, and it was a world of which Bea had been a essential part. She and Rod had been in this nest together for seventeen years. Now people were slowly coming to realize that in Jack's sleek, professional new world, Bea might not fit. Not only were the days of the old office numbered; so, perhaps, were Bea's.

Bea seemed to know it. One day Jack invited the staff to look at the samples for curtains and carpets and wallpapers and to comment on them. Bea held herself off to one side, huffy, wanting to take part but at the same time deploring the whole idea of new offices—Jack's idea—which symbolized to her everything that had gone wrong since her world was invaded. Jack asked her for suggestions on the design of the part of the office she was going to use. She stonewalled him.

After it was all over and Barbara and Bea were alone, Barbara said gently, "Bea, I don't think you're going to make it to moving day."

Bea replied, "I don't think I am either."

19.
Six Years Pregnant

Mother's Day was a particularly great day for that notable mother-to-be, Karen Bongiorno. Her pregnancy had passed the twenty-seven-week mark. Her quintuplets were out of the danger zone.

Still, every day inside the womb was a plus. The doctors were now able to make fairly close estimates of the babies' weights. The smallest was now one pound, ten ounces, and the largest almost two pounds. Through Karen the babies were receiving steroids to develop their lungs, vitamin K to prevent bleeding in the brain, and other specialized medications, as well as general vitamins, and iron, and other supplements.

The year before the pregnancy began, the Bongiornos had been thinking of selling the large house they'd bought out in the country in hopes of a having a family, and moving into a smaller home, closer in. "It's a good thing we didn't," she said, "because now we're really going to need the space."

As small as they were, the babies had become vigorous kickers. "Sometimes they do it all at once," she said, "ten little feet stomping away. It can be a little uncomfortable, but it's nice to know they're so strong."

Releasing a breath, she laboriously adjusted her position in the bed she'd scarcely left in the past six weeks. "We aren't sure about their sexes," she said. "There are a few boys, and we're not sure about the girls. It's hard to tell on the ultrasound. It's just a jumble of arms and legs. There are so many of them, and they're bigger now, and you can hardly tell what belongs to whom."

She pulled the blanket back up over her swollen belly, the repository of five miniature human beings. "I know that when they're born they're going to have to go into special care," she said. "They'll have a fight ahead of them, even at twenty-eight or thirty weeks. So I'm doing all I can to get them ready for that fight. It's all I can think about: keeping those babies inside."

•   •   •

Three weeks to go. Susan had stopped work and told her boss that contrary to what she'd said when she first announced her pregnancy, she would not be coming back. She now saw that she intensely wanted to be with her baby during its first year at least. She and Tracy had talked it out and decided they could make it on one salary for twelve months. After that, they'd see.

What until the week before was just one end of the MacGregors' upstairs hall was now the baby's room. A Sheetrock partition had been erected, and a door. Susan had just finished the curtains for the baby's room, a landmark in her struggle to get things ready. Now they could imagine the whole scene vividly—the crib over here, their baby in it.

"It all looks so pretty," Tracy said. "I assume the baby will have better manners than to throw up all over it."

"I wouldn't count on it," Susan said.

•   •   •

For two days Susan had been cooking and cleaning. "Today's the big day," she told Tracy over the phone. She'd slept a little later that morning and missed seeing him. "My project is to see if I can clean under the bed and still manage to get out. I've gotten so round I'm afraid I'll get stuck."

She was kidding about the getting stuck, but during the day Tracy kept thinking of it. He was almost surprised when he got home and approached the kitchen door to see Susan vertical, moving around, making dinner.

•   •   •

Seeing the MacGregors as they arrived at the office, Barbara felt they looked entirely different. Tracy was wearing a knit shirt, shorts, white socks, and sneakers; Susan a blue pregnancy smock. "You two look sweet," Barbara said, "so nice and casual. It's the first time I've seen you that way."

"No more briefcase," Susan said. "I'm a lady of leisure now."

Bea calculated Susan's total weight gain for the pregnancy at twenty pounds. Now, at last, Susan seemed to accept that she wasn't going to get fat. "That means I can put on four pounds in a couple of weeks," she said. "Let's go eat!"

Susan's blood pressure was somewhat lower. "That's the way it's supposed to be," Bea said. "Late in the pregnancy we watch blood pressure pretty carefully."

Elevated blood pressure, along with protein in the urine and swelling of the face and hands, can signal one of the real obstetric emergencies for women in late pregnancy: preeclampsia—dangerously high blood pressure and excessive swelling. It develops, sometimes suddenly, in 5 percent of pregnant women—most often in first-time mothers-to-be, teenage mothers, mothers over forty, women carrying twins, and women who work, no matter at what. The cause remains unknown, and there is no treatment that works for everyone. In its later stage, eclampsia, it can kill both a mother and her baby.

"How do you feel, Susan?" Jack asked when he came in.

"Ready to get it all over with."

"That's pretty common after the first two or three ninety-degree days of the summer. A touch of heat and everybody over seven months is ready to call it quits."

"Can you tell how long she's likely to go?" Tracy asked. "Will we go another three weeks?"

"Only going with the numbers and what I see here tonight, there's no reason to believe you won't. No evidence yet that the head is trying to come down into the pelvis or if you're dilated at all. You probably won't be, but sometimes we're surprised with the first baby; a few weeks to go and we get a few centimeters of dilation."

Jack placed his hand at the bottom of Susan's swelling abdomen, putting his thumb to one side and his fingers to the other. He then closed them around a grapefruitlike ball and moved it slightly from side to side. "The head," he said. "It's down, in good position. The back at the moment is lying along your right side.

"It weighs about five and a half pounds now," he went on. "It's going to put on two pounds, maybe a little more, in the next couple of weeks."

Susan had talked with Rod about the episiotomy, but she brought it up again now with Jack. She was still leery of it. She'd read about the vagina-stretching technique used by midwives called "ironing the perineum," claimed to make episiotomies unnecessary.

Jack didn't think much of it. "The muscles of the vagina," he said, "can stretch only so far. They're like a piece of elastic; when you stretch and stretch and stretch it, it never comes back all the way. And so the mother's muscles become loose, and she can have real problems. Maybe you escape an episiotomy, but you may get a thirty-year-old woman who dribbles urine down her leg every time she laughs or sneezes." Obstetricians did some gentle muscle-stretching too, he added, but they didn't rely on it. Beyond a point they used episiotomies, and the patient preserved her elasticity.

Susan had one more question. "Is it okay to have intercourse?" she asked quietly. "I mean, at this late stage of the pregnancy?"

"Definitely," Jack said. "No problem. You can't hurt the baby. In fact we sometimes recommend it to patients to get the baby moving along."

"In that case," Tracy said, "we can wrap this thing up in a couple of days."

•   •   •

May seventeenth. Karen Bongiorno's twenty-eighth week of carrying her quintuplets. The quints were fine but Karen was in danger. She had preeclampsia. Her blood pressure was rising, her protein levels were low, and her blood-clotting factor was nil. The doctors would have to deliver her babies immediately. Because of the preeclampsia, the anesthesiologist could not use a method that would knock her out just from the waist down, as he preferred. He would have to use a general anesthetic—not good for the babies, because it would affect them too, slow down their hearts and responses. They would have to be removed very rapidly, before the general could reach them in full strength.

Before the cesarean began, Karen's principal doctor, perinatologist David Hollander, assembled teams of nurses and doctors in the operating room, each of which would stand ready to take a baby as it was brought up out of Karen's body and begin the regimen of emergency care that premature babies received.

"There were so many people in that OR," one doctor said afterward to another, "it was a circus."

"Yes," said the other, "but a very coordinated circus."

There were twenty medical professionals in the room. Three doctors would operate and remove the babies, assisted by three circulating nurses. Five pediatric specialists, one for each baby, were standing by, and each specialist was accompanied by a nurse. There were two anesthesiologists and two anesthesiological nurses.

Dr. Anthony Quartell and Dr. Hollander performed the cesarean. Three minutes after starting the incision they reached and opened the uterus. The first baby out, at 9:41 A.M., was the one later named Katelyn. A minute later, together, came a pair of boys, Matthew and Daniel. The next minute came another pair of boys, Travis and Zachary. As they emerged they were handed to the support teams. The babies were touchingly thin. Their skin was transparent.

The tricky thing was to make sure that the blood samples drawn from the babies' umbilical cords were marked for the correct baby. As they were born, each baby was given a letter of the alphabet, from Bongiorno A through Bongiorno E; was labeled accordingly with an ankle band; and was footprinted. Each pediatric team evaluated its baby. The scores were good. All the babies were strong and healthy for their stage of development. Their weights were appropriate, ranging between a pound and a half to two pounds, and on average they were thirteen inches long. The combined weight of the five babies was nine pounds, less than the birth weight of some single babies. The extra pounds Karen carried were in large part those of the extra fluid and placentas and umbilical cords for the five—the support system.

One by one the babies were swaddled, placed in special bassinets equipped with oxygen, and taken to Neonatal Intensive Care. Karen, who had gone under the anesthetic a childless woman and now, still asleep, was the mother of five, was taken to the recovery room.

Karen's uterus was bleeding alarmingly. So much of the uterine wall had been covered by placentas, four of them, that the placental bed—the area they'd been attached to—was exceptionally large. Once the placentas were removed, finger-sized blood vessels freely poured out blood. Normally, the contracting muscles of the uterus would have pinched off those vessels, but since Karen's uterus had been so drastically stretched, the muscles weren't up to the task, and she was given medication instead. Dr. Quartell stood by her bed for an hour, massaging her belly.

The birth of the quintuplets took place on a Friday. Not until Sunday evening was their mother well enough to be wheeled down to Neonatal Intensive Care to see her babies.

While the six of them had been fortifying themselves in the hospital, family and friends organized themselves into baby-tending shifts. A close friend had written to dozens of baby supply companies telling about the quints and asking for free merchandise. Some companies had declined, but most—Gerber in particular—had come through with everything from baby food to bassinets and strollers. The uniqueness of the quints, their star quality, had drawn help in a way that ordinary babies in need seldom did.

Karen stayed in the hospital for three weeks. "It'll be tough at times," Dr. Hollander said as they said goodbye. "But for someone who could survive what you've already been through, the rest should be relatively easy."

•   •   •

On May twentieth Rod delivered the child of the alcoholic woman who in October, early in her pregnancy, had appeared so dull and lifeless. Back then it had seemed likely that this baby might be afflicted with fetal alcohol syndrome. But during that October visit Rod had taken her into his office and talked turkey about what her drinking could do, and his remarks had apparently had an effect. She had started attending AA meetings. Her new baby, a boy, seemed to be normal in every way.

The day after that, Jack delivered Lois Geller, who had longed for a daughter, of her fourth son.

•   •   •

It had happened—Jack and Bea.

One afternoon he'd gone into an examining room to look at a patient and found her crying. Inquiring among Bea and the staff, he pieced the story together. The patient had phoned and said she was in pain, and someone had told her that there were no appointments left but if she came to the office they'd slip her into the schedule.

Bea did not like having people slipped into the schedule. She also did not like hypochondriacs. "You're always complaining," she told the young woman. "How will we ever know when you're really sick?"

The patient burst into tears. She was in fact something of a hypochondriac, but to Jack that wasn't the point. A grim resolve welled up in him. "Let's go outside," he said to Bea. They went to the parking lot.

"She's always bellyaching," Bea said. "She's no more sick than you or I am."

"Even if she's not sick," Jack said, "she thinks she's sick. She's allowed to think she's sick and to come here and tell me about it because that's my job. I'm her doctor." There was a moment of heavy silence. "Bea," he went on, "I've had it. I'm sick of you abusing my patients, I'm sick of trying to be nice to you, I'm sick of cajoling you. I can't do it anymore. So would you just please leave and go home."

Bea walked back into the office and worked out the rest of her day. She didn't want to be thought of as the kind of person who didn't finish the day.

Rod was on vacation. The next day was Bea's day off. Jack felt that he had been vague with her, merely telling her to "go home," and he wanted to nail it down. He phoned and told her not to come in anymore. When Rod came back, he said, they would be in touch with her.

Several days later Rod returned home and, as was his custom, phoned Jack to see how things were going. "Would you come down here right now?" Jack said to him. "I really need to talk with you."

"Can't we talk tomorrow?" Rod asked.

"Get in your car," Jack said, "and come down here right now." That got Rod's attention. Jack had never talked to him that way before. That night at the office, after hours, Jack told him what had been going on.

Rod was caught in the middle. On one side was Jack, his partner and friend, gifted doctor, upon whose business and managerial skills he had come to depend. On the other side was Bea, gifted nurse and old friend, who knew him as well as anyone outside his family. When Rod's wife's mother was dying, Bea had sat up the night with her. The O'Driscolls and the Perezes saw each other socially. The O'Driscoll family dog was a present from Bea and her husband.

Rod told Bea he hoped to engineer a two-week cooling-off period: She would stay out of the office, and things would calm down, and she could come back. But one day he called her up and said, "Beasie, I can't do it. Jack just won't go along with it." And that was that. Rod sent her a Waterford crystal vase with a sentimental note of thanks. Bea called and thanked him and started looking for work.

The shock in the office was massive. Yes, Bea had been asking for it. Yes, it had seemed inevitable. But, for the staff and also for many of the patients, once she'd gone, the vacuum left by that enormous personality was intense and disorienting. Barbara, Eleanore . . . everyone in the place had fought with her at one time or another, or been nicked by her tongue. But life without Bea?

First Genevieve had gone and now Bea. Something that had animated their lives and made them come to the office every day almost eagerly, looking forward to the friendship and the fun, was gone now. The sorority had been disbanded.

•   •   •

"Is anything *happening?*" Susan asked Jack in exasperation. It was Thursday, the sixth of June, four days before the delivery date Frank Conte's ultrasound had foretold.

"Apparently not," said Jack, completing his internal examination. The baby's head hadn't moved into the pelvis, and the birth canal was still blocked by the cervical plug, a deposit of mucus in the neck of the uterus. Patients got pelvic exams their last four weeks, and Susan had had two, but at this stage there was seldom much to see.

He examined the base of Susan's abdomen, taking the rounded protrusion there between his fingers and squeezing slightly. Then he moved his hand to the top and squeezed again. "Well," he said, straightening, "I can't tell if that's head down there and butt up here or head up here and butt down there. It makes a difference. I think we'd better do an ultrasound."

Susan's belly, sharply defined, looked like a giant tortoise. There were no stretch marks, and there was no brown line down the median, but the skin was somewhat darker than the skin on the rest of the body. The navel stuck out a third of an inch. Just above it, Jack squeezed out a ribbon of blue gel.

"You can do an ultrasound without making her drink all that water first?" Tracy asked.

"No need for the water now," Jack said. "The baby's so big we'll have no trouble seeing it. This isn't like looking for tiny details on a four-month fetus."

He pressed the ultrasound probe to Susan and saw the fact of the matter immediately: the little globe at the top of the big globe was a baby's bottom. He put more gel at the bottom of the belly and applied the probe, and a luminous circle appeared on the screen—the baby's head. "He's making it easy for us," he said. "Everything looks good." He turned off the ultrasound and wiped the gel off Susan.

"And there's no chance of him turning around?" Susan asked.

"Yes, there's still a chance. He still could just go off and do it. But it's extremely unlikely."

"Where do we go from here?" Tracy asked.

"Okay," Jack said. "If we don't have a baby by, say, next Thursday, I'll do a nonstress test. We'll attach you to a fetal monitor and see how the baby's heart rate responds to the baby's own movement. When the baby moves the heartbeat should accelerate. That tells us that the baby's well oxygenated and the placenta's functioning."

Susan touched Tracy's arm. "You were going to talk to him about . . ."

"Oh, yes. We decided we want him circumcised."

"No problem," Jack said, smiling, "assuming it's a boy."

"Well, according to our pediatrician," Tracy said, "that's what it's going to be." They had gone to meet their new pediatrician last week, John La Conti, recommended to them by Jack. At the end of the visit Dr. La Conti had said, "Okay, now let me guess what you're going to have." He'd stood up, ceremoniously extended his hands and put them on Susan's stomach, and after a pause said, "It's a boy, and I'm right 80 percent of the time."

"Have you got some boys' names ready?" Jack asked.

"Actually, no."

"I guess maybe we should try harder to think of some," Susan said.

"So go make an appointment with Eleanore for next Thursday," Jack said.

"I'm sure I won't need it," Susan replied. "I've got to have this baby before Thursday."

"That's what they all say," Jack said.

As they went back through the waiting room Ahava Podhorcer, a young woman who'd attended the childbirth classes at St. Barnabas with the MacGregors, entered it and was shown right into an examining room. She was having contractions. The next day she'd have a six-pound, nine-ounce son.

•   •   •

Jack phoned in from the hospital to report a notable birth. The staff was all ears; they knew this was the day that Julie Birchler, mother of eight, would go for her ninth.

All of the eight had been vaginal deliveries, and Julie had wanted a vaginal delivery this time too. Jack, on duty alone because Rod was taking a short vacation, had determined that the baby was in what is normally considered a bad position for a vaginal birth: it stood in the womb, ready to exit feet first, the so-called footling breech position. Footling breech generally means an almost certain cesarean. Julie, with her tried and tested pelvis and its proven ability to pass large babies, would have been a good candidate for vaginal breech delivery, but not this time. While she was in labor, Jack had an ultrasound scan done, and looking at it he was shocked. This was a *really* big baby. That fact added to the poor birth position made vaginal delivery a recipe for disaster. So he had done a cesarean.

"It's a boy," Jack reported to the office. "Eleven pounds, six ounces, no less. Everybody's doing fine." A sizable baby indeed for the practice's most populous family.

Of her thirty-nine years, Julie Birchler had been pregnant a total of six years, nine months, and twelve days and had produced eighty-five pounds of human being.

•   •   •

It took a few moments to realize what it was about the young woman in the waiting room that was so distinctive. She was pretty, with white skin and black curls, but that wasn't it. She was unusually small, but that wasn't it either, or her air of vitality and good humor. Two crutches rested against the wall next to her chair. That was it: She had only one leg.

Her name was Eva Burd. She was Jack Bonamo's patient. To Rod and Jack she symbolized something important to them both, the role that a sympathetic and encouraging obstetrician could play in helping a disabled woman to motherhood.

When she was nine years old, Eva had been diagnosed with bone cancer in her left leg. She underwent eleven operations. Each time the doctors would take away the cancerous portion only to see the cancer recur. By the time she was sixteen she had lost not only her leg but, in an operation called a hemipelvectomy, much of her pelvis. She had also lost some of the nearby muscle and half the feeling on her left side.

Her doctor had told her she could never have children. Without a pelvis, there would be little to resist the growing weight of the fetus, and, much too prematurely, the baby would come rushing out. She must give up any idea of bearing a child. She went to another doctor, who said much the same thing, and two others after him, with the same result.

The amputation had been so drastic that there was nothing to attach an artificial leg to, but a prosthesis was created nonetheless, a special harness that strapped to her body. Unimpeded, she got herself a demanding job as head of the word processing department in a large Morristown law firm—120 attorneys. She also met the man she wanted to marry, a young accountant for the water company, George Burd. He wanted a family, and she was determined to give him one. With new resolve she renewed her search for an understanding obstetrician. Someone recommended O'Driscoll and Bonamo.

Jack examined her and said, "I don't see why you can't have a baby. You've got everything you really need to do it." The baby, Jack reasoned, would be kept in the uterus by the cervix; muscular and tight when not dilated, it could restrain the baby very well. There seemed to be no "absolute contraindication" against her having a baby.

Eva soon conceived. As the weeks went by she had more and more trouble keeping her balance on her crutches. "My stomach feels as if it's almost on the ground," she told Jack. "It keeps pulling me over, as though I were leaning forward all the time." Once, carrying laundry down the stairs, she fell, but no damage was done.

Later, looking back on the experience, she remembered a problem no one had predicted. "I realized that if I gained too much weight, I ran a risk of straining my leg, and if I did it might not be able to hold that weight. That leg was important to me, so I drove myself crazy trying to watch everything I ate." There was another surprise. "The heavier I got, the funnier I looked, a big round ball on top of a stick—like a candy apple." As she grew heavier the prosthesis no longer fit, and she had to give it up and use crutches.

Eva kept the same schedule of obstetrical visits as the other patients—once a month and then, in the last trimester, once a week. She wanted very much to have a regular pregnancy, and she did. It went well. She felt wonderful. She carried the baby into the ninth month.

As the time of birth approached, neither she nor Jack knew exactly what to expect. With some of the muscles on her left side gone, and with partial numbness there too, how would she push the baby out? But Jack was confident he could manage the situation as it developed, and his confidence helped Eva stay calm.

He told her that at the very first moment she felt labor she should go directly to the hospital. Since she had no pelvis to delay the process, it was possible that any sort of contraction would shove the baby right out. As it happened, though, the birth was not quite that precipitous. Her contractions were ineffective. Jack ordered a drug for her that stimulated contractions, and soon the delivery began.

What Jack then saw amazed him. The vagina and cervix, which were not enclosed by a pelvis but exposed to view, began to bulge. Then they opened widely, and a baby plunged through, born not by slow degrees, as is normal, but all at once—head, shoulders, body, legs, the whole works. It was like a cesarean birth, the free and rapid delivery of the entire baby. As in a cesarean, the baby, not having had to crowd through the tight, bony pelvic passage, was unbruised, and its skull was round and well formed.

Instead of the agonies of delivery, what Eva did feel was intense pain from an unexpected place, the leg that was gone, echoes of the cancer pain of years before. Somehow the process had triggered long-dormant nerve connections, producing "ghost" sensations. But they were soon over.

"My God," she thought that night as she lay in Recovery, her newborn daughter at her breast. "What if I'd accepted the word of those doctors who said I couldn't do it!"

Eva waited four years before having another baby so that her first child would be old enough to take care of herself to some extent. In her fifth month of pregnancy she quit her job; raising two children and working would be just too difficult. Her labor was slower and more difficult; the baby was large, about a tenth her own weight. She had to have a lower-body anesthetic. Her baby was a second girl. She had the family she'd dreamed of.

Two years later now, on the day of this gynecological visit, she'd accumulated a lot of experience at being a handicapped mother. "Some people want to deny parenthood to people like me," Eva said. "When my first child was a baby, I had to figure out how to carry her when I walked on crutches. I had to compensate for what I didn't have. I slung her over my arm in a special way. It was fine, but one day a woman in the mall said to me, 'I can't believe you'd actually have children!' When I was pregnant with my second, we were at a party and a woman said to me, 'What are the chances of your child being born with only one leg?' And I said, 'Probably the same as the chances of your child being born with three.' Some people just don't get it."

She believed her children instinctively wanted to help, even as babies. When her husband or mother picked them up, they'd wiggle all over the place, but when Eva picked them up, they'd stiffen their bodies to make it easier for her. They wouldn't move their heads or arms or legs until she was able to sit down and get herself into a comfortable position. And then they'd wiggle. It was as if they knew.

"They're six and two now, and they still go a little bit beyond what you'd expect of children. They don't leave their toys around because they know that Mommy will fall on them. The older one, she knows that when you see a disabled person in the supermarket, you don't stare and make a scene. She waits until we get in the car to ask what happened to that man."

She and her husband tried to maintain a normal atmosphere at home. He never treated her like a cripple. She did the laundry, cleaned the house, got the children ready for school. They refused to use the handicapped parking space, leaving it for someone who really needed it. "The kids know I'm different, but it's part of their life, and we think dealing with it has made them into deeper, richer people.

"You can see it in the mall, their reaction to other children. Some people let their kids make a big scene when they see me. Last week in a store a little boy lay on the floor so he could look up my dress and find my other leg. His mother thought it was funny. I just bit my tongue and looked at my six-year-old. Her whole reaction was 'That's my mommy, and that's that.'

"I try to look beyond how strangers react to me," Eva said, "like when I'm in the supermarket trying to get the two-year-old into the front basket. I may do things a little differently, but I'm not harming my child in any way. I just do the best that I can. I look right through those people. I'm not about to stop my life because of what they think. I look at my children and thank God for them and remember I'm just lucky to be here."

Eva was Jack's last patient for the morning, and when she left he went to the coffee machine. Barbara was there. "That woman," he said.

"Really something, isn't she," Barbara said.

"There are patients who complain about this and that, the trials and the tribulations of taking care of a baby, but not Eva. She never once says, 'Poor me, how hard it is to raise a child with this disability.' That never enters her mind. When I ask her about the baby, she talks about how good she is, how she never cries when she's going down the steps with her, how she knows Eva has to go slowly, how she fits herself into Eva's disability."

Still thinking about Eva, he poured himself a cup of coffee, not daring to put sugar in it in front of Barbara. "In this business you see some brats," he said, "but you also see some pretty terrific people."

Destiny had not yet finished testing Eva. One day several months later the office would be shocked to hear that Eva's husband had been killed in a motorcycle accident.

•   •   •

On the eighth of June, Rod O'Driscoll was called to help Grace Findley, the woman who had been badly burned by a New York doctor, deliver her second baby. He was named Tucker James Findley, and his weight was a robust nine pounds, fourteen ounces.

•   •   •

June had become a series of ninety-degree days, hot and airless. The edges of the shimmering, orange sun were diffused by the steam in the air. At night, lightning would fret the sky, but if rain came, it wasn't the kind that broke the weather. The spring blossoms that had covered Maplewood just a few weeks before were largely gone now, withered early. Too hot. Hard on everybody but especially on women who were nine months pregnant.

Cars rolled by with tight-shut windows enclosing private zones of chill, but no one was on foot, not on the sidewalks or in the yards. For a while, despite the temperatures, Susan had taken five- or ten-minute neighborhood strolls, sometimes all the way into Maplewood village. But she'd had to give her walks up. They were taking too much out of her. Lacking an air conditioner, she retreated to the screened porch on the side of the house. The porch was painted white and had a cool stone floor. The cushions on the white wicker furniture were covered in a pastel floral chintz. Begonias and impatiens trailed from pots suspended from the ceiling, and a ceiling fan kept the air moving. This was where she and the baby would spend their first summer together.

The baby was moving a lot more, not kicking so much as squirming. There was more pressure, too, low in her belly. Sometimes she had cramps, but none of it ever amounted to anything. There was no real sign that anything was happening, but somehow she felt that something was. She was sure she wouldn't be keeping that Thursday obstetrical appointment.

She'd spent some of June seventh, her original due date, the one Dr. Bonamo had given her a million years ago, in the garden. She couldn't get over far enough to pull a weed, but she could water plants and drag a rake. She felt absolutely no activity inside her that day, and she remembered her mother saying that babies can be quiet just before labor starts.

Joking, Tracy told her she wasn't doing enough laundry and cleaning to be about to deliver. She hadn't yet had the burst of energy they said you got just before the baby came, the one that sent you into a frenzy of housework. She remembered what Roseann, her childbirth instructor, had said about the rush of vigor: Resist it. Save the energy.

They'd decided to have the baby sleep in their bedroom at night, so they could be sure they'd hear if it needed them and so Susan could breast-feed easily. Her mother brought over the family bassinet, and they put it near their bed. Her brother Gordon arrived in town, hoping he'd get there while she was still pregnant. It was a sight he had to see.

Looking back on the pregnancy, she was amazed how quickly it had all gone by. Things had moved right along. But now they weren't moving fast enough. She was eager to meet the baby, to see what it looked like, to see if it was a boy or a girl. She and Tracy felt the nine months had changed them from kids to adults. Sometimes they felt they already were parents.

The things she was taking to the hospital were all laid out on the guest room bed, with her bag, a quilted calico satchel, beside them. In that respect, at least, she was ready. The hospital was so close. They'd be there in ten minutes.

Tracy tried to keep calm, for Susan's sake. He'd found himself wishing he could have a glass of wine; as a gesture of support, he hadn't had anything to drink since Susan got pregnant. She wouldn't be drinking while she was breast-feeding either; Tracy hadn't yet made up his mind if solidarity went that far.

His boss at AT&T, knowing he was going to be out of the office, had given him projects that had to be done soon. Some mornings when he left the house he felt nervous about leaving; he didn't want to go, thinking he might have to turn right around and come back. He'd wanted to wear a beeper, but his office was too far away, out of beeper range.

Nothing to do but wait, so they waited, trying to read Susan's body's signals, trying to find some portent in them. Somehow, at some moment, the mechanism was going to start.

The baby waited too, head down, tucked like a diver with arms and legs clasped to its body, eyes shut, a traveler poised and ready for a journey which, though just a few feet long, would take it from one world into another.

20.
Stirrings

When a baby achina, a species of Australian anteater, is ready to be born, its mother gets the message. Achinas have spines on their backs like the quills on a porcupine, and the spines start growing before birth. By the time the baby reaches the appropriate degree of maturity, he's so prickly that his mother can't stand it anymore, and she ousts him from her pouch. Human babies send messages too, when they're ready, but the messages are often harder to read.

On Monday evening, June tenth, Susan's estimated date of confinement as revised by ultrasound, she went to bed with no particular evidence that anything major was about to happen to her—she felt crampy, but there was nothing new in that. Just after two on Tuesday morning, however, she was awakened by a new sensation.

Getting to this point had been a slow progression. It had begun weeks before with the Braxton Hicks contractions, which felt like gentle fingers pressing on her abdomen. Gradually the fingers had begun to press harder, and then they had slowly changed from fingers into constricting iron bands—bands of pressure. They hadn't hurt at first. The bands were flat, not on edge; they weren't cutting. When the bands tightened, her stomach became rock-hard, a granite boulder. She felt she could crack an egg on it. Tonight the progression had brought her to a new stage. The constrictions had changed from discomfort to pain. She was approaching labor.

The pain rose and fell. When it had gone, she touched Tracy's shoulder, and he came to consciousness immediately. "I'm having contractions," she said. "I think they're the real thing."

"Oh my gosh," Tracy said. They both were silent for a moment. "Do you think we ought to time them?" he asked, and then answered his own question. "Let's time them."

When the next swell of pain began, she let him know, and he looked at his watch and wrote down the time on the pad on the night table. She lay on her back, hands spread on her stomach, eyes closed, concentrating, and then the pain wore down. Tracy wrote the time down. "Okay, tell me when you're getting another."

Over the next forty minutes, the intervals between the contractions seemed to fluctuate. Usually they were about ten minutes apart, but sometimes they were six or five, even four.

"Should we call the doctor?" Tracy asked.

"Not yet. They have to be five minutes apart, and they have to be regular."

"I wonder how long that will take," he said. "Can you sleep?"

"I think I can," Susan said. "I'm tired." And then she did more or less manage to sleep, in the old brass bed where it had all begun, nine long months before. The contractions went on through the night, each of them picking her up, clenching her, putting her down, but seldom breaking through her fatigue.

In nine months the fetus within Susan had grown from a one-celled fertilized egg into a human being made of billions of cells. Today the being was ready to be born, and a mysterious process had given the uterus its long-delayed command to contract. The muscular uterine walls would close upon the fetus, sporadically at first and then, if all went well, rhythmically in concert. By pressing the fetus from every direction but one, the uterine bear-hug would make it follow the line of least resistance and send it inching headfirst down through the dark.

The way was narrow and tight, and the deeper the baby went, the tighter the passage would become. The passage also twisted. It was a serpentine hole through flesh and bone whose irregular contours would make the baby keep pivoting and changing course. Toward the end, the contractions alone would not be enough. Susan would have to use all the strength in her body to drive the baby through.

The last major barricade would be the cervix. A cone of thick, strong, fibrous tissue projecting from the bottom of the uterus, it would have to open enough to pass an object with a diameter of at least four inches. Before it could open it had to be thinned by a process called effacement: pulled and pressed to membrane thickness.

The tool would be the baby's skull. The uterus would extrude the body, driving the head before it. The skull—despite the nature of its primary job, to protect the soft brain—was still pliant, yet it was strong enough to thin the cervix by stretching it and butting against it. The MacGregor baby, like most other babies, would be born through an act of force, shoved into the world.

•   •   •

The bedroom was on the east side of the house, and the sunlight reached it early on June eleventh. The summer solstice was less than two weeks away, and at six-thirty, when the alarm went off, the sun was high and the room already glowing. Tracy was usually the one who stopped the alarm and got up first, but this morning Susan swung her arm over and stopped the noise. "You're not going anywhere," she told her husband. The moment she'd awakened, she said, she'd known that things had progressed. The contractions were more intense, and she thought she was leaking some water.

Amniotic sacs don't leak; like balloons, they're intact or they're broken, though not all the fluid may escape the uterus at once. If one breaks high up, it may take a little while for the split to reach the lower sac; until it does, there may be a bit of early fluid. What women take to be leaking water is likely to be mucus.

Susan's contractions still seemed to be mainly ten minutes apart. They decided not to call the doctors' answering service. Not yet. "Let's just hang out a while," Susan said, "until regular office hours."

It seemed like a very long wait. The contractions grew closer, and there was more fluid. The contraction rate didn't yet qualify, they knew, but the fluid worried them. At nine forty-five, Tracy stood up and said "Let's do it" and made the momentous call, the one that might set the whole march of events in motion.

Barbara Valente answered. "She's been having contractions all night," Tracy told her.

"Oh, that's exciting. Dr. O'Driscoll's on duty. Wait just a minute and I'll get him."

Rod was full of enthusiasm when he came to the phone. "Hey, that's great," he said. "How often are the contractions coming?"

"About every eight minutes," Tracy said, "although they vary a little. And she thinks she's leaking some water."

Rod asked to speak to Susan, and he took her through all her signs and symptoms. "I tell you what," he said, as if he were about to suggest a walk in the park. It was the opener he customarily employed when he wanted you to do something and wanted to make you think it was going to be a piece of cake. "Why don't you come on over and let's take a look."

Susan went into the guest room, scooped up all the things she was taking to the hospital, and packed them into her satchel, wondering if she had everything but finding it hard to think systematically. Her main needs were her toiletries and two nightgowns and a robe and slippers to wear after she got to Postpartum. She snapped the bag shut and Tracy grabbed it and headed down the stairs. He was headed out the door when he remembered his camera. He came back in and found it and pressed the battery-check button. It failed to light.

"Let's go by my parents and borrow theirs," Susan said, and they phoned the Spragues and said this probably wasn't it, but it could be, and could they borrow their camera?

The Spragues lived eight blocks in the wrong direction, which made Tracy nervous, but he resisted the temptation to speed. When they got there, they saw Betty and David waiting at the head of the driveway, David with the camera in hand. Betty, eyes bright, leaned through the open car window and kissed Susan and said, "I'm so proud of you." David shook Tracy's hand. The Spragues stood there in the heat of the morning, watching as the green Saab climbed Mountain Avenue and turned right onto Wyoming, taking their daughter toward the great recapitulation of life.

Jane Rissland was the nurse on duty. She led Susan and Tracy down the narrow, winding hall, past the thousands of tiny blue eyes staring out from the baby photos on the walls, into the farthest examining room, the one with the stuffed satin stork hanging from the ceiling. Out of habit, Susan headed for the scales to be weighed in, but Jane laughed and said, "We're not going to weigh you. That isn't what's on our minds today." She led Susan to the examining table and gave her a yellow paper smock to wear when she removed her clothes.

When Susan was ready, lying on the table, Jane wrapped a broad, elasticized band around her abdomen. It was the fetal monitor, whose purpose was to gauge Susan's contractions and the fetus's heartbeat. Rod appeared promptly, his smile reassuring the Mac-Gregors.

"The monitor looks fine," he said, after the first contraction had faded. He put on gloves and performed an internal examination, slipping his index and middle fingers into the vagina. Maneuvering them with the sureness and economy that came from having performed tens of thousands of such examinations, he immediately found the cervix. As they told medical students, it was like touching your nose—firm but not hard, soft but not mushy, with a dimple in the middle: the opening. There was practically no dilation; the cervix was nearly closed.

"Obviously something is happening," Rod said, "but not really a lot, at this point. Now let's test the fluid with nitrazine. It's a simple test, sort of like the litmus tests you did back in high school chemistry. It's a little slip of paper with a chemical indicator that detects pH. If there's any amniotic fluid in the vagina, the slip will turn blue."

Rod studied the moistened slip. "Nothing much to see there. Okay, you've probably got a while yet, maybe about twenty-four hours. I tell you what. Why don't you go home and get some rest? Both of you. This may be your last chance."

Looking at Susan and Tracy, Rod saw the expression he had seen on the faces of so many young couples in this situation—part disappointment, part relief. "In a couple of days," he said to Susan, "you'll be eating French fries and milkshakes." Then he turned to Tracy: "And you'll be changing diapers."

Half an hour after the MacGregors had gone, Jack phoned in from home to see how things were going, and Rod updated him. They confirmed the plan for the rest of the day. Rod had to be in the operating room at one-thirty. Jack would be at the office for afternoon and evening hours. "You'll be the next to talk to the MacGregors," Rod told Jack.

"Wouldn't it be nice if she didn't have to be induced?" Jack said. Induction with Pitocin might be called for if she failed to go into labor by forty-one and a half or forty-two weeks. There was another possibility—that Susan's labor might begin but be erratic and diffuse, failing to produce the good, strong contractions that would move the baby down through the birth canal at a steady rate. The kind of experience that Susan had been having all day, with confused and disorganized cramps, brought this possibility to Jack's mind. The condition is called dysfunctional labor, and the treatment is augmentation. It also involves use of Pitocin, a bit of which can regularize and focus the contractions and make them effective.

The doctors' preference is for nature to start things rolling, requiring them merely to jump aboard and guide them. But if nature is delinquent, they have means at their disposal.

·   ·   ·

The MacGregors drove back to the Spragues and gave them the news: false alarm. The Spragues, so eager to be grandparents, were disappointed; they'd been sure labor was starting and that the next time they heard anything it would come from the hospital. But they tried not to let on. When the MacGregors got home, Susan said, "No point bringing the bag in the house. Let's leave it in the car."

Time on their hands. Susan went into the yard and puttered in the rock garden. It was very hot, over ninety. Some of her new plants looked thirsty, so she watered them, keeping the water off the foliage so it wouldn't cook in the sun. Then she came in for a nap. Tracy paid bills.

When Susan awoke, at about four, she was having what felt to her like genuine contractions. Tracy came up and they timed them. The frequency was about eight minutes.

"Should we call?" Tracy asked Susan. "To keep them up to date?"

"Dr. O'Driscoll told us to," she said. "Go ahead and call."

Tracy phoned Barbara, "just to touch base," he said. Barbara said she'd tell Jack and was sure he'd phone back soon.

"What can we do to step things up?" he asked her. Barbara smiled, recognizing the impatience of the father-to-be. "Well, now," she said, "I can't tell you to do twenty jumping-jacks and then her contractions will be four minutes apart."

Tracy laughed. "I was thinking, maybe a walk."

"Ordinarily I'd say yes. One of the advantages of living near the hospital and not having to go there until things are pretty far along is that you get to stay active, but not on a day this hot. Do whatever feels right to her, but I think a walk in this heat might exhaust her. I'd say, just stay indoors with the air conditioner. Save the strength."

"We don't have air conditioning," Tracy said, "but we're okay." The heat was a problem, though. It was tiring both of them. "This thing isn't going to go on much longer, is it?"

"You're just anxious," Barbara said. "You've got nothing to do but wait, so you're anxious. You've just got to relax."

Barbara spoke with Susan. "I'm afraid I'm getting wiped out," Susan said. "I mean, I've been having contractions for fifteen hours now. Ever since two this morning."

"Well, do whatever makes you comfortable," Barbara said, "and I'm sure Dr. Bonamo will be calling you back soon."

Twenty minutes later, before Jack was able to return the call, Tracy called the office again, a touch of excitement in his voice. "Some of the contractions are three to four minutes apart," he told Jack.

"But they're not all that way?" Jack asked.

"No, the others are mainly eight minutes."

Jack talked to Susan. "You're coming along," he said, "but it's still sporadic. In terms of progress, it doesn't mean a great deal until a pattern is established; a woman can have contractions three minutes apart for twenty minutes or so but then go back to a stretched-out pattern. But you live so close—why don't you come over and we'll take a look and see what's happening?"

After he hung up the phone, Jack said to Barbara. "She's just kind of nowhere. Just holding. The problem is the weather. And fatigue. And being anxious. She's counting her labor from two o'clock in the morning, and I think that's making her anxious."

The MacGregors arrived and sat in the waiting room, on the couch by the window. To Barbara, observing them through the glass-doored speak-through, Susan seemed dazed. She was wearing a little lipstick, which made her seem all the paler. Tracy was fidgeting and she was patting his knee. Looking at Susan with an experienced eye, Barbara guessed that real labor was some time off. It wasn't hard yet. It wasn't heavy.

Back in the examining room the bright green lines on the fetal monitor soon made Susan's plight graphic: her contractions were erratic and inconsistent—seven minutes, four minutes, eight minutes. Jack inspected her cervix and found that it had not dilated at all. Her water had not yet broken.

"I want you to try and forget the whole thing of whether or not you're in labor," Jack told Susan. "Not easy, but give it a try. It would be wonderful if you could stop concentrating on it, because this business of waiting by the door can drive you crazy. You've got to get your mind off it. Go out to a restaurant. Watch a movie or something on TV. Try and get some sleep."

In the car going home, Susan was so disheartened she could barely speak. She was tired of waiting, tired of nothing going on. It seemed like forever.

As soon as Susan was in the house she started feeling different. The contractions were about seven minutes apart now, like clockwork, and they were more uncomfortable. They felt like menstrual cramps multiplied by fifty—strong, comprehensive tightenings, as if her body were in the grip of a giant hand, except that the force was from within. It was real pain but not sharp, shooting pain; more like extreme, overpowering pressure. On the way home from the doctors' they'd rented a videotape, but she couldn't watch the movie. She couldn't eat anything. At nine o'clock she went to bed.

It began to rain, rain beating down hard on the slanted roof just above her head, and there was some lightning. She couldn't sleep. The pain in her back, which the doctor said was caused by the baby's head pressing against her spine, was awful.

At a quarter past eleven she called to Tracy and they timed the contractions. The first pair were three minutes and thirty seconds apart, and all the others were almost exactly three.

"That's it," Tracy said.

"Call the doctor," Susan replied.

Tracy phoned the doctors' answering service, gave his message, and hung up. Neither of them said anything. Within two or three minutes the phone rang, and Tracy grabbed it.

It was Dr. O'Driscoll. "How're we doing?" he asked, his voice as fresh as if it were midday.

"Three minutes apart," Tracy said.

"How long are they lasting?"

"A minute and a half."

"Okay, this sounds like it. Let's go for it."

"The hospital?"

"Absolutely. But take your time. There's no hurry."

"We'll meet you there?"

"Absolutely, when things get a little further along. Just go on over. Go to Admissions and they'll take it from there. I'll be getting reports from the people in Labor and Delivery, and when they've got some idea of how you're dilating, they'll put out the word and either Dr. Bonamo or I will be there, depending on who's on call at the time. You'll be taken good care of."

While Tracy was on the phone, Susan dressed. She chose a white cotton pullover and her dark blue-green Laura Ashley jumper. In a way she felt she should be dressier for this important occasion, but what was the point? Whatever she wore she'd soon be taking it off.

They went downstairs, and when they reached the door Susan turned and looked back at the living room. It occurred to her that this was one of life's watersheds, and that when she saw that room again, everything would be different. She'd no longer be living the extension of her honeymoon, just the two of them encapsulated in the privacy of this house. She'd be a mother, and there would be a third person, and life would be lovely and satisfying in a whole new way.

An impressive contraction caught Susan just as she climbed into the car, and she had to sit there—her legs still out the door and her feet on the driveway—taking deep breaths, until it passed through. Tracy drove north on Wyoming Avenue, past handsome houses whose fading white azaleas were just visible in the headlights. Then west on South Orange Avenue, a four-lane road that went up a low mountain and down the other side, winding in esses down through the wooded preserve. In ten minutes and two more contractions they had reached Old Short Hills Road, and a few seconds later they were turning into the vast, illuminated parking lot of the former St. Barnabas Hospital, now St. Barnabas Medical Center. As Tracy stopped at the entrance to the lot to pick up his ticket, he realized that the ticket, stamped with the time, would clock the coming ordeal. It was just a few minutes after midnight—Wednesday, June twelfth.

The automatic doors of the brand-new east wing swept open, and Susan and Tracy entered the sleekly designed reception lobby. Even at this hour there were people in the corridors—doctors in white cotton coats and with stethoscopes dangling from their necks, nurses in pink or green sanitary coveralls.

"Now you just sit here for one minute," the woman at the information desk said, not needing to ask them why they were there, "and I'll phone for a wheelchair."

"I don't think I'll need a wheelchair," Susan said. "I can walk."

"I know, dear," said the woman, "but it's the rule. Everyone gets a wheelchair." Patients in guided wheelchairs didn't get lost and wander into brain surgery.

The wheelchair came after only a few minutes, but to the MacGregors it seemed like a very long time. The chair was propelled by a woman in a starched pink coat—a "transporter"—who wheeled Susan down an endless white hall. Tracy followed. He had to walk behind the chair, since traffic in the hall prevented him from walking beside it, and because of that he felt somewhat out of touch with his wife—that he'd given her over to strangers.

In the admissions office there were no other incoming patients.

Susan had preregistered weeks earlier, one night after a childbirth class, as the instructor had suggested, so the admissions procedure now was a simple affair. Just two papers to sign. Another contraction, a real teeth-gritter.

The transporter pushed the wheelchair into the elevator, which was very large, big enough for two stretchers on wheels. Susan, her chair placed in the center of the car, felt small.

The elevator doors opened at the third floor in the hospital's old wing. On the wall was a sign saying Labor and Delivery. From a bin the transporter pulled a yellow cotton gown and asked Tracy to put it on. They resumed their trip down the corridor, stopping at a pair of closed swinging doors. The transporter tapped a square metal plate on the wall, a switch that made the automatic doors fly open. Susan's heart quickened. This was Labor and Delivery.

The reality was not what Susan had envisioned. She'd expected a scene of frantic action, a chorus of screams from women in labor. But all was still. The opened doors revealed a large foyer with gleaming green linoleum and a white, U-shaped formica desk at the center: the command post called the nurses' station. Six video monitors were mounted near the ceiling, and the screen of each was divided into two separate displays. In the course of the past year the bright green electronic lines on those twelve displays had traced the heartbeats of five thousand new babies and the contractions of their mothers, but now they were all flat and motionless. So far tonight there were no babies, no expectant mothers at all in Labor and Delivery.

A half dozen nurses and attendants were sitting around the nurses' station chatting quietly. Several looked up as the wheelchair rolled in, and one popped to her feet and came over.

"MacGregor?" she said warmly.

"Yes," Tracy said.

The nurse took the admissions papers. "Susan MacGregor," she read. "Dr. O'Driscoll's and Dr. Bonamo's patient."

"Yes," Susan said. She indicated Tracy. "This is my husband."

The nurse smiled; she'd already figured that one out. She was in her thirties, with curly blond hair and a gentle manner, pretty. "My name is Tracey," she said, helping Susan out of the wheelchair.

Susan and Tracy laughed and explained that Tracy's name was Tracy too, and nurse Tracey said hers was spelled with an E.

"This could get confusing," Tracy said.

"You're the only mom up here at the moment," said the nurse, whose last name was Kitchin. "So we're going to put you in Room 6, because it's right here next to the nurses' station. Make yourself comfortable, and put on this hospital gown, and get into bed. As soon as you're ready, I'll hook you up to the fetal monitor, so we can have a continuous picture of how the baby is doing. Then the resident will come in and check you out and see how you're coming along."

Room 6 was one of nine birthing rooms. They all contained birthing beds, the main reason patients could stay in the same room all the way through, from the moment they arrived until, as triumphant new mothers, they were wheeled off to Recovery. Rather like a conventional bed in appearance but higher off the floor, the birthing bed was patient-friendly. Various parts of it could be raised or lowered to improve the patient's comfort. In ways not obvious to the lay person, however, the bed was crafted to the needs of the doctors and nurses. At delivery time, for example, the nurse could instantly remove the bottom third of the bed, including the footboard and the end of the mattress, to allow the doctors close access to the birth site. All around, it was a marvel of parturitional mechanics. Each bed cost $15,000, more than some automobiles.

Not when she first arrived but later, during the waiting, Susan noticed and appreciated Room 6. It had lavender wallpaper covered with small white fleurs-de-lis arranged diagonally. There was no separate bathroom—nurses didn't want mothers to be able to lock doors that might prevent the nurses from quickly coming to help, or to get out of their sight for long; instead there was a curtained-off toilet, and that curtain, like the curtains on the windows, was done in a pattern of thin vertical stripes of alternating lavender and peach. The floor was a gray linoleum flecked with blue. Between the window and the bed was a large reclining chair, for an exhausted husband to sprawl on.

On the wall opposite Susan's bed was a broken electric clock whose hands were stopped at five of five—a fitting symbol for the eternal waiting that most labors involved. Beneath it was a picture that seemed appropriate too. It was a pleasant watercolor of a large white goose waddling left to right with eight goslings padding along behind her. Geese were among nature's champion maternal bonders; baby geese fastened on whomever they first glimpsed as they broke from their shells. If what they glimpsed happened to be a human being, they'd follow that person everywhere. Here, in this room where so many human hatchlings first saw their mothers, the geese were an apt symbol.

Susan undressed and put on her gown and got in bed. In a few minutes Tracey Kitchin came in. "Now let's put on the monitor belts," she said, delicately turning back the covers. "This band goes around you here, on top of your belly. . . . There. Good. And now this band goes at the bottom of the belly. . . . That's perfect."

She looked over at the monitor on a stand by the bed. It wasn't video; it was a machine that sent an endless strip of graph paper scrolling along horizontally. As the strip travelled, two slender metal arms, driven by electronic signals from sensors on the bands, flicked up and down, inking erratic but continuous traces. The machine had come to life. The top line, which recorded the baby's heartbeat by ultrasound, jittered along in a tight, healthily irregular pattern, and the bottom line, which displayed the contractions like occasional mountains on a plain, undulated slowly. "That's good," Tracey Kitchin said. "It's a good display." She turned a knob and a rapid, rhythmic thumping filled the room, the by-now-familiar syncopation of the baby's heartbeat. "If you decide you want some quiet, you can turn it down with this knob."

She took Susan's temperature and blood pressure and pulse. "Okay," she said. "The next thing is, you'll have your first examination and we'll see if there's been some dilation. I'll call Doreen."

A minute went by and then a young woman in green scrubs, with a floppy green scrub cap over her hair, came into the room. She was very small, barely five feet tall. Her scrubs were too big for her; she was drowning in them, as if she were wearing men's pajamas. The pants were so long they covered her shoes, and she had to shuffle when she walked. She was attractive in a pixieish way. Dark blond hair sprouted from under her cap. Her ginger eyebrows were peaked and her cheekbones were high, which gave her face a permanently mischievous expression. She looked like a high school cheerleader, the little one they put at the top of the pyramid, except for one thing: she was pregnant.

"Hi," she said in a soft young voice. "I'm Doreen DeGraaff, the chief resident."

21.
Fingertip

The MacGregors shared with most parents-to-be a special dread: that when the crucial moment arrived and the baby was coming, their own doctor would get caught in traffic or break his leg on his front walk going out to his car, and their baby would have to be delivered by a doctor they'd never met. In their view there could be only one thing worse: that there wouldn't be any doctor available at all, only "some resident."

Few patients knew what residents were or what they did. It was generally assumed they were some kind of unqualified, inexperienced medical student who was hungry for patients to practice on. Like all residents Doreen DeGraaff was very accustomed to walking into a patient's room and announcing herself only to see that desperate look on the patient's face, the look that shrieked, "I want my doctor!"

Doreen was twenty-nine, the same age as her patient in Room 6. Her youth, however, and her misleading appearance—her severest professional problem was finding scrubs that were small enough for her, and tonight she hadn't come even close—belied her status. Among the staff of Labor and Delivery, a chief resident was a figure to be reckoned with.

She had been born in Secaucus, which was notorious across the river in Manhattan, where comedians made jokes about its stinking pig farms and slaughterhouses. In Secaucus, people had no illusions; life was real and life was earnest. She was the first member of her family to go to college. In her junior year her roommate, whose father was a doctor, said, "Doreen, why don't you apply to medical school?" It was one of those offhand remarks that change lives.

During med school she spent some time in obstetrics, and she fell in love with it. For the most part OBs dealt with healthy patients who came in and had their babies and went home smiling. It was a happy specialty. Even gynecology seldom involved insurmountable medical problems.

At the end of medical school, Doreen's training would be only half over. Lying ahead would be residency, an intense, four-year professional honing for new doctors during which the classroom learning of med school would be grounded in extensive practical experience. And where she did her residency, Doreen knew—a good teaching hospital or a mediocre one—would have a great influence upon her entire career. She wanted St. Barnabas, the best teaching hospital in the state. St. Barnabas received five hundred applications for five places. Doreen got one of them.

OB residency takes a year longer than do some specialties—internal medicine and pediatrics, among others. The first year is the internship, and for Doreen, looking back upon it, it was a blur. The five interns—Doreen was the only woman—had the job of looking after all the normal labor patients in Labor and Delivery: some 3,500 women. They admitted them all and examined them all, started their IVs, delivered most of them under the supervision of the patients' doctors, and followed them through Postpartum. For weeks at a time the interns would work thirty-six-hour shifts: thirty-six hours on, twelve off, thirty-six on, twelve off, and so on and on. It was particularly hard on the three married interns, who seldom saw their families—Doreen had married her high school sweetheart and, during med school, had had a son—but when the year finally ended, all three were somehow still married, and another was engaged.

People sometimes disparage the residency system as a form of hazing. What possible good, they ask, can come of subjecting young doctors to that degree of fatigue and stress? Jack Bonamo's answer: "Obstetrics is an unusual business in that you're called upon to make life-and-death decisions when you've been awakened in the middle of the night and you're totally exhausted—when somebody might say a few words to you that signal a life-threatening emergency for a woman or her child. The only way you learn to act and react under that kind of strain is by having done it."

If anything, the second year was worse, but in the third year

Doreen and her fellow residents got a chance to act for the first time as full-fledged doctors. For eleven weeks each worked in another hospital in the area, usually a big public hospital. Doreen was sent to Elizabeth General Hospital, where she was in effect *the* doctor for what was called the "service population," meaning the impoverished patients who weren't paying their own bills and therefore had to accept whichever doctor walked through the door. For almost three months she saw the clinic patients, did vaginal deliveries, and performed cesareans and other surgery. Doctors from the hospital were on hand, but basically she was on her own. When her stint at Elizabeth General was over, she returned to St. Barnabas with a new level of skill, capable of making independent decisions.

She found it difficult to blame patients who were leery of having residents fiddling with their vitals. She herself used to feel the same way: she hadn't wanted residents practicing on her. ("I would never advise any one," said Henry Bracken, an eighteenth-century English obstetrician, "to employ a *young* physician.") But now she knew that view was simplistic. For one thing, residents in a good teaching institution are carefully and elaborately supervised until it is clear they are able to function well alone. For another, unlike the attending physicians, who may have become a little rusty, their procedures perhaps a bit antiquated, the residents have recently been instructed in the latest procedures and saturated with the most up-to-date medical information.

It is said that the presence of a resident is an important deterrent to laxness and malpractice; the doctors know that the residents know. If the resident objects to what the doctor is preparing to do, the attending thinks twice about doing it. One resident was overheard saying to an attending over the phone, "Well, if you want it done, then you come in and do it yourself, because I disagree with it, and I'm not doing it."

Doreen had seen many times that when there was a real emergency, one that couldn't be delayed to allow the attending to get there, the residents were a godsend; between the four residents on duty, they could handle almost anything. Without residents, patients would have received a lot less doctor attention.

The year before, when she was a third-year resident working late one night on the high-risk obstetrical floor, she sensed that a patient was having trouble. She put her on the fetal monitor, and there was nothing wrong—not really wrong, just subtle things about the fetal monitor tracing she found disturbing. She was afraid they might be signalling that the patient was having an abruption—that the placenta was tearing away from the wall of the uterus, in which case the baby would quickly die.

The nurse looked at the monitor strip and failed to see anything alarming. It was a difficult spot for Doreen. A third-year resident doesn't casually override an experienced nurse, one she works with all the time. Doreen thought about calling the chief resident. That was daunting. What if she was wrong? But she couldn't just let things go; she couldn't risk the baby. She placed the call. The chief resident said that he'd be right up and that in the meantime Doreen, since she was the one who had seen the tracings, should phone the attending at home. That was the most daunting step of all.

She gave the groggy OB her report. "If you're worried," he replied, "set up a cesarean. I'm on my way."

"A cesarean?" Doreen asked. It was scary. On her say-so, just because she didn't have a good feeling about a tracing, a baby that really needed another two months inside its mother was going to be born prematurely.

"That's right," the doctor said. "If you're this worried, we're doing a cesarean." Her reputation was on the line. It turned out, though, that she was right. There *had* been an abruption. Half the placenta had already come loose. A longer wait and the result would have been tragic. A resident had saved a life.

Now Doreen was just entering her fourth year of residency. It was a whole new world. All fourth-year residents are called chief resident—chief of the other three residents on their shift—and they have substantial clout and numerous perks. For one thing, at St. Barnabas they had The Palace, which is what they called their luxurious chief resident's suite, with an attractive bedroom known as the on-call room. The bed came in handy because Doreen was seventeen weeks pregnant and needed a place to rest once in a while, on those marathon shifts that the chiefs had to work.

As chief resident for this night shift, Doreen had started work at six o'clock yesterday morning and would be on call until four this afternoon—a total of thirty-four hours. An hour ago she had done a hysterectomy, and before returning to the chief resident's suite she had dropped by Labor and Delivery just to see how things were going. Things were quiet and the intern was grabbing some sleep, and when Susan arrived Doreen had told the nurses to let the intern sleep awhile; she'd take care of Susan. Chief residents, who for two years have been doing mainly high-risk obstetrics, often volunteer for deliveries and other routine procedures as a refresher for their upcoming first year in practice.

"I'm going to examine you, to see how you're coming," Doreen said to Susan, "and then I'll phone Dr. O'Driscoll and give him a report." Rod was on duty that night.

"You're a fingertip," Doreen said when she was done. "Your cervix is dilated the width of a fingertip. That's actually not very much, but it's a start. The cervix hasn't effaced at all; it hasn't started to thin out. That's because the baby really hasn't moved down into the pelvis yet. I think we've got at least twelve hours to go."

"Twelve hours," Tracy said. "It seems as if it's been forever already."

Doreen smiled sympathetically. "It won't be so bad," she said. "This is how it goes with a first baby. If you like," she said to Susan, "you can get up and walk around."

"I'd like to," Susan said. She gestured at the fetal monitor. "But aren't I connected to this machine?"

"Whenever you're ready," Doreen said, "the nurse will disconnect you."

Doreen went out to the nurse's station and dialed Rod O'Driscoll's number. "Hi, Dr. O," she said. "It's Doreen. How are you? . . . Susan MacGregor's here. She's contracting about every four or five minutes, and she's only a fingertip, thick, and high. The FH looks fine. . . . Okay, we'll let you know if we need you. . . . Alrighty. . . . Bye, bye."

She put down the phone and turned to Tracey Kitchin. "We'll let her do her thing," she said, "and if she gets really uncomfortable, we'll check to see if she wants her epidural." *Her* epidural, Doreen had said, as if it were not just a medical procedure for Susan but an entitlement, an obvious need, an inevitability—like *her* dinner.

Across the nurse's area was a white plastic bulletin board, about four feet by five, mounted to the wall. Called "the board," it gave the status of every patient on the floor. "MacGregor" had been written in black marker, followed by "O'D/Bon" for O'Driscoll/Bonamo and "40+" for the number of weeks of pregnancy. A zero was entered to record the number of children Susan had had. The column for nurse was marked "Tracey." Doreen wrote the time of her examination, 1:00 A.M. In the column for thickness of the cervix, she wrote "closed"; the cervix had not yet thinned at all. For dilation she wrote "FT" for fingertip. Under the column recording whether or not Susan's amniotic sac had ruptured, she wrote "I," meaning that the membranes were still intact. She drew a small black arrow pointed up, which meant the baby was still high in the birth canal. There was a space to list medications the patient had received, and Doreen left that blank; if Susan received an epidural, it would be entered there.

On a little board next to the big board, Doreen wrote "5874," the extension number of her room in the chief resident's suite. "Call me, whatever," she told Tracey Kitchin, "if you need anything done or if it gets busy." Then, the bottoms of her scrubs covering her shoes, she scuffed off down the hall.

In Room 6, the mood was dejection. Tracy sat on the edge of the bed near Susan, reaching over her to brush her thick brown hair from her white forehead.

"How can the baby not be doing anything?" Susan said, exasperated.

"Well," said Tracy encouragingly, "you're dilated a little. You're 'fingertip.' "

"Yes, but which finger?" She held up her little finger.

"Maybe it's the thumb."

Susan sighed. "It's so discouraging. Hardly any real sleep for twenty-six hours already, and it looks like another twelve." A contraction started, and she began taking deep breaths and exhaling them.

On the Room 6 monitor at the nurses' station a jagged green line traced the contraction, and Tracey Kitchin reflexively kept glancing at it as she sat chatting with the other nurses. They talked mainly about the job—problems they had with this or that, what you did for what. The staff wasn't used to this much inactivity. It was the quietest night any of them could remember.

Tracy came out of Room 6 and spoke to Tracey Kitchin. "She'd like to take a walk," he said. "Could you come unhook her?"

Tracey Kitchin came in. "I think a walk is a great idea," she said. "This floor is like a big circle. You can go see the babies in the nursery. You can go visit the new postpartum wing." She removed the monitor belts. Arm in arm Susan and Tracy slowly went off down the hall, through the swinging doors they'd entered by. They stopped at the big plate glass window of the nursery, fascinated by the rows of new babies in their plastic, chrome-legged bassinets. There were about twenty of them, all swaddled identically, all lying on their left side, propped there with a folded cloth under their back. The tops of the fuzzy little heads poked out of the swaddles. They looked like trays of cocktail sausages en croute. The premature nursery was a shock: tiny, bluish gray babies with transparent plastic tubes dangling down and taped to their limbs or inserted in their mouths and noses. The jaundiced babies under ultraviolet phototherapy lamps looked purple.

"Well, that's one thing," Tracy said. "We're not going to be premature."

As they returned to Labor and Delivery, Susan's belly grew taut with pain, and her hands went down to cradle the heavy dome. The intern, a tanned, serious young woman with dark hair, was nearest to her and noticed.

"Contraction?" she said, taking Susan lightly by the elbow.

"Yes," Susan said between clenched teeth.

"Are they getting stronger?"

"Yes."

"They're stronger," Tracy said, "but she's weaker."

Tracey Kitchin assisted Susan toward her room and into bed. After the contraction was over, the nurse asked, "Are you comfortable now?"

"When I'm lying on my back," Susan said, "I feel like a fish out of water. My stomach feels like a big weight that could flop me one way or the other."

"Here, let me raise your bed." The nurse pressed a button, an electric motor hummed, and the head and foot of the bed rose slightly, supporting Susan in a shallow V. "There, that's better."

She pulled Susan's covers back and examined her large, hard belly, listening with her stethoscope at several places. Then she smiled at Susan and said, "The heartbeat sounds fine. Want to hear?" She turned the knob on the fetal monitor, and the headlong throb of the baby's heartbeat filled the room.

"It sounds faster than last time," Tracy said.

"It *is* faster than last time," Susan replied. After a minute she tightened and looked at the ceiling and said, "Contraction coming . . ."

"Back pain too?" Tracey Kitchin asked.

"Yes . . ." Susan began to take deep breaths. When the contraction was over her forehead was wet. "I've had back pains before, but I haven't felt anything quite like this."

"The baby's coming down," Tracey Kitchin said, "and at this particular time, as he's coming down he's looking up, and the back of his head is against your spine. What you need is some sleep. Why don't we give you something to help you?"

"Some kind of pill?" Susan asked.

Tracey Kitchin shook her head. "Not a pill. The pill we give is Seconal, but we don't give it to people in pain; it just makes it worse. No, what we'd give you is morphine. It works in two ways. It makes you relax, but it also takes away the pain. You'd be able to get some rest. You've got a big day ahead of you."

Susan turned to her husband. "What do you think?"

"Will it hurt the baby?" he asked the nurse.

"No. We never give it to someone who is within two hours of giving birth, because it really does affect the baby's respiration. We never give it to someone who's past three centimeters. But you're still in very early labor. And if you could get a couple of hours sleep, it would do you a lot of good. We call it 'therapeutic rest.' You shouldn't go into delivery absolutely exhausted."

Susan thought for a few moments. "Well, I'd like to get some sleep tonight . . . just because I'd like to put my energies into labor instead of staying awake."

Tracy nodded. "It's been such an awfully long time since she's had any rest."

"Well, think about it," Tracey Kitchin said. "If you want morphine, I'll speak to the resident and she'll call Doreen and check it with her." Nurses always called the residents, both male and female, by their first names.

"If you stay awake the rest of the night," Tracy said to Susan, "you'll really be bushed by the time the baby comes."

"Why don't I speak to Doreen about the morphine?" Tracey Kitchen suggested. She left the room and soon returned with the intern, Gail Loewenbach. "Do you want to go for the morphine?" she asked Susan. Calling the chief resident in the middle of the night was not something an intern did matter-of-factly, and before she did she wanted to make sure the patient completely understood and that she hadn't changed her mind.

"No effect on the baby?" Tracy asked again.

"No, there's no effect on the baby, as long as the baby isn't born within two to three hours. What the morphine will do is relax you. It will let you rest. It would be different if the contractions were less than every four to five minutes. If they were every two minutes and very strong, that would be something else. But now the contractions aren't giving you rest, but on the other hand, they're not changing the cervix that much either."

Susan shut her eyes. "Okay," she said almost inaudibly. Five minutes later, Tracey Kitchin returned carrying a syringe.

"Can my husband sleep here too?" Susan asked.

"Of course. That chair over there is a recliner. It goes right back. I'll get you both some blankets."

"Before I sack out," Tracy said, "I'd better call my office and tell Joyce to cancel my meetings. I'll put a message on her machine." When he came back he saw that Neil Russo, the second-year resident, a tall, husky young man with dark curly hair, was wrapping himself with a blanket. "It's cold," Russo said to Tracy.

"It *is* cold," Tracy said, noticing it for the first time. "Why is it so cold?"

"This place is kept that way on purpose," Russo said. "It's for the sake of the patients in labor. They have to work so hard, and if the temperature were normal they might pass out from the heat of their exertion. But it sure does make it cold for the rest of us."

•   •   •

It was three in morning. In the staff lounge, leftover pizza had congealed in its box. At the nurses' station, Tracey Kitchin and five other staff members, all of them blanketed, huddled in a circle like Indians around a dead campfire. And in Room 6—six years after the Lynchburg mating dance, nearly three years from the vows in the little church, and nine months from the early movie and early-to-bed and the sperm Olympics that had sent a champion to claim the golden egg—a fully realized fetus was moving toward the implicit goal of it all, free being.

22.
Bonnie

At a quarter past four, a patient was put in Room 5, wall to wall with the MacGregors. She was a small woman with a bearded husband who stood about six foot six, and the board said she was dilated seven centimeters—almost three inches. Her cervix was 90 percent effaced. It was her second baby, and she was moving right along.

Two hours later, just after six, Tracey Kitchin woke the MacGregors. "You slept pretty well," she said to Susan with satisfaction. "I was watching on the monitor. You slept right through your contractions."

"Yes," Susan said, "I guess I did."

"I didn't sleep at all," said Tracy. He looked it. His face was colorless.

"How are you feeling?" the nurse asked Susan.

"I can really feel the baby's head has moved," Susan said. "It's farther down. Less pressure on the back. Definitely more manageable."

"When you dilate more,"the nurse said, "we'll be able to tell which way the baby's looking." It was possible to feel the pattern of the bones in the baby's skull through the unbroken amniotic sac. These patterns would provide a sort of map of how the head was aligned.

She took Susan's temperature. "It's time to check your progress again. Doreen is coming up to do the examination."

Doreen arrived on the floor, studied the board for late information, and went into Room 6. While she examined Susan, loud cries came through the wall from Room 5, part moan and part shriek.

"We have neighbors," Tracy said, startled.

The cries grew louder. "Good grief!" Susan said. "What's happening to her?"

"She's fine," Doreen said. "She's just having a baby."

Susan and Tracy looked at each other, mouths agape.

The doctors and nurses had their own theories about who screamed and who didn't. First-generation Haitian, Filipino, and Greek women tended to scream, they agreed, and Poles and Portuguese and Ukrainians from the Ironbound section of Newark—women who had old-school husbands who didn't want to take part in the birth and didn't want their wives doing Lamaze. Far from joining in, these husbands sat outside and smoked and waited and left their wives alone, sometimes sending a female family member in to see how things were going. Having a baby was women's work.

But another folkway was involved, Jack Bonamo believed. Especially among Hispanics and Italians, the wife screamed partly to show the husband how much pain she was enduring to have his baby. The German and Chinese women, on the other hand, could be in incredible pain yet never make a sound.

Some women said amazing things while in labor. One patient, as Jack tried to ease her back pain by putting pillows under her knees, yelled, "I f****** hate you!" The nurse, to whom Dr. Bonamo was a respected figure, gasped. Later Jack told his wife that afterward, when he visited the patient in the recovery room, civility had returned. "You never would have known she'd ever done that," he said. "Butter would have melted in her mouth."

These days, nearly all fathers chose to be with their wives. Some hung back at first, but then, near the end, as delivery approached, they'd change their minds and ask to come in. Jewish fathers, the theory went, were the most attentive, but Italian fathers were the most enthusiastic, the most emotionally involved. Once in a while, when wives began to scream, husbands would panic and command the doctor to "Do something!" Someone would have to take them out in the hall and soothe and explain.

"You've made progress," Doreen said to Susan when she'd completed her exam, "While you slept, you dilated some more. The morphine was a good idea. You're two centimeters now."

"How big is that?" Susan asked. "A half dollar?"

Doreen smiled. "A nickel," she said, "but getting bigger all the time. And your cervix is 70 percent effaced. The baby's head has come down a bit too."

"How about that!" Tracy exclaimed.

"You'll probably do some more dilating before too long," Doreen went on. "Especially for your first baby, you need to efface before you'll finish dilating."

On the wall in the nurses' area was a molded white plastic display that showed what dilation and effacement really looked like. Tracy had studied it earlier. There was a row of life-size representations of the cervix, arranged progressively from zero to ten centimeters. Ten centimeters of dilation—the target amount, the calibration that the whole process was working toward—wasn't much larger than an orange. It seemed impossible to Tracy that a baby's head could squeeze through that passage.

There was also a series of cross-section views of the cervix at each stage, to give a visual idea of effacement. An uneffaced cervix was about an inch thick. A completely effaced cervix was paper-thin. In just hours, a cervix had to undergo drastic stretching.

Doreen did a nitrazine test and determined that Susan's water hadn't broken. She replaced the bedcovers. "It looks like this afternoon, and since we can't let you eat, and we're afraid you'll get weak and dehydrated, it's time for the IV. You'll feel much better, and you won't get as tired. You can suck on hard candy and ice chips. That'll be about it."

Susan picked up on Doreen's steady use of the pronoun "we," as in "we're going to give you an IV." Had Doreen become her obstetrician? "When will I see Dr. Bonamo?" she asked.

"Dr. O'Driscoll has been on call tonight," Doreen said, "and I've been phoning him and filling him in. There's no point in him being here now; there's nothing for him to do. But he's coming in this morning, and you'll see him then. He's an early bird, so it will probably be soon. Dr. Bonamo will be here later this morning. Don't worry. When things start moving, he'll be here."

Doreen left, and Tracy, as was becoming his custom, went out in the hall to grill anybody he saw about what lay ahead for Susan. The area had become suddenly busy. The board showed that a third patient had come in. A nurse's aide rolled an isolette, a wheeled bassinet, toward Room 5.

Doreen was at the nurse's station, writing a report. "So how's it going?" Tracy asked her, seeking double confirmation.

"The baby's engaged in the pelvis. It's at the top, but it's where it needs to be. The big question is the contractions. Her contractions will pick up again as the morphine wears off. What needs to happen is for her contractions to get into a decent pattern. They're still where they were when she came in—four to five minutes apart. They'll have to grow longer and stronger to push that baby down and out. But the contractions she's having now at two centimeters aren't any stronger than the ones she was having last night."

"How long do you think it'll be?" Tracy asked.

"Well, you can figure it this way. There aren't any rules in labor, but it's generally true that once a patient gets to four centimeters, the dilation proceeds at one centimeter an hour. So once she gets to four, it'll be about six hours after that." She turned back to her report.

Fresh screams burst from Room 5.

"Wow!" Tracy said.

Gail Loewenbach, though she was only in her first year of residency, was already used to the cries of the battlefield, and she couldn't help but be amused at Tracy's shock. As he hurried back to be with Susan, the screams ebbed.

Tracey Kitchin brought in the IV equipment. Quickly and painlessly she found a vein in Susan's arm and inserted the plastic-sheathed needle. She removed the needle itself, leaving the sheath, to which she attached a socket. Through that socket she took blood samples. In a moment, four color-coded vials of Susan's dark red blood lay side by side on the tray. She hung a large bag of clear IV solution from a steel rack suspended from the ceiling, then connected the IV tube to the socket in Susan's arm. "There," she said. "Perfect."

The patient in Room 5 began to scream in earnest, and at intervals there was another woman's voice, shouting "PUSH! . . . PUSH! . . . PUSH!"

" That's Nancy," Tracey Kitchin said. "When Nancy's the nurse, you can always tell: it sounds as if Nancy herself is having the baby. Dr. Bonamo says Nancy could get a woman to push out the Empire State Building." Nancy's credentials were good: the mother of five, she once had a twelve-pound baby.

Through the wall came, "PUSH! . . . PUSH! . . . PUSH! BEAR DOWN! PUSH DOWN ON YOUR RECTUM! PUSH!"

"Once," Tracey Kitchin continued, "another nurse said to her, 'Nancy, you've got to stop. We're all beginning to have rectal pressure.' "

Several voices, one of them male, cried out at the same time, "DON'T PUSH!" Minutes went by, then a chorus of jubilation.

Susan and Tracy braced for more, but no more sounds came through the wall. That, evidently, was that.

"Whew!" said Tracy, exhaling, as if he'd just given birth.

Ten minutes later a little procession emerged from Room 5: first a nurse wheeling a bassinet that held a ball of blankets with the top of a tiny head just visible, then the gigantic father, looking joyful.

•   •   •

At six forty-five, the shifts began to change. Sister Regis, the head nurse, arrived and started sizing things up. In the nurses' lounge, night nurses Tracey, Evelyn, Yvetale, and Nancy briefed day nurses Flo, Gloria, Karen, and Bonnie. Eight residents sat on and around a desk outside the recovery room discussing every patient, one by one, talking about their progress during the night, reviewing their signs and what had been done for them. When the last patient had been covered, they all stood and moved off, some to work, some to bed.

Tracey Kitchin went into Room 6. "Hi," she said. "Are you feeling some energy from the IV yet?"

"I think so."

"How's the baby? Does the baby feel it too?"

"I think the baby's asleep."

"Well, we'll wake him up when we're at ten centimeters."

Susan stiffened. "Oh, wow . . ."

"Contraction?"

"Yes. . . ." Now the contractions seemed massive and comprehensive. They made her feel as if her whole body was being ground into the bed. She couldn't fight them, she had to go with them.

"Do your breathing."

"Tired . . . of breathing," Susan said between breaths, and Tracey Kitchin smiled. The breathing regimens that Susan had learned in the St. Barnabas childbirth program took a lot of energy. And the amount of water they removed from the body, as vapor through the lungs, was huge.

When the contraction was over, Tracey Kitchin patted Susan's brow and cheeks with a cool, damp cloth. She pointed to the fetal heartbeat monitor, which had just etched a craggy alpine profile onto the chart. "You see there? They're three minutes apart. That's progress. Now hopefully they'll get stronger." She took Susan's hand between both of her own. "Time for me to say goodbye," she said. "My shift is over."

The MacGregors looked stunned and alarmed. Somehow they never had imagined that they would lose their wonderful nurse halfway through the process.

"You'll be fine," Tracey Kitchin said. "You're doing beautifully, and your new nurse is a doll. Bonnie Bergman. A real pro. She's one of my favorites. One word of advice?" she added almost shyly.

"Yes?" Susan said, totally attentive.

"Just this. If you get tired, don't be afraid to take the epidural."

"I don't want to miss out on the birth," Susan said, "I want to deliver my baby. I don't want to be numb."

"You won't go numb, you'll just be relaxed. You'll never feel pain, but you will feel pressure. Nearly all our patients have epidurals, and afterward they all say they're so glad they did."

"She's already been a trouper," Tracy said, "so far as I'm concerned."

"She's been terrific," Tracey Kitchin said. She looked out the window. The sun was up, and the early light was coming in. "It's a nice day to be born," she said.

•   •   •

"Hi," said the new nurse. "I'm Bonnie."

Bonnie Bergman was something altogether different. She was tall and very tan, with dramatic makeup and long black lashes. Her hair was blond, blown, and tipped. Her fingernails were over an inch long and painted fuchsia. After the homespun Tracey Kitchin, this was pretty high-octane stuff. And in contrast to Tracey Kitchin's easy manner, Bonnie Bergman's seemed impersonal. The MacGregors were mute as they watched her quickly and efficiently checking this and that, sizing things up for the new shift, getting on top of the situation.

She took Susan's temperature, and when she examined the thermometer, one perfectly crafted eyebrow lifted. "Ice chips?" she asked Susan, who nodded. "Okay," Bonnie said, "I'm going to take it again in fifteen minutes, and in the meantime, no ice chips, okay?" She began probing Susan's belly. Her hands were dark against Susan's white skin, and her nails were vivid. "Are you feeling the contractions more in front or in back?"

"Front, but there's still some back pressure."

"The baby's moving down."

"How can you tell?"

"Look over here at the fetal monitor," Bonnie said. "Here's the baby's line on the top; it traces the baby's heartbeat. And here's your line; it traces your contractions. It's flat with intermittent bumps or peaks. As the contractions have gotten stronger, they've gotten taller."

Another contraction came on, and Bonnie bent down to Susan and guided her through it, her hand on Susan's belly. "That was a big one," she said, looking at the chart.

"You're telling me," Susan said and smiled weakly. "Do the contractions get more intense than that?"

"These are good contractions," Bonnie said, "but they'll have to get stronger. The muscles in the upper uterus have to contract and pull on the lower uterus, and the lower uterus pulls on the cervix, stretching it. I predict this baby's coming sooner rather than later; don't ask me why."

"Why?" said Tracy.

"Don't ask," Bonnie said with a smile. They all laughed.

"I predict it's going to be born at five of five," Tracy said. The two women looked at him, and Tracy pointed to the electric clock, its hands stopped at five of five. "I've been staring at it all night," he said.

"You have to have this baby before I leave," Bonnie said. "I hate to leave before a baby's born. Yesterday I left a woman at nine centimeters. I hated to do it."

"I'll do my best," Susan said. There was warmth in her voice. Bonnie had won her over.

Bonnie was, as Rod would have put it, the salt of the earth. The mother of three, she would soon give one of her kidneys to her husband, who needed a transplant. She was also funny. And versatile. Nursing was her third career. She had started as an English teacher, then gotten her real estate license, then entered nursing. Even as a nurse working double shifts, she had continued to sell condos on the side. There were college tuitions to be paid—at the moment she had a daughter at the University of Pennsylvania who was majoring in intellectual history. Emblematic of Bonnie's versatility and her singular combination of glitz and competence was that to the amazement of all, those long fuchsia nails in no way interfered with her giving patients expert and comfortable internal examinations.

"Are you going to have the epidural?" Bonnie asked.

"I'm not sure. I'm trying to decide. I really didn't want one, but . . ."

"But now you're thinking about it?"

"It'd be different if I hadn't already gone through a whole day of this."

"Well, it's your decision," Bonnie said. She removed the absorbent cloth Susan was lying on. Childbirth was a wet business. The room had been supplied with three stacks of absorbent Chux pads, and ever since Susan got in bed, the nurses had been spreading them under her, regularly pulling out soggy ones and replacing them with dry.

A voice came through the open door: "Bonnie, Dr. O is on the phone." She left the room and gave the doctor her report, and he said he was on his way. She looked at her watch. It was 7:40.

Labor and Delivery was bustling now. There were patients in five rooms, and the staff were busy caring for them. At times there were a dozen people or more around the nurses' station—obstetricians, pediatricians, anesthesiologists, residents, nurses. Nurses aides wheeled beds and replenished supplies. Sister Regis, tall, erect, with a courteous executive manner, moved among them all, giving quiet orders and solving problems.

The atmosphere on Labor and Delivery was purposeful and at the same time congenial. Most of the people on the floor knew each other well, from many long shifts together, and as they went about their business they exchanged light remarks. Only rarely would things grow tense, as when complex measures had to be taken swiftly.

Bonnie stood observing the Room 6 monitor, faintly concerned, oblivious to the conversation of the two residents nearby who talked as they wrote their progress notes. She peered at the upper line, which represented the baby's heart rate. Just possibly, she thought, it might be starting to display a particular variation called the sinusoidal pattern. If it was, that might not be good. It could signal Rh incompatibility problems, or an abruption of the placenta, or fetal anemia.

Bonnie spoke to Doreen and they both watched the monitor. Doreen wasn't as worried. "With an external monitor," she reminded Bonnie, "you can't be sure it's sinusoidal. If she had an internal monitor on and the tracing looked like that, I'd be much more concerned. If it continues, I'll put on an internal."

Just before eight, Rod arrived. He was wearing a tweed sports jacket and a jaunty tie. He talked with Bonnie and Doreen and looked at the chart from the fetal monitor. "I'm not too alarmed about that pattern," he said. "I see what you're talking about, though, and we'll keep an eye on it."

When he entered Room 6, the weary MacGregors both came to alert. One of *their* doctors was here—he was like a visiting celebrity doing a turn, and his street clothes looked exotic among the bland and baggy hospital garments.

"Next time," he said to Susan, using his tried-and-true tension reliever, "we'll have your husband bring a baby home from the store, okay? It's easier." He laughed, at the same time surveying the young couple. As tired as she was, Susan looked fresher to him and calmer than her husband. It seemed that with the approach of delivery, nature's child-bearing instinct was giving Susan inner strength and endurance and a serenity that was sustaining her through it all—as if the apprehensions of nine months were being overridden by the sense that she had work to do.

Rod looked at Tracy and noticed he was slightly haggard. "Have you had any coffee, Tracy?" he asked. "We could get you some." Tracy declined. He was twitchy enough already.

Rod brought back the covers and examined Susan's belly. Then he put on rubber gloves and performed an internal examination.

"I'm checking to see if you're ready for me to break your water," he said. Piercing the amniotic sac could regularize an erratic labor. And if the sac was broken, then he might be able to reach through the opening of the cervix and attach an internal monitor directly to the baby's scalp. That would make the monitoring much more reliable.

His touch was cautious and gentle, but as he probed her cervix Susan winced. "Nope," he said, shaking his head. "I don't think I could do it. If I could do it easily, I would, but I see now that it would make you grossly uncomfortable. The act of getting to it, trying to force the cervix—you're not quite that far along." He stood up and removed his gloves. "I'm hoping we can move you out of this latent phase of labor pretty soon. The latent phase is what they call the first four centimeters. When people go through what you've gone through since yesterday, the question is, are they having a prolonged latent phase, or are they in false labor?

"It certainly didn't appear to be false labor," he continued, "the way it's been going on. The test was when they gave you the morphine. If it'd been false labor, the morphine would have gotten rid of the contractions, knocked them right out, and you wouldn't be having any now. I would have been very surprised if that had happened, because I've been pretty sure this was the real thing. Now we know. This is the real thing. So this isn't false labor; it's dysfunctional labor. That's all you can call it. Prolonged latent phase with a dysfunctional labor."

"How long will it be until the baby comes?" Susan asked.

"This afternoon sometime."

"Before three," Bonnie directed. "Before my shift ends."

"I wouldn't count on that," Rod said. "But you know what they say: the first four centimeters are the hardest."

He buttoned his jacket, ready to leave. "Dr. Bonamo will be in pretty soon, and between the two of us we'll keep a close eye on you, all right?"

"When I called you last night," Tracy said, "we thought Susan was about to deliver. She had very strong pain. Strong contractions."

"The back pain," Susan said. "I couldn't stand it."

"You did the right thing to call," Rod said. "You had no way of knowing whether or not it was for real. I know how it is—the embarrassment factor. You hesitate to look like a worrier."

"We'd been in the office twice that day," Susan said.

"You did the right thing," Rod said. He paused, thoughtfully. "You know, I think it's about time to give you a little Pitocin, to get you into productive labor." It was dangerous to use Pitocin too early, before the baby was in the proper head-down position, except in an emergency situation. But Susan now met the conditions.

At the nurse's station he spoke to Doreen and Bonnie. "It's a long one," he said. "I'm telling you. I can't remember a patient having so much dysfunctional labor. It's craziness." Craziness was one of his pet words. "But the Pitocin should do the trick."

Bonnie came back into the room carrying a small bottle of clear liquid, the Pitocin. In an IV bag she mixed five units of it with 500 cubic centimeters of D5W, a blend of dextrose and water. She hooked the line from the IV bag to a bright blue infusion pump mounted on a vertical chrome pole. Then with another tube she connected the pump to the IV socket in Susan's arm. She set the dial on the pump to 12 cubic centimeters an hour. "Pitocin," she said as she worked, "is a fairly natural substance. It's the synthetic version of the same hormone the body produces to bring on the contractions. But this way we can control it."

When Bonnie turned on the Pitocin pump, red digital numbers blinked to life on its control panel, and she adjusted the controls painstakingly, setting them to two milliunits per hour. She would increase the dose every fifteen minutes until the contractions were two to three minutes apart. "You won't feel anything for a little while," she told Susan. "The Pitocin is titrated, so it takes about twenty minutes for one drop of it to have an effect. But before long it will start to make a difference, and your contractions will develop a good, regular pattern, and things will begin to move along."

Afterward Susan lay waiting awhile, not sure what to expect. "I could use one of those hard candies," she told Tracy, and he opened a decorated tin and handed Susan a small orange lozenge.

A contraction gathered and climaxed. "It's a good one," Tracy said, watching the monitor. "Best one you've had in a while."

"Good. . . ."

"You're coming down . . . coming down . . . there. Feel better?"

"Yes," she said, releasing breath. "I was lying on my side. It was better. Maybe it gets gravity to help."

Bonnie, who had stepped out of the room before the contraction, popped back in. "Ah," she said, "you're on your side. That's why the contractions looked different on my monitor. They trace differently when you're on your side."

"It was a strong one," Susan said. "Is that the Pitocin?"

"Not yet."

Susan sighed and looked at the apparatus around her—the IV and the tubes and the blue pump with its jittery red numbers.

"Pretty high tech, huh?" she said.

Bonnie smiled reassuringly. "You'd be having a tough time without it," she said.

Tracy maintained his vigil, ready for the next contraction and at the same time rubbing Susan's back. Her eyes began to close. "If I snore," she said, "wake me up." She slept for a few minutes, then was gripped by a strong contraction.

Twenty minutes later, Bonnie looked in. "Guess what. We're getting a reasonable contraction pattern. You really haven't had that much Pitocin yet, and yet you've already got a good pattern." A contraction came along, and she watched as the tracing on the monitor wove up and down, a mechanical device creating a precise depiction of human pain. "Good," she said. "That was pretty good on the Richter scale. You're making real progress."

The tracing gradually subsided, then quivered, as if in anticipation of the next jolt.

23.
Epi-lite

Shortly after ten A.M. Jack Bonamo walked into the room. He smiled at Susan. "You *are* pregnant, aren't you?" he said, kidding.

"I think so," Susan said, trying to smile back.

"I think so too," Jack said. He drew on a pair of pale yellow rubber gloves. "The morphine was a good idea?" he asked.

"Yes, but I'm still real tired."

"I know you are. But you look much more comfortable than you did this time yesterday." He did an internal exam to check the cervix, then gave a little nod to Bonnie, the signal that he was ready to perform the procedure that was logical at this point. "I think you're ready now for me to break the sac," he said. "It'll help things along. You're going to feel uncomfortable for one minute, but then it'll be over."

From Bonnie he took a small beige plastic instrument that looked like a crochet hook. Then he bent over Susan. Bonnie put her hands on Susan's belly and pushed on the fundus, the very top of Susan's uterus. That was meant to squeeze the baby all the way down and push its head tightly against the cervix. The head would act like a stopper so that when the sac broke and the water rushed out, the umbilical cord couldn't rush out with it, slithering through the cervix.

That condition, in which the cord gets ahead of the baby's head, is called prolapse of the cord, and it is an extremely serious, classic obstetrical emergency, a factor in almost 1 percent of births. If any part of the cord should precede the baby, the cord can be pinched between its own body and its mother's. Pinching the cord for even a short time cuts off the baby's supply of oxygenated blood, with calamitous results.

When a cord prolapses, the patient must be raced to the operating room for an immediate cesarean. To prevent the head from coming down en route, putting pressure on the cord, the intern is assigned to put his hand up the patient's vagina and hold the head back. The patient is not transferred to a stretcher but rolled in her own bed, and since the doors are just wide enough to let the bed through, the intern has to climb up onto it with the patient, crouching over her with his hand in her body. The two of them together are covered in sterile drapes; the rolling bed with its shrouded hump makes an eerie sight as it races past the nursing station and across the crowded hall.

When the bed arrives in the operating room, the drapes are yanked off. There is no time to prep the patient carefully, swabbing her belly with Betadine, the iodinelike antiseptic. A resident pours out the whole jug of Betadine onto the belly, prepping not only the patient but the intern as well, staining them both brownish orange. There isn't time, either, to attach monitors, so the intern serves as the monitor, palpating the cord as it passes his hand and calling out the fetal heart rate to the doctors—not exact numbers but high, low, good, bad—so they have some idea how the baby is doing. The intern has to hold his position, hand restraining the head, throughout the operation, until the doctors remove the baby through the cesarean incision.

Everyone in Labor and Delivery knew what cord prolapse entailed and worked hard to avoid it.

Jack snagged the diaphanous sac with his little hook, and Susan's lower body flinched.

"Are you okay?" Jack asked. "I hurt you, but it's all done."

"I'm okay," Susan whispered. Then she stirred and brought her legs together. "I feel water . . ."

"Good. Your sac is broken. We should see some progress now, and now we can install an internal monitor on the baby. Internal monitors are much more accurate than the fetal monitor we strap around your abdomen."

Patients suspicious of the instrumentation of childbirth sometimes told Jack they'd heard that internal monitors were unnecessary for routine deliveries. Jack's reply was generally, "Yes, that's true, but the problem is knowing for sure which births will be routine." He'd go on to explain that with almost half of babies who experience fetal distress—any serious, perhaps life-threatening condition in the womb—there is nothing to alert the doctors and nurses. By the time the medical staff becomes aware of it, the baby may well have died or been disabled. In many of those situations, however, an internal fetal monitor can detect the danger while there is still time to do something about it.

Bonnie held out a sterile paper packet to Jack. He opened it and withdrew a long clear plastic applicator. Within its tip was a cylinder about half an inch long, the electrode of the internal monitor. From one end of the electrode ran a long thin cord made of red and green wires intertwined. On the other end was a spiral of silvery wire so fine it was hard to see. This curl would screw into the baby's scalp, fixing the monitor to its head.

Jack put his first two gloved fingers into the vagina to examine the baby's skull. Now that the amniotic sac had been broken, he could touch the skull through the cervix. It was important not to place the monitor along the joint between two skull bones or in the soft triangle where three bones converged. Keeping his fingertips against the skull, he took the applicator with his other hand and moved it into the vagina, using his examining fingers as his guide. When the applicator and electrode touched the skull, Jack turned the applicator clockwise. There was a click, which meant that the electrode had implanted and was free of the applicator, which Jack then withdrew.

"You won't see any mark on the baby from this," Bonnie told Susan, "the wire is so fine." She taped the cord from the internal monitor to Susan's leg and plugged the other end of the cord into the place on the recording machine where the external had been connected. The display promptly began to record signals sent directly from the baby's body. Messages from the unborn.

Bonnie felt relieved. Now that the internal monitor was in place and providing a true reading, she could see that there was nothing amiss with the pattern on the monitor. It was a good pattern; the heart rate had good variability.

Susan worked her way through three contractions, dozing between them. After the fourth she looked at the ceiling and said, "I'm so exhausted. I wonder if I should have an epidural."

"We can give you an epidural at this point," Jack said. "It would help you relax. My friend Richard Fain, he's another obstetrician here, calls it a second wind to get you over the mountain."

"Should I wait?"

"Nah. No reason to wait."

Bonnie straightened the covers. "We can always give your contractions back to you," she said. "But you're really tired."

"I really am tired," Susan said softly.

"I know you are," Jack said.

"If I had an epidural, could I have just a small one?"

Jack smiled. "Epi-lite? Sure."

"I've been doing my breathing off and on for thirty-eight hours now. I'm beginning to think I could use some help."

"Absolutely," Tracy said.

Susan brooded, her cheek against the pillow, then said out loud but as if to herself, "I just want to feel the baby."

Jack reassured her. "You'll feel the baby and you'll push it out. It won't stop the push, just the pain. At the end, when the baby's ready to be born, we'll cut back on the anesthetic enough to bring you back a little pain, just enough so that you'll feel it and can deliver."

Susan sighed. "Okay," she said, resigned. "Let's do it."

"Thank God," said Bonnie. She went out to the nurse's station, and soon her voice sounded over the intercom. "Dr. Fox, I need an epidural in Room 6." When she returned, Susan and Tracy looked glum. Too much waiting and too little sleep, Bonnie thought. And they probably were feeling a bit guilty, afraid that by agreeing to the epidural they'd caved in and somehow diminished the birth experience.

Sensing that the MacGregors' spirits could use some lifting, Bonnie turned to Jack and wagged her finger at him and said with mock gravity, "She *will* deliver before three. Before my shift is over. I hope that's understood."

"We'll do our best," Jack said, laughing. He knew what Susan was going through. He'd seen many patients who struggled through a prolonged latent phase, hours and hours of almost-labor-but-not-quite. Early on, they tolerated pain a lot better than they did toward the end. There usually came a point when they just couldn't take it any more.

"This baby has to be born this afternoon," Bonnie went on, "because I want to be here for it, and tonight is Nail Night. Once a week my friends all get together and we have our nails done. Actually, I had my nails done last Saturday—I had a nail emergency. But I've got five girls lined up tonight for Nail Night, and I can't let them down." Susan managed a smile, and then Tracy smiled a little too.

A boyish, friendly-faced man in his early forties, wearing gold-rimmed glasses and dressed in green scrubs, came into the room wheeling a small metal cabinet. It was Craig Fox, the anesthesiologist. "Here he is," Jack said, "the man the patients all love. We obstetricians take care of the lady for nine months, but when the pain starts, she forgets us. Once the pain starts, the only doctor she cares about is the anesthesiologist."

Bonnie laughed. "That's their favorite person," she agreed.

Dr. Fox tried to be deadpan as he made his preparations, but he was visibly pleased at being a favorite person. An anesthesiologist at St. Barnabas for ten years, he did about seven hundred epidurals a year.

"I'm going to explain what we're doing every step of the way," he told Susan. "This procedure is basically like having a shot in the physician's office, except in this case we're not injecting a muscle but putting anesthetic into the space around the spinal cord." But not into the cord itself, he made clear. Spinal injections were now rare at St. Barnabas. At that hospital, at least, spinals and the other methods of anesthetizing a woman in labor had been all but replaced by epidurals.

The spinal cord, he said, is the bundle of major nerves that run up and down the back, through the stack of spinal vertebrae. That cord is contained in a sac filled with fluid. The outer skin of that sac is the dura. Between the dura and the muscles of the back is the so-called epidural space. That was where Susan's anesthetic would go. It would bathe the dura, seeping harmlessly through it into the spinal fluid. Once in the fluid, it would bond to the receptor sites on the cord, blocking the transmission of pain messages from Susan's lower torso to her brain.

Dr. Fox asked Tracy to leave the room for a few minutes; observing the epidural procedure was more than most husbands could take. Bonnie, preparing her patient, went around to the other side of the bed. "We want you to sit on this side," she said. "Face this way, toward me, away from the doctor." She helped Susan swing her legs around until they hung over the side of the bed , then sit up. "That's perfect," she said. "Now lean toward me. Bow your head and put it on my chest." She drew Susan forward until the top of her head rested against Bonnie. "Drop your shoulders and round your back as much as you can. Good. That stretches your spine and separates the vertebrae, to give Dr. Fox plenty of room."

From his side of the bed Dr. Fox parted Susan's hospital gown, revealing her back. The first step was to numb her skin so that she wouldn't feel the epidural injection. He took a syringe with a very fine needle and, finding his spot between two vertebra in the lower back, injected a little novocaine just barely under the skin. The liquid raised a small welt. Fox knew that once he'd raised that welt, he had numbed that area of the skin; the novocaine would work fast. Through that welt, he would inject the larger needle that would travel to the epidural space.

The needle itself didn't deliver the anesthetic. That was done by a catheter. The catheter was just a plastic tube, so fine and flexible it would never go in by itself. It had to be led in through a tunnel—the needle.

The crucial thing was to reach the epidural space exactly. If Fox went too far, he would penetrate the dura and unintentionally give Susan a spinal; since the anesthetic was too strong for a spinal, it could give Susan a seizure or stop her breathing. If, on the other hand, he fell short of the epidural space, the anesthetic would fail to numb her pain. A delicate business—yet he couldn't see where the tip of the needle was; it was a blind procedure. There was just one way to know.

"I'm going to insert the needle now," he said. "You won't feel any pain, just a little pressure." He touched the long, hollow needle to the novocaine welt, then carefully, steadily pushed it in. He moved it only a short distance and stopped. "Are you feeling any pain?" Fox asked Susan.

"No," she said in a small voice, holding tightly to Bonnie. As Fox had predicted, she felt merely the sensation of someone lightly nudging her.

The syringe did not contain anesthetic, nothing but air. Very slowly, just a few millimeters at a time, Fox advanced the needle through the tissues. As he went, he gently tapped on the syringe's plunger. He knew that as long as the needle was moving through tissue, he would feel resistance to the plunger; there would be no place for the air to go. He advanced and tapped, advanced and tapped. Then suddenly, as he tapped, the plunger slid into the syringe. The air had found a place to go, and that place was the only open space, the epidural cavity. He was there.

Leaving the needle in Susan's back, he disconnected the syringe from it. Then he tore open the square, transparent plastic envelope that contained the catheter, the long thin tube that would carry the actual anesthetic into Susan. It was calibrated, and by watching the calibrations as he inserted it into the needle, he could tell exactly where its tip was. When the catheter reached its correct depth, Fox removed the needle, retracting it back up along the catheter, a larger tube sliding over a smaller one, leaving the catheter in place.

Without the needle, the catheter looked innocuous, an almost clear plastic tube, so fine it was hard to notice, emerging bloodlessly from the lower back. Susan felt no pain from it at all. When the catheter had gone in she'd felt a tiny electric tingle in one leg, a funnybone feeling—a common reaction, the doctor said. That was all. Her one difficulty had been that while the needle was still in she'd had a contraction. She'd been uncomfortable and wanted to breathe heavily and move her body to lessen the pain. But she hadn't dared. Not with a needle in her back.

Fox dabbed a liquid adhesive onto the area around the catheter and painted a path of it up her back. The adhesive had a strong but not unpleasant smell, a familiar odor; it was tincture of benzoin, which her mother had put in the vaporizer when she was little and had colds. When it dried it left a tacky surface. Then Fox took a small white square of plastic sponge from the envelope and placed it on Susan's back right next to the catheter. The sponge had a groove in it, and he laid the catheter along the groove. He taped the catheter in position on her lower back, then taped it right up the path of adhesive on her back and over her shoulder.

At Susan's shoulder Fox connected the free end of the catheter to a small socket: the attachment for the line from the infusion pump that would deliver the anesthetic. But before he hooked up that line he drew some anesthetic into a syringe and injected it directly into the connector. "I'm giving you a dose to begin with," he said, "a slightly higher concentration, to give you some prompt relief. Then I'll let the analgesia recede to a lower level, which we'll probably maintain until you're all dilated and ready to start pushing."

Bonnie helped Susan swing her legs back up onto the bed and lie down, then brought the sheets over her.

Fox hooked the connector to the line from a second blue infusion pump, which stood on the same chrome pole as the Pitocin pump.

"Okay," he said, "we're all set. Now there are three things I want you to remember. First, when you move around in bed, don't drag your back across the sheets, because if you do, you could pull the catheter loose and we'd have to do the whole thing all over again." He knew he'd taped the catheter on very securely. Still, it was a useful caution.

"Don't worry," Susan said, by no means eager to do it all over again.

"Second, you can lie on your back or on either side, but if you lie on your side, you have to remember to change positions at least twice an hour, so that you don't tend to get numb only on one side.

"And the last thing to remember is my name—Dr. Fox—and that's important, because if you need more anesthetic or something, you can tell Bonnie who to call. Otherwise she might bring you the janitor." In tense situations, every doctor knew, even the lamest attempts at humor could be therapeutic. Susan smiled.

Fox turned the dial on the infusion pump until the red digital counter read 10: ten cubic centimeters an hour. It was a low dose, the average dose. "There you are," he said. "You won't have any pain at all from now through the rest of your labor. Yet at the same time you'll be alert." The whole installation of the epidural had taken four minutes.

"That's wonderful," Susan said. "Thank you so much."

"The first thing you'll feel will be a tingling sensation in your feet and legs," the doctor said. That would be from the test dose. "Pretty soon your legs will be pretty numb. You'll be able to move them, but you won't be able to stand up. And then you'll be numb from the ribs on down. I'll be checking on you regularly, and we'll adjust the pump to give you just the amount you need. When it comes time to push, we'll see to it that you can do it very effectively, but without real discomfort."

Fox, in his quiet, circumspect, matter-of-fact voice, had just described a miracle that childbearing women throughout the existence of the human race had never dared hope for: labor and delivery nearly free of pain but conscious and alert—an active, fully participating childbirth with the terror and agony gone.

Fox left the room and returned several minutes later, bringing Tracy with him. "Can you move your legs?" he asked Susan.

"Yes," she said, "but they're pretty numb."

He stood by for a while, inconspicuously observing the monitor, watching as Susan went through two contractions. Each time the tracing peaked, he checked her face for reactions. When the third reached its climax, he said to her, "How do you feel?"

"I feel fine," she said. "That stuff is great."

"Are you feeling contractions?"

"No, I'm not having any."

"You're having one right now. Look at the monitor. You're right at the peak."

"That is amazing!"

A nurse came in the room and said, "Dr. Fox, you're being paged." He went out to the nurses' station and made a call.

Several hours later, in the doctors' lounge, Fox would talk further about the pros and cons of the epidural. "It's more than a matter of avoiding pain," he said. "Epidurals have real benefits for the baby. We've found that if the mother is calm, she avoids hyperventilation. That actually improves the blood flow into the placenta and makes for a smoother time of it for the baby."

As an anesthesiologist, Fox not surprisingly believed that only anesthesiologists should perform epidurals. "Untrained people are giving epidurals," he said gravely, "and there have been problems—patients who've had respiratory arrest or seizures when the needle went through the dura into the spinal fluid; patients who've had cardiac arrest or lack of oxygen to the mother or the baby. I've had patients who have been given epidurals by obstetricians in small hospitals, and more often than not these women say something like 'They had all kinds of problems, they stuck me a half a dozen times, and then they got it in and it didn't work. It took them forty-five minutes, and finally they had to give me something else for pain.'

"One more advantage of the epidural," he added, "is that oftentimes the patients don't need an episiotomy. The epidural makes it easier for them to push properly, and they're more relaxed. There's enough relaxation from the epidural that they can avoid the episiotomy."

•   •   •

In Room 6 a half hour after installing the epidural, Dr. Fox looked down at his patient with a practiced eye. "Do your legs feel warm and tingly?" he asked.

"Yes."

"You're nicely relaxed."

"What a relief," Susan said. "I just needed to rest." She was very pale now, her skin like wax, but the strain was gone from her face.

•   •   •

Susan now had six lines tethering her to various devices—one for the IV, one for blood pressure, one each for the epidural and the

Pitocin, and one each for the internal fetal monitor and the external contraction monitor. A perfectly healthy woman rigged up like a lab experiment, she looked in mild amazement at the web of tubes and cords leading from her body. "I feel like I'm getting ready for space travel," she said to Tracy.

"It's a great day for it," Tracy said. Outside the hospital window, big white clouds were moving west to east against a clear blue sky. The labor was taking a long time, but it was by no means the chaos that the jumbled slide show at the first childbearing class had led Susan and Tracy to anticipate. High-tech procedures like epidural sounded frightening when described but could be a godsend when the need arose.

Susan was resting comfortably now. She looked like a cameo, or a Renaissance painting. Over and over, in quiet moments, she seemed to fall naturally into the classic mien of the pregnant madonna—head lowered and to one side, skin pale, her expression slightly ethereal, faintly sad. From time to time Tracy became part of the tableau, standing over her like the biblical father, looking down with love and solicitude. They had fallen into ancient patterns, function dictating form.

In truth it was Tracy who was strung out. He fidgeted and fretted.

At ten past twelve Doreen examined Susan again.

"What do you think?" Tracy asked.

"You've got maybe six more hours. You'll be a father by dinnertime."

Tracy popped a lozenge into his mouth. "You remember when we all picked dates?" he asked Susan with satisfaction. "You know who picked the twelfth, don't you?"

Susan patted his hand. "You did."

"You're moving right along," Doreen said. "The cervix is almost completely thinned out." She systematically nudged Susan's belly. "The baby's head is coming down."

She went out to the board and changed the information. On the space after "Cx" she wrote "5–6"; the cervix was dilated between five and six centimeters—a little over two inches. The number after "Eff," for effacement, was changed to 90; the cervix was thinned to 90 percent of the goal. The stout wall had become membranous.

There was a column headed "ST," for station—a way of describing where in the birth canal the baby was. If the station was zero, that meant the baby's head was at the midpoint of its journey through Susan's pelvis. If the station number was a minus, that meant the head was approaching the midpoint but not there yet. Station minus-two, for example, meant that the baby's head had not yet engaged in the pelvis. Station minus-one, which is what Doreen now wrote on the board, meant the head had entered the pelvis and was fully engaged.

When Doreen next returned to Room 6, she had two people in tow: her husband, Kevin, a tall, athletic man, and their son, Christopher, a little fellow with freckles and a button nose and straight blond hair falling into his eyes. Though only six, Christopher was at home in Labor and Delivery. Residents' children didn't see them much, because of the hospital hours, so for the past four years Kevin had often brought Christopher to St. Barnabas to keep his mother company and to hang out. He had the run of the place. He knew everybody and had picked up a lot of knowledge about childbirth. A staff obstetrician who was a special pal of Christopher's had even cut a yellow gown down to Christopher's size.

Doreen introduced her guests to the MacGregors. "They're here for my ultrasound scan," she explained. "We're due down the hall in about five minutes. I'll see you in half an hour. Dr. Bonamo is nearby, so you'll be covered."

After they'd left, Dr. Fox appeared, and after asking Susan his usual questions and finding her comfortable, he turned the dial on the pump from ten to six. She was nearly dilated and wouldn't need as much pain relief for a while. As delivery drew near, he could turn it up again.

Jack came in, wearing cranberry-colored scrubs. He had a gynecological procedure to perform, a D&C, at one o'clock at the same-day surgical center across the street.

"So you're actually doing it," he said to Susan lightly. "Looks like the Pitocin did the trick. People impugn Pitocin. They say, 'I was fine before the Pitocin.' I say, 'You were fine, but you were never going to have the baby.' "

Jack spread his hands on Susan's lower belly. "What do you feel when you have contractions?" he asked.

"Just a little pressure."

At one-thirty, his gynecological surgery over, Jack was starting a quick lunch in the doctors' section of the hospital's new cafeteria. He had just taken a bite of his tuna sandwich when, from a speaker in the ceiling, he heard a voice call out, "Dr. Bonamo. Dr. Bonamo. Please call five-three-five-two." It was the number of the nurse's station in Labor and Delivery.

He went to the phone on a nearby column—there were phones all through the doctors' section—and dialed the number. Doreen, who had returned from her ultrasound, answered and said, "She's fully dilated." In three minutes Jack was in Room 6.

"Wonderful," he said. "That's the end of the first stage of labor. After thirty-six hours you got there. How do you feel?"

"I feel . . . different."

"Okay," Jack said, "let's see if you can push. We'll let you try to push a while and see what that accomplishes, and then we'll go on from there. If you can't push, don't be upset. We may need to let the epidural wear off a little. If that's the way it is, we'll just let you rest a while and try again."

He and Doreen stepped outside the room. "I've got to stop by Breen's office for a couple of minutes," he told her. "I'll be right back." Dr. Breen's office was thirty seconds away, down the hall and around the corner.

Bonnie now prepared Susan for the final effort—stage two. The pressure of the baby's head against the rectal nerves would make Susan want to push, to bear down with each contraction until the baby left her body. With a first-time mother, stage two could take hours.

Bonnie raised Susan's legs, letting them rest on the wooden side rails of the bed. "I want you to try just one good push," she said. "Not too much, don't strain. Just one push."

Susan closed her eyes and gripped the rails with her hands and flexed her lower body.

Bonnie watched intently. Suddenly she opened her eyes wide. "Oh, my gosh!" she said. "This is amazing! I think the baby's coming."

There it was, a tiny patch of wet, hairy scalp. For the first time, emerging from its lair, the new MacGregor had been sighted. For the first time its skin had been touched by the earthly air in which it would spend its life.

"Where's Dr. Bonamo?" Tracy asked anxiously.

"He's right down the hall. He'll be here in a flash. Don't push. Give me two minutes to get everything ready, because you're about to have this baby." She dashed out of the room.

Doreen was still standing just outside the door. "The baby's here!" Bonnie told her. "I saw the head! Where's Dr. Bonamo?"

24.
Sam

Since Susan MacGregor was making progress, Jack had decided to leave her with Bonnie a little while to try to do some pushing. He wanted to let Bonnie teach her to push before the pressure got strong, let her learn the mechanics of it while she was still comfortable. That was normal procedure: to give the patient a test run. A trial push would tell Jack approximately how fast it was going to go and when the main action, requiring his presence, might occur. In the meantime, on the principle of using every golden moment, he'd drop some reports on his boss.

As he walked into Dr. Breen's office, the secretary was just putting down the phone. "Oh, Dr. Bonamo. They want you back in Labor and Delivery," she said, her voice reflecting the tone of exigency she'd heard on the other end of the line.

He ran back down the hall, afraid that something had happened to the fetal heart beat. He burst into Room 6, and Bonnie said: "Dr. Bonamo! The baby is right here. It couldn't be better. We couldn't even get through one push!"

Doreen said, "The head is *there*."

"It came down with *one* push," Bonnie said. "It came right down. While we waited, the baby came down on its own."

"Wow! That's good!" Susan said, amazed.

"Good?" Jack said. "It's terrific. We're going to have a baby before we know it, folks."

"You almost missed it," Tracy said to Jack, only half kidding.

"Not on your life," Jack said, pulling on gloves. "I wouldn't have missed it for anything."

"Is she all right?" Tracy asked Jack.

"She's terrific," Jack said. "Some people are lucky; they can get that motor force going even though, thanks to the epidural, they don't have the pain." Susan was indeed fortunate, he thought. The baby probably wasn't large, and its position was good; it was following the path of least resistance, just as it was supposed to. The epidural had relaxed Susan and the Pitocin had kept her contractions regular. A textbook case.

Bonnie said to Susan, "All right, now we're going to shorten the bed. Bring your feet up next to your body for a minute." She lifted and removed the footboard and stood it in the corner. Then she lifted off the whole bottom third of the bed, including that part of the mattress. She swung up the stirrups and locked them in place.

"Now Tracy and I are going to move you down the bed," Bonnie said. "Come on down, honey." Bonnie held her under one arm and Tracy under the other, and Susan lifted her weight on her elbows and heels and, taking care not to rub her epidural tube, eased her torso along the mattress until her bottom was even with the end of the truncated bed. The baby would be born right off the end of the bed into the doctors' waiting hands. Bonnie put Susan's feet into the stirrups.

She rolled in a small, blue chest of drawers with a white enamel tray on top—the birthing cart. On it was a sterile kit that contained everything needed for a delivery: surgical instruments, scissors for the umbilical cord, a suction bulb, some needles, a needle holder, and a red plastic box to put used needles in. In one of the drawers were numbered plastic identification bracelets for the MacGregors and their child and also the equipment she'd use to footprint the baby.

According to the system, the doctors's gloves were kept sterile and the nurse was considered unsterile. That way, the nurse could handle all sorts of unscrubbed objects in the room—equipment, furniture, the patient, bed linen, and so forth. But that meant it had to be Jack and Doreen who now covered Susan's lower body with sterile disposable paper drapes. They put one across each thigh and one over her abdomen. There were sterile towels in the kit, and Jack put several under Susan, with a sterile drape over them.

Against the wall, near the headboard, Bonnie positioned a rolling bassinet, the warmer. It had heat lamps in its hood to protect the baby against the chill it would feel when it passed from the 98.6 degree temperature of Susan's body to the much cooler room. Making sure the baby could be warmed was one of Bonnie's most important predelivery tasks. Another was to see that the suction device fitted into the wall, next to the warmer, was working; the anesthesiologist would use it to suck mucus from the baby's mouth and nose and stomach during his examination.

Finally came the spotlight. It was mounted on a shaft, like a floor lamp. Bonnie placed it near the end of the bed so it could illuminate the forthcoming action.

Susan said, "I feel water."

"Good," Bonnie said. "That means your contractions are getting stronger. They're pushing out the fluid."

Her legs now drawn up in the classic posture of modern childbirth, her feet in the metal stirrups, her thighs high and spread, her eyes open wide, Susan turned and looked at Tracy. "This is it," she said. "Can you believe it? Nine months!"

"This is it," Tracy said softly, and kissed her brow.

Susan moved her head back to center and focused her attention. "More water again," she said.

Tracy jumped up, overcome by the power of suggestion. "I have to go to the bathroom," he said, and dashed out of the room.

Susan smiled and said to Bonnie, "This is worse on him than it is on me."

At ten of two, all was ready for the final episode in the drama. Tracy was back and standing by the bed, holding Susan's hand.

Jack moved up to the side of the bed and stood by Susan. "Let me explain what's going to be happening now," he said in his warm, informal voice. "That one time you pushed, your baby's head became visible. When the push was over and the pressure stopped, the head withdrew—you know, like toothpaste being sucked back into the tube; the vaginal muscles pushed it back in. Now you're about to push again, this time in earnest, and with every push the head will come down a little farther. In between pushes it'll withdraw, but never quite as far back as it had been. Each time it'll make progress.

"The big moment will be when the head gets so far down that it can't be sucked back in—when it doesn't withdraw but stays where the last push brought it. From then on, there'll be no stopping it."

Susan nodded. She was totally centered on what was about to happen.

Doreen was sitting on a stool at the end of the bed, inspecting the scene of impending action. The vagina had opened slightly, and, as Bonnie directed the bright light, Doreen opened it more with her fingers. "I think I'm seeing the baby's head," she said. "Yes, it's the head. It's lined up perfectly."

Looking into Susan's body and glimpsing the head, Doreen had noted something important. From the position of the fontanel, the soft place where three plates of the skull met in a triangle, she could tell that the baby's head was looking down, toward Susan's spine and toward the floor. That was the ideal starting position for a smooth trip through the pelvis. Soon, responding to the pelvis's internal contours—which, as Dr. Smellie had found two centuries ago, were something like a bent oval cylinder with a twist—the head would make a one-eighth turn to the left. That would mean that the long diameter of the head was lined up with the long diameter of the pelvic opening at that point. The head would be following the easiest, most logical course, not wedging itself into a cul-de-sac. Later the head would turn back to center, looking down again. Things would match up.

Bonnie glanced at the monitor. "Okay, honey, we've got a contraction starting. I want you to take a cleansing breath, all right?" Susan took a deep breath through the nose and held it, then released it through the mouth. "That's fine," Bonnie said. "Now, let's do three breaths for each contraction. A breath before each push, and hold it. Put your chin to your chest and hold it. You'll be fine. Tracy, you do the counting." Tracy began to count out the breaths, and Susan followed.

"You're starting!" Doreen called to Susan, peering in. She could see the red-green cord of the internal monitor slowly moving toward her and the vagina separating, starting to give way. And then she saw the top of the baby's head with the internal monitor attached to its scalp.

"Okay!" Bonnie called out, like a track coach at the starting line. "You're going to get behind this contraction. You're going to take a breath and hold it to a count of ten. *Take your breath!* And *push!*" The count was a way of ensuring that the push was sustained. Short pushes didn't do the job. Each contraction was to be held for three ten-counts, with breaths in between.

Susan drew air, her chest rising. She shut her eyes and compressed her lips, and color came into her face.

"One . . . Two . . . Three . . . " Bonnie and Tracy counted together but not quite in synch.

"Just one of you count!" Susan gasped. Bonnie told Tracy to do it.

"That's it," Jack said to Susan. "You're doing fine. Keep pushing. Keep pushing. Beautiful."

When the contraction was finished, Bonnie had Susan take a cleansing breath and then asked, "Are you feeling pressure in your rectum yet?"

"Not really."

"You will."

By rectal pressure she meant pressure on the nerves of the rectum, which lie parallel and immediately adjacent to the vagina. Pressure in the vagina would cause a response in the rectum, the same sensation as in defecation—the urge to expel the large form that was travelling through. "We don't want them to push anteriorly, on top," Doreen said later, "because then they'd be pushing the baby into the pubic bone. We want them to push on their bottom, their rectum, as if they were having a bowel movement. It pushes the baby's head down and out, so it doesn't get jammed up against the pubis."

Bonnie kept an eye on the monitor, noting the frequency and strength of the contractions. If they started to space out, she would increase the Pitocin.

Since Susan was pushing so well but not really suffering, the epidural level seemed just right. Susan had needed more sensation in order to push effectively, but the extra pain caused by the baby's head coming down, pressing against the rectal nerves, was providing it.

Another contraction. "Chin on chest," Jack said. "Chin on chest. Hold it! That's right." Many women, straining to push, directed the force against the wrong place. They would shut their eyes and puff out their cheeks and press air against their face or throat—pushing "in their face." Or they'd arch their back and push their belly up in the air. Jack always made a point of having them hold their chin against their chest, because that focused the pushing where it did the most good, way down, on the rectum. It was easy to spot patients who hadn't pushed effectively. The next day their eyes would be bloodshot and their cheeks red, because the pressure would have burst capillaries.

"We're going to have a baby soon," Doreen said. "The latent phase went on forever, but it sure did bring the baby down." She covered a finger with Surgilube and slipped it into the bottom of Susan's vagina. Gently, back and forth in a U-shaped motion, she massaged the perineum, the area between the vagina and the anus. The massage would stretch it and make delivery easier. It would also help Susan target where to push.

A new series of pushes began. "I see hair," said Doreen, sitting on her stool at the end of the bed, Susan's feet in the stirrups above Doreen's shoulders.

"Eight . . . Nine . . . Ten . . ." said Tracy, and Susan let a gust of tightly pent air explode from her lungs.

"And just relax," Doreen said. Susan's taut limbs slackened and settled.

"Good girl!" Bonnie said. Having given birth three times, she knew firsthand how important to the patient encouragement was.

"Way to go!" Tracy said, his voice full of excitement and admiration, as if he'd just seen a brilliant athlete make an incredible play.

Dr. Fox had returned, and off to the side as Susan continued to push he was working ahead of the action. He had prepared a syringe of Pitocin and was now inserting its needle into the stopper on the IV bag. He wanted the syringe to be ready for the moment right after the placenta was delivered. At that point he would give her one last jolt of Pitocin to make her uterus sharply contract, closing off the big blood vessels in the uterus that were now serving the placenta. When the placenta broke free, they would pour blood into her uterus. The contractions would pinch them off. They would also help clean out the uterus by expelling any surplus tissue that hadn't come out with the placenta.

With Tracy at her side, steadfastly counting, Susan began a new push. She drew a breath and, groaning, held it. Her legs jerked, making the stirrups clatter in their sockets, and her shoulders lurched from the mattress. Through it all came cries and moans of heavy strain, as if she were wrestling with a gigantic animal.

"Keep it going!" Bonnie cried. "Keep it going." Jack smiled. Bonnie always yelled "Keep it going."

"Six . . . Seven . . . Eight . . . Nine . . . Ten . . ." Tracy counted. "Now take a quick breath."

"Beautiful," Doreen said. "It's right there."

"Beautiful," said Jack. "I love to see that head." If the obstetrician could see the head, that meant he wouldn't have to go in after it with forceps.

"Get a mirror!" Susan shouted at the end of the push. "I want to see."

"Could we move the pump over," Jack said, "so we can get the mirror in here?" Bonnie moved the stand with the Pitocin and epidural pumps and then placed a large rectangular standing mirror so Susan could observe. Tracy, torn between wanting to stay by Susan and the desire to glimpse his child, moved down the side of the bed as far as he could without taking his hand from her wrist.

Susan felt a fresh contraction building. "I'm starting!" she cried out.

"Down on your rectum!" Jack commanded. "Concentrate your push on the rectal area." In Jack's experience many patients, when they saw the head crowning, lost their concentration and stopped pushing well, and the head would go back in. It was hard to keep concentrating on pushing in the right place. So the staff had to keep coaching. But Susan was doing it exactly right. "Beautiful!" Jack said.

Tracy completed his count. "Nine . . . Ten . . . take a breath."

As Doreen watched, the pink tissues at the opening of the vagina turned slightly blue, as if they were being bruised. There was some blood, not a lot; mothers didn't bleed much unless there was a problem. The tissues of the vaginal lining, now puffed up, began to squeeze forward, pushing ahead of the baby, moving with it as the baby came through. Susan's tissues weren't especially swollen, because she hadn't been pushing for long. When there'd been a long siege of pushing, things could look a lot worse.

"The head is crowning," Doreen said. There it was, a semisphere of gray scalp filigreed with fine, dark, wet hair. The head had not retreated at the end of the push. It was holding its ground.

There were four professionals in the room: the obstetrician, the resident, the nurse, and—because birth was imminent—the anesthesiologist. Though each had seen thousands of babies born, they too, along with the MacGregors, stared at the little gray patch, awed.

"My baby," said Susan, full of emotion. Tracy, looking in the mirror too—his mouth open, astonished—was beyond words.

"Slow down the count," Doreen said to Tracy. "You're too eager." Fathers had a tendency to count too quickly as birth approached, perhaps on the theory that the sooner they could get their wives to ten, the better. But the women needed the full count to do their work. Rushing didn't help.

"When are we going to say her labor began?" Bonnie asked. Tracy looked over and saw that she was writing on a clipboard, calmly filling out a form. It slightly alarmed him that in this wild moment, when his child was being born, she was doing her paperwork. But a moment that seemed frenetic to Tracy was tranquility itself to Bonnie and the doctors. Everything was under control. There certainly were plenty of personnel, more than enough to deliver that one little baby. And there was so much paperwork for the staff that they had to get it done when they could.

Bonnie had eight forms to fill out before the baby was taken to the nursery. Two of them asked how many hours of labor Susan had had. Jack could choose to consider labor as having started when Susan's contractions became regular or when her cervix began to dilate. There could be a big difference between those two times. So Bonnie asked Jack the usual question: When did this patient's labor begin?

"Nine this morning," Jack replied. Jack went by the standard definition of labor: "progressive dilatation producing cervical change." Bonnie wrote "9 A.M." on the two forms and hastily filled in several other blanks. As she well knew, once the delivery took place, her whole attention would have to go to the baby.

"Two more pushes," Doreen told Susan, "and you'll have a baby."

"Do you feel much pain?" asked Jack.

"No," said Susan, smiling.

"What did I tell you?" Jack said. "Dr. Fox knows what he's doing."

Susan's knees were starting to come together. At this stage, like most women, she was naturally afraid of being torn apart by what was coming through, afraid to let the baby out. She was following the instinct to protect herself. But closing the legs could push the baby's head back up. "Just relax your legs out," Jack said. He had an effective way of combatting the knees-together syndrome. He had Susan grab the back of her thighs just below her knees and pull against her legs. In addition to keeping the necessary separation, it would give her something to do with her hands. The maneuver also bent the body, lifting the shoulders off the bed and moving the chin toward the belly. It was a much better birthing posture than the flat-on-the-bed mode.

Susan strove to get a push going, but she couldn't quite manage. She'd had a little cramp, not a real contraction, and the pushing wasn't effective. "That was a false start," Bonnie said. "Nothing to worry about. Why don't you just rest through this one? Breathe a little and get some strength, and let's wait for the next string of contractions."

Bonnie looked at the monitor and saw the baby's heart rate decline and not come back up. That was normal—a sign of an impatient baby. "The baby's saying, 'I don't want to rest; I'm coming out now!' " she joked. "The baby wants *out.*"

With the next push the vagina slowly opened and the top and back of the head emerged from Susan's body. "The head is halfway out!" Doreen exclaimed. She guided it with one hand while the fingers of the other kept dipping into the Surgilube and massaging the vaginal tissues to keep them from tearing.

"Don't push now. No pushing," Jack said. "The rest of the head will come out by itself. The vaginal muscles will squeeze it the rest of the way, all by themselves."

"Don't push," Bonnie said. "I want you to pant. Fast little breaths, one a second." If Susan was panting, she couldn't hold her breath; she couldn't push. Pushing now could cause an explosion and a perineal tear that would require an elaborate episiotomy. Panting gave her something to think about besides that relentless urge to expel. Susan conscientiously began to pant.

The head emerged from the vagina—soft-looking, slightly collapsed, smaller than a man's fist, facing the floor. It was an incredible sight: a miniature human head, gray as slate, protruding from a large white human body.

With her lower birth canal now full of baby, Susan felt an almost overwhelming urge to push down and expel. "Don't push!" Bonnie said. "Don't push now! Keep panting!"

"Don't push!" Jack said emphatically. "Stop pushing!"

"I'm trying," Susan grunted between pants.

Though the baby's head was born, its body was still squeezing through the convoluted birth canal. At this moment the shoulders were navigating the pelvic straits. Their widest dimension, shoulder tip to shoulder tip, had aligned with the largest dimension of Susan's pelvic passage, an action that had turned the body to the left. Susan and Tracy, not quite understanding that, were amazed and slightly unnerved by the eerie thing that happened next.

The head had been facedown toward the floor as it cleared Susan's body, but now it slowly and smoothly rotated to the left, and suddenly its face was visible. It was as if, conscious of an audience, it had turned to take them in. The process was called restitution; the head, now free of constraint, was lining itself normally with its body.

For the first time, in the mirror, Susan saw her child's eyes and nose and mouth. "Wow!" she gasped, then tried to pant again.

The baby had been absolutely silent. Not a wail or whimper. But not because of a sweet disposition; the baby had no choice in the matter. Later Doreen recalled how frightened she'd been as a student the first time she saw a delivery. "I thought the baby was dead," she said, "because when the head came out it was pale and colorless and it didn't cry. I said to myself, 'Oh, no, it's a stillborn.' I soon found that it was colorless because it hadn't breathed yet; when its body was still in the vagina its rib cage was compressed by the vaginal muscles, and it couldn't expand its lungs. In a moment it was born and it starting crying and turned pink, and everything was fine."

This period before Susan's baby took its first breath, while it was still getting oxygen from her blood via the umbilical cord, gave Doreen a brief chance to do something important. She grabbed the suction device from the delivery tray and inserted its slender tube in the baby's nostrils, one by one, and in the mouth and throat. Pumping the rubber bulb on the device, she drew out mucus. If the baby was allowed to breathe before that task was done, the mucus might be taken into the lungs and interfere with breathing.

Tracy, filled with curiosity as to the baby's sex, studied the little face. But it was frustrating. There was nothing in the baby's flattened features to suggest its gender.

Jack said, "Okay, we've got the head, now we're going for the shoulders."

Tracy was itchy. "Should she push?" he asked.

"Not yet," Jack said, talking as Doreen continued with the delivery. That was one of the advantages a doctor had who worked with a resident: he had time to explain things to a patient. "I know what you're thinking, that since pushing got the head out, she should keep pushing to get the rest out. But that's not the way it works." Doreen had taken the baby's head in her fingers. Even in her small hands, the head looked tiny.

"The shoulders are obviously bigger than the head," Jack went on, "so what you want to do is bring them out one at a time, first one and then the other. But which one first? Okay, the baby is on its side, so that means one shoulder is up and the other is down. The uppermost shoulder comes out first, and to get it out we have to lead it down, to get it out from under the pubic bone. So we take the head and put just a little traction on it." Doreen carefully drew the head down toward the mattress. "Like that. And the little shoulder slides right out. There.

"If Susan had pushed," Jack went on, "she'd have wedged that shoulder behind the pubic bone. But she didn't push, because she's so terrific, and the shoulder came right out."

Doreen changed the position of her hands.

"The other shoulder, called the posterior shoulder, is simple. When Doreen lifts the baby's head and neck—like that—that shoulder comes right through." And it did. "Now you see why we didn't want Susan to push," Jack concluded. "It was important for us to have that control."

Doreen smiled down at the baby. Its shoulders were out but its arms, still crossed, were tightly bound to its chest by the vagina.

"Well done, little MacGregor," Jack said. "Well done. Now let's get you born."

Doreen cradled the baby's neck in one hand and held out the other, ready to support the emerging body. "Now give me one nice little push, not too big," she said to Susan. "Are you ready?" Her voice rose. "Let's go for it."

Susan gathered the force in her body and pushed. The baby plunged into Doreen's hands. Arms, back, buttocks, legs—out it all came in one liquid rush, to a clamor of cheers and happy laughter.

"There it is!"

"Hooray!"

"Wonderful!"

"Honey, look!" Tracy said, choking with emotion.

"Oh my gosh!" Susan said weakly, her voice full of exhaustion and wonder, as if after a very long ordeal she'd just seen heaven opening to her.

Doreen held up the child. It was streaked with fluid and mucus and rich red blood.

"Welcome to the world, young man," Jack said.

"That's two-oh-nine," said Bonnie, recording the time of birth.

Outside his mother's body but still linked to it by the three-foot-long umbilical cord, the baby received one last surge of nutriment-laden blood. And then it was time to end his status as a tethered parasite and embark on independent existence, like a diminutive astronaut disconnecting from the mother ship for an eighty-year walk in space. With a white plastic clip from the delivery kit, Jack pinched off the cord about an inch and a half from the baby's stomach. Then he took a metal clamp and placed it on the cord nearer Susan.

When the cord was clamped, the baby's old supply of life-giving oxygen was shut off, and so was his means of getting rid of carbon dioxide. As a result, that poisonous gas began building up in his bloodstream. When the buildup reached a certain concentration, it chemically stimulated the respiratory center of the brain. The center sent signals to the muscles of the rib cage, telling them to contract. That pulled the diaphragm down, which in turn made the lungs, airless until then, balloon—the baby's first breath. When the baby exhaled, he howled, adding his own new sound to the earth's cacophony. It was a good healthy wail, a cry not of pain or terror but discomfort and surprise. Almost immediately the gray of the baby's skin began to yield to pink. He was "pinking up."

To Bonnie and the doctors, that first wail was sweet music. They knew from experience that the drawing of the breath needed to make that inaugural wail would be the most critical action this baby would ever take. It was the most important indication that all was well with the newcomer in Room 6.

"A boy!" Susan cried in joy. "Oh, Tracy!"

"I can't believe it," Tracy said.

He bent down to kiss Susan and she took him in her arms. "Our baby," she whispered, looking into his face. "Our son!" Then both turned back to look at the miracle in Doreen's gloved hands.

"What's his name?" Bonnie asked.

"His name is Samuel!" Susan declared, lifting her head and shoulders back off the mattress as she called it out.

Tracy, clearly caught off guard, looked at her. This had come as a complete surprise. "Samuel?" he asked. "His name is Samuel?"

They'd chosen girls' names but couldn't settle on a boy's—none of the boys' names had sounded right to Tracy, not quite right for his son—so they'd put off the decision. Now, at the moment of birth, the decision had been made.

"Do you like it?" Susan said, eager for a yes. "It's my great-grandfather's name."

"I love it," Tracy said. "It's a good basic name. Are we gonna call him Sam?"

"Does he look like a Sam?"

Tracy considered his son. The little face was puffy and distorted from the compression. "Sam?" he said. "Absolutely."

25.
Nines

"All right, Tracy," Jack said. "The time has come!"

"For what?" asked Tracy, still somewhat dazed.

"It's time for you to cut the cord."

In the past decade or two, as men escaped the fathers' waiting room and made it to the childbearing bedside, the cutting of the umbilical cord had come to be considered one of the rites of male parenthood, a mark of the truly involved husband. A month before, Jack had asked Tracy if he wanted to do it, and Tracy, some of whose friends had done it, said yes. Now, however, looking at the cord, he had flutters of doubt. It was a slick, sinewy tube about an inch thick. Just under its bluish white surface, two arteries and a vein spiralled like the red and blue stripes of a barber pole.

"How do I do it?" he asked uncertainly.

"With these scissors," Doreen said. "It's tough and rubbery, so you have to be decisive about it." She took the baby's end of the cord and held out the section on the other side of the plastic clip. "Right here."

Tracy, who despite his heartiness tended to be somewhat squeamish, was nervous about cutting something so intimately attached to his own new son. But he began to work the scissors. It was unsettling: here he was, deliberately cutting blood vessels belonging to his wife and his new child. He got halfway through and paused to get a better grip on the scissors, which were slippery now with blood.

"Keep going," Bonnie said encouragingly.

"A little more," said Doreen. "You're almost there. It's hard to do if you're not used to it."

The scissors severed the cord. There were cheers, and Tracy looked up from his labor, his expression a blend of pride, fluster, and astonishment. It was such a dramatic action and, if one looked for symbols, a significant one. The father had come between the mother and the child and cut their connection. Or maybe the father was giving the child freedom, an act he would have to repeat many times in various ways over the years to come.

Sam was on his own. It was an abrupt change that now demanded prompt and drastic changes in his life systems. Respiration had already converted, and digestion and elimination weren't major problems. For five months Sam had been getting part of his nourishment by drinking the fluid in which he swam—which contained some proteins and sugars—just lately as much as eight pints a day. Now he would simply take all, instead of just some, of his sustenance by mouth. For the same length of time he had been urinating, a bit, into that same fluid; the kidneys, though immature, were fully formed and functional.

Nature's real tour de force, though, was what was already happening to Sam's circulatory system. When Jack applied the first clip to the cord, it choked off the torrent of blood. That was a crisis indeed, the equivalent of a cooling-water failure during a nuclear meltdown. Major measures had to take place at once—switches thrown, valves opened and shut. One such adjustment was nothing less than an impromptu restructuring of Sam's heart.

Before birth, there had been no need for blood to be sent from his heart to his lungs for oxygen; Susan's lungs were providing oxygen for two. So the blood was allowed to bypass the lungs, through a special hole between two major blood vessels from Sam's heart. When the umbilical cord was clamped, that hole immediately began to close, and for the first time blood was shunted to his lungs. Until the hole completely sealed, when he was about three months old, fresh blood and waste-bearing blood would mix, and he would tend to look a bit blue. Perfectly normal.

Soon after Sam was born and after the cord was cut, Bonnie had taken him from Doreen and quickly cleaned and dried him with a towel. Then she put him under the radiant heat of the warming table. Like most babies Sam was born with some insulation, a layer of what was called brown fat. But if he was allowed to chill, the brown fat would swiftly burn off and his temperature would begin to drop. The warming table would prevent that.

Bonnie now engaged herself in giving Sam his official identification. She opened up an ink pad and pressed Sam's tightly curled foot to it as flatly as it would go. Then, twice, she pressed the foot to footprint sheets. One copy would go into Susan's hospital records. That copy already had Susan's fingerprint on it, which Bonnie had unobtrusively taken during delivery, between pushes, when she knew that the birth was imminent and she'd be the delivering nurse. The other copy of the footprint sheet, the one that said "Happy Birthday!" on it in plump blue letters, would go to Susan for the baby book.

Bonnie fastened white identity bracelets around both Sam's ankle and Susan's wrist, and she banded Tracy with an orange one, which he would have to wear until the baby left the hospital. For reasons of security Tracy, without his band, wouldn't be allowed to fetch Sam from the nursery to bring to Susan.

When Bonnie was done, Dr. Fox took over. "Okay, little guy," he said, "here we go." It was time to check Sam out.

The procedure that Sam was about to experience was the inspiration of Virginia Apgar, a pediatric anesthesiologist. Dr. Apgar perceived that in the bustle and celebration that followed delivery, the babies themselves weren't always looked at closely, and serious problems, such as breathing difficulties, sometimes went unnoticed. What was needed, she felt, was a simple, uniform procedure for examining new babies to reveal trouble instantly. So in 1952 she invented one. It became standard all over the world, giving this quiet, modest person a satisfaction few ever know, that of having saved the lives of innumerable human beings.

Twice in the first few moments of his life, at one minute and at five minutes, a newborn is judged by the five objective Apgar criteria: heart rate, breathing, muscle tone, reflexes, and color. For each, the baby is given a rating of 0, 1, or 2, which are added up to give the Apgar score. A pink baby—all babies are pinkish early on, especially their noses and ears—with a heart rate over 100 beats a minute, strong breathing, lively arms and legs, and a quick response to irritation of the skin gets five twos . . . a perfect ten.

But tens are very unusual. The baby has to breathe to get pink; after one minute it is unlikely to have breathed enough to become pink all the way to its fingers and toes—they're still blue. Nothing to worry about, at this point. The old joke is that the only baby who ever got a ten was a lawyer's kid.

Dr. Fox took a towel and rubbed Sam's spine vigorously. Sam squirmed and fussed, indicating good nerve response. Fox suctioned Sam again, running a tube into his nose and mouth and this time Sam's stomach as well. One reason was to get out any remaining mucus or amniotic fluid, which might impair his breathing. Another was to make sure those passages were normal—that, for example, he didn't lack an esophagus. Sam didn't like that process either, and howled.

"What a big voice for such a little guy," Jack said.

"I know!" Bonnie said. "Listen to him scream."

"What good lungs this baby has," Tracy said.

Dr. Fox thought so too and gave them a score of 2. Sam's heart rate was 140, well over the 100 mark—another 2. By picking Sam up and seeing how well he supported his body, and by pulling his arms and legs out straight and seeing how readily they snapped back to the semifolded position babies prefer, Fox could see that Sam's muscles and reflexes were working well: two more 2s. As for color, although Sam was generally a robust pink, his hands and feet were a little bluish—totally normal, but it rated a 1.

Fox called out the Apgar to Jack and Doreen—"It's a nine," he said—and entered it in Sam's medical records. Bonnie swaddled Sam in two blankets and put a tiny stocking cap on his head for warmth. Then she gave him to Jack, who placed him on Susan's chest. "There he is," he said to her.

"Hi, little fella," she murmured, glowing. She held Sam to her and kissed his head again and again.

"He's got nice color," Jack said.

Sam began to bawl. "Waa! Waa! Waa!"

"Listen to you!" Susan said in tender mock reproof. Sam kept crying.

"Honey, it's a boy!" Tracy said, reconfirming. Susan smiled and hugged little Sam.

"I *said* it was going to be a boy," Jack said lightly.

So spellbound had Tracy been by all that was happening that he had neglected to perform perhaps the most important task assigned to the father. "Oh, you know what I forgot to do?" he said. "Take some pictures."

Susan, a good sport, laughed a little.

"No problem," Bonnie said. "You can take some now." The dramatis personae posed in several combinations, always with Sam at the center, like an Oscar at the Academy Awards. Susan took the photos of Tracy holding his son. Bonnie made Tracy sit down before taking the baby. It was a rule. Already that week Bonnie had had two fathers faint on her, one from the sight of blood and the other from excitement. When the last picture was snapped, Sam went back to the warming table for his five-minute Apgar—another nine: very good and fortunately very common.

"Now we deliver the placenta," Jack said.

Doreen pressed a stainless steel tray against Susan's bottom. Jack took up the slack on the umbilical cord and then tugged a little. "I'll just stay over here," Doreen said to Jack with a smile, moving slightly to one side, "not that I don't trust you to do it gently." From experience she knew that if she stood too close when the placenta came down, she would get drenched. A hazard of the profession.

Blood gushed out. The gush told Jack that the placenta was detaching and ready to come out. The cord suddenly went slack again and seemed to grow longer in Jack's hand—the familiar "lengthening" phenomenon, which signalled that the placenta had completely detached. Torn from the patch of uterine wall it had clung to for nine months, it was moving down. Jack tugged the cord again, and Susan groaned in discomfort. Swiftly and wetly the placenta slipped from Susan's body and plopped into the tray.

Doreen held up the tray for the MacGregors to see. Here was the ineffably marvelous device that had acted as the essential link between Susan and her child. Like the umbilical cord it was a thoroughly practical apparatus, designed for use, not for show. Yet in its way it was beautiful, another extraordinary sight for the MacGregors in a day of extraordinary sights. Not gory. Spectacular. Everyone in the room, even the professionals, paused for a moment to look at it.

It was oval and floppy, like a big omelet or a flattened football—the ancient Chinese called it the "fetal pillow." It was about seven inches long and an inch and a half thick. It weighed a pound and a half. The side that had been attached to Susan was dull, but Sam's side was a intricate mesh of brilliant red and blue blood vessels—a painting by Jackson Pollock, or an infrared satellite photo of the Amazon delta. Down through those gaudy tributaries had come the vital stuff Sam needed, oxygen and nourishment, and back through them had gone carbon dioxide and waste.

Attached to the baby's vivid side of the placenta was a filmy membrane, the amnion, the inner layer of the amniotic sac. "See that?" Jack said, pointing to it.

"Yep," Tracy said, half curious, half leery.

"It looks like a dry-cleaner's bag, doesn't it," Jack said. He put his hand through the place where the sac had been ruptured and expanded the diaphanous sphere. It was one of his favorite little demonstrations. The sac was so light and delicate that it seemed it might float to the ceiling. "That's where Sam has been living," Jack said.

"Wow," Susan and Tracy said in unison, their eyes wide.

The placenta wasn't discarded. First Jack examined it carefully to make sure it was complete, with no tissue torn away; it was, so he knew that no fragments had been left in the uterus to cause complications. Bonnie put it in a plastic box—the one that the surgical sponges had come in—and carried it out of the room to be put in the placenta freezer. It would go to a company that would make blood products and extract hormones from it. Tissues from the placenta would also be used as temporary grafts for burn victims. The umbilical cord, if it was the right size, would go into the freezer too, to be used as a replacement artery in a heart bypass operation. It had recently been discovered that both placenta and umbilical cord, frozen and saved for years if necessary, could be used as a source of blood cells for bone-marrow transplants; it was hoped that when perfected, this technique would obviate the extremely painful operation by which bone marrow was presently extracted from human donors. In short, the organs that Susan and Tracy had created to sustain Sam's life would go right on sustaining lives long after Sam was done with them.

"My guess is he weighs six-eleven," Jack said.

"When I lift him up, I can tell you," Bonnie said, winking.

"She used to work at Shoprite, in the deli department," Jack said to the MacGregors, keeping the joke going. "When she lifts that little roast beef of yours, she can tell you to the closest ounce. She's weighed so many of them she doesn't even need the scale."

"You're really lucky," Doreen told Susan. "No episiotomy, and no major tearing, either. All we've got here are some periurethral lacerations. We'll sew them up pretty easily, and you'll probably never feel the stitches later."

"That's wonderful. You never had an epis," Bonnie said, using the delivery-room patois—"ep-*eez*."

"How come I got off so light?" Susan asked.

"Well, I think part of it was that the epidural relaxed you, and maybe the massage we gave the perineum helped," Doreen said. "Also, you did a really good job of pushing; you knew *where* to push and when *not* to push."

Tracy was standing by the warmer, looking down at Sam, who wasn't crying at the moment, just making little alive noises. Tracy murmured back at him lovingly.

"He's cute," Jack said from the end of the bed, where he was following Doreen's progress with the stitching. He did no sewing himself but assisted Doreen, dabbing the area with gauze to keep it clear of blood, tying the ends of her sutures for her, holding the free end of her suture up out of the way, holding tissues back so that Doreen could see where she was sewing.

"Were you tired?" He asked Susan.

"Yes . . . tired."

"Are her parents out there now?" Bonnie asked Tracy, who nodded. "Great, great. Don't tell them, and we'll all go out to see them together."

The thought of telling her mother made the event freshly real to Susan. "I can't believe it," she told Tracy.

"I can't either," Tracy said.

Sam was still crying, and Susan cooed to him. "Oh, he's got the hiccups," she said, enthralled by the lilliputian burps. "Look, he's pulling his little ears!" She studied him. "He's got so much hair! It looks like red hair."

"Red hair could be from you," Tracy said.

"It could be black," Jack said. "At this stage it's hard to tell."

"Hate to cover it up," Bonnie said, replacing Sam's cap, which had come off during the picture-taking. It gave him a certain air. "Sam MacGregor," she said.

"Isn't that great?" Tracy said. "So cute."

"Sam MacGregor sounds like a character in a spy novel," Jack said.

Tracy said, "I thought it sounded like a bartender."

"A baseball player," said Doreen.

Doreen was still suturing. "We're almost done," Jack said. "That place is fixed."

Dr. Fox came in, and with Susan lying on her side, he carefully removed the tape on her back and then the epidural catheter. The hole left by the epidural catheter was so fine that once the catheter was out it disappeared. No Band-Aid was necessary.

Tracy took Sam in his arms. He put his cheek next to Sam's, and Susan took a picture. "Funny face," she said affectionately.

"Him or me?" Tracy said.

"Both of you."

It was 2:21, just twelve minutes since the birth. "Okay," Bonnie said, "I think I've got everything tied down here. Let's take him down the hall."

•   •   •

When Sam's visit with his grandparents was over, Bonnie wheeled him into the Admitting Nursery, where the scale was. She unwrapped him and placed him on the scale. "Now you're going to hear from him," she said to Tracy. Sam, yanked from his warmer and cross about it, obliged with a squall.

Jose Santo Domingo, a neonatologist, happened by and watched as Bonnie unwrapped Sam. "How much, Bonnie?" he asked with a smile. Bonnie's guessing the weight was part of the game.

She hefted Sam thoughtfully. "I'd say about . . . six-fifteen, six-fourteen."

Carol Gongla, the Admitting Nursery nurse, put Sam on the scale. "Six-thirteen," she said.

"You're good, Bonnie," Dr. Santo Domingo said.

"Aw, shucks," Bonnie said, feigning irritation. "An ounce off." She went through the rest of her procedure, then handed Tracy a sheet of paper with "It's a boy!" written across the top. On it was Sam's footprint, hardly bigger than a kitten's, and his length and weight. "Okay," she said, preparing to leave. "Sam will stay here in this room for a while. He's cold now, because we've had his blankets off, but Carol will warm him up. Then she'll bathe him, and he'll get cold again, so she'll warm him up again."

"It's like microwaving leftovers," Tracy said.

"By the time that happens, maybe an hour and a half from now, Susan should be almost ready to leave Recovery. So, near the time she goes to Postpartum, you should be able to take the baby to her."

Tracy needed one more reassurance. "Everything okay?" he asked Bonnie as they walked out into the hall.

"Everything's fine. You've got a great baby."

"Bonnie, thanks so much for everything."

"You're welcome," Bonnie said and disappeared down the hall. She was moving fast. Her shift was over, and this was Nail Night.

•   •   •

Tracy went back to Room 6. Nurses aides were stripping it, and people from Housekeeping were washing it down. Susan wasn't there.

When Doreen had finished the sewing, Jack had bathed Susan's lower body. Most OBs wouldn't dream of washing the patient, but Jack, if he was the person who was free, was always glad to do it rather than just leave the patient waiting there wet and bloodstained. Bonnie had come back in time to change Susan's gown and help her onto a stretcher and roll her into Recovery. Tracy visited her there and found her tired, sleepy, and very, very happy. The recovery room nurse had placed an ice pack on Susan's bottom to reduce the swelling and soreness, although since Susan hadn't had to push long, the swelling was minor. Every fifteen minutes the nurse took Susan's blood pressure. She had shivered a while after the birth—no one really knows why women shiver at that point, though there are plenty of guesses—but that was over now. Just before four o'clock she was moved to her room in Postpartum, Room 3309.

There was another young woman in Room 6 now, and a twitchy prospective father. "You deliver somebody," Jack observed, "and when you come back a few minutes later there's somebody else in that room. It's a hot-bed hotel."

And so it would go, shift after shift, day after day, year after year, in Labor and Delivery, and for all the hi-tech it would essentially be as it had always been.

26.
Three

Ith it was seven A.M., but it looked like high noon. The lights in the nursery were on full force and had been all night long. The nurses liked their patients well lit. They needed to be able to observe them closely and to quickly detect anything untoward—a change in color, for example. Some researchers believe that the brilliance of nurseries hurts newborns' eyes—lighting intensity has increased nearly tenfold over the past twenty years—but most studies have failed to find a connection. Babies, some say, have an extraordinarily sensitive blinking mechanism that protects their eyes. Whatever the case, the illumination in the St. Barnabas nursery this Thursday morning didn't seem to be hurting anyone's sleep. Twenty-three swaddled tenants buzzed away in their Plexiglas bassinets, recuperating from their recent exertions.

Sam MacGregor's bassinet, or crib, was in a group of a half dozen arranged three-and-three, a six-pack of neonates. All the babies were in identical positions, lying on the right side, propped there by a tucked blanket. At the top of each swaddle the crest of a fuzzball head was just visible; only one baby had its stocking cap on. Out of the other end of each bundle stuck a ruddy foot, so that the ID bracelet around the ankle could be checked without a complete unwrapping.

The nurses did not tiptoe; they did not whisper. As they went about their duties they talked to each other at regular volume about their lives and loves and lunch plans. The babies didn't seem to mind. The nurses moved among them, unswaddling, bathing, changing, and reswaddling them with graceful, practiced motions. Each baby would cry or whimper a moment during the routine. The nurse would pick it up; kiss it or touch cheeks with it; give it a bit of soft, brushy affection; and set it down and give it a pacifier. It would drop back to sleep. The newborns slept two hours for every hour they were awake. Babies crying—in short spells, anyway—didn't alarm the nurses at all. They expected it.

Shortly after seven, Doreen DeGraaff appeared at the Postpartum nurses' station, which was just outside the nursery window, and reviewed the chart for MacGregor, Susan. Then she headed down the dim corridor, still on its night lights, for Room 3309. The room faced east and the daylight was flooding in. Both Susan and her roommate were awake. Propped up against her pillows, Susan looked thoroughly ready for her first full day of motherhood. The change in her appearance was striking. Her eyelids were still shadowed in plum, but the tension and fatigue were gone from her face. Her bedjacket was pink decorated with big red roses, with pockets and sleeves of cream-colored lace, and the pink of the jacket was exactly the pink of her cheeks.

"How was your night?"

"Good. Restful. I got some sleep. And I had the baby in with me about two hours."

"Any trouble urinating or anything?"

"No, no."

"Good. That was the only thing we were worried about. There was a little tear by your urethra."

"It's a little swollen, so I had ice on it last night."

"Your legs are finally feeling normal again, right?"

"Yeah, my legs feel normal; my back is fine. And I don't feel too groggy. I guess that epidural was a really good idea."

"That's good. Now I'm going to press just a little bit on your belly. . . . It's nice and firm, like it's supposed to be. You'll notice today when you get up the first couple of times, the bleeding might be a little heavier, because you've been lying in bed. Are you breast-feeding?"

"Yes."

"You'll also notice that when the baby nurses, your uterus will contract, and you might bleed a little more. Some bleeding is normal, so you don't need to worry about that. Later in the day it really should slow down a lot."

"Okay. Good. Well, I already notice that today's better than last night."

"Alrighty?"

"Yes."

"So I'm going to come by later and see the baby."

When Doreen left, Susan lay back and thought how lovely it had been to be alone with her baby. It was nice just to get to know him. His skin was like hers, very pale. His features were changing from visit to visit. He was so cute. When he'd been in with her last evening, when Tracy was there, Tracy had said half-humorously, "You don't even know that I'm here!" She'd replied, "Well, no, I know you're here."

Tracy was coming again in the afternoon. Her parents were coming over this afternoon too. They'd been so happy about the baby's name, because it was the name of Great-grandfather McLeod. His middle name was Reel, which was Tracy's grandmother's married name and Tracy's middle name as well. This kid would be Scottish right down to the ground.

She remembered how astounded she'd been to see the little head come out of her body—that was wild. And the sight of the placenta. Just amazing, how complex it was. An exciting day.

The round, smiling face of Rod O'Driscoll, senior cherub, appeared at the door. He was wearing a dark greenish tan double-breasted gabardine suit and a flowered tie. "Receiving visitors?" he asked jovially.

"Yes," Susan said happily.

"Congratulations," Rod said. "Super. It was six pounds what?"

"Six-thirteen. A little smaller than I thought."

"That's okay."

"He looks great."

"Your latent stage of labor was weird, really weird. So prolonged, you know. I didn't think you'd deliver until around four o'clock. But once you got going, once you got jump-started, you went like gangbusters. It was a good trade-off—long labor, short delivery."

He pulled some hospital forms out of the side pocket of his sports jacket. "Okay," he said. "Jack had all the fun, and I'm doing all the paperwork." He asked Susan a string of questions and then answered the questions she had for him.

"Okay, my dear," he said at the end, "I think that's it. Let's see. Today is Thursday. Home for you on Saturday. It'll be Dr. Bonamo who sees you tomorrow. I probably won't see you again in the hospital. So, enjoy your baby."

. . .

Just before nine, Jack came into the nursery office and hung his jacket on a chairback. It was time for him to perform once again the surgical procedure he had performed so often before, the most common operation done on males, and the oldest—circumcision.

The wisdom of the operation had been debated for millennia. Two years before, the American Academy of Pediatrics had reversed the negative position it had taken in 1971 and declared that circumcision had "potential medical benefits and advantages." It noted that uncircumcised male infants suffer eleven times more urinary tract infections, which can be serious, and that circumcision virtually eliminates cancer of the penis and probably reduces sexually transmitted diseases and cervical cancer in women. Not all doctors agreed; one pointed out that the rate of postcircumcision infection and other complications runs about 1 percent to 3 percent.

In America the proportion of males circumcised has varied widely—from 5 percent a century ago to 95 percent in the 1960s to about 60 percent by the end of the 1980s. (In modern Britain it is less than 1 percent.) Tracy and Susan had talked it all over with Rod during one of their last OB visits and had decided that Sam should be circumcised, on the familiar theory that if Dad was, the baby should be too. Sometimes the pediatrician did the job, but the MacGregors wanted Jack to.

Jack put on a sterile yellow gown and entered the long narrow room that connected the nursery office with the nursery itself. Along one wall of the room was an elbow-high, stainless steel countertop. The nurse, Debra Scism, had already brought Sam from the nursery, undressed him, and put white cotton leggings on him to keep him warm. She had placed him on his back on a blue, padded plastic form, an Olympic Circumstraint, which was lying on the countertop. Shaped to a baby's body, it had Velcro bands, with which Debra bound down Sam's arms, legs, and abdomen. Furious to have had his nap disturbed, he squalled, his eyes shut tight, face pink, tongue waggling in a wide-open mouth the size of a quarter. *"Noisy* baby," Jack said to Sam affectionately. Sam quieted down at once as if he had understood.

The challenge of performing a circumcision is of course to remove the foreskin without cutting the penis. The modern answer to the challenge is a bell-shaped metal cup fitted exactly to the proportions of the head of the penis. The cup slips between the penis head and the foreskin. The scalpel cuts against it.

Debra Scism showed Jack a cellophane envelope containing a shiny steel shaft, on one end of which was a metal cup that seemed big enough to cover a raspberry. "One-point-three," she said.

"Hmm, no," Jack replied. "You're being generous." He didn't think Sam's penis was as big as Debra did. Already, size was making a difference in Sam's life.

"One-point-one?" she asked.

"Yes, I think so."

Jack pulled pale yellow gloves up over the sleeves of his gown. Then he swabbed the penis and testicles with the red-brown disinfectant, and at the stimulus the little penis stiffened. The first step was to loosen up the foreskin. He took a slender pair of tongs of the sort that opened when squeezed instead of closed, and he put it gently into the opening of the foreskin. He moved the handles together, and the tongs parted, stretching the soft flesh. Then, to make additional slack, he took surgical scissors and made a slit in the foreskin lengthwise, from its tip almost down to the place where it joined the shaft of the penis. Sam, who had started crying again, now, as Jack cut, stopped crying.

With the fingers of one hand, Jack squeezed just behind the head of the penis, to make it protrude; it looked like a purple marble. With the other hand he took the metal shaft with the bell-shaped cup at one end and held the cup against the penis, trying to fit it over the head. He had trouble.

"You know what?" he said to Debra, enjoying his own embarrassment. "I think I need a one-point-three."

The nurse smiled. "I knew I wasn't too generous on that boy," she said, and they both laughed.

"Well," Jack said, "I should have known better. You people around here know your penises."

Sam fretted, and Jack soothed him. "All right," he said softly, "you're all right." Sam returned to his snooze.

Jack pushed the cup of the one-point-three onto the head of the penis until it enveloped it. A perfect fit. Then he drew the foreskin back up over the cup. "Now for the tricky part," he said.

With a special clamp he encircled the foreskin near the rim of the cup. It would serve as a guide for Jack's scalpel. If it held the foreskin snugly all the way around, and if Jack's scalpel didn't falter, Sam would never need to blush in any locker room.

It was time to remove the foreskin. Jack picked up a small scalpel and moved it deftly around the foreskin where it met the clamp. The foreskin, a tiny doughnut of flesh, fell away. There was no blood. Sam whimpered, then stopped. Jack took Vaseline-coated gauze and wrapped the entire penis. It would keep Sam's diaper from sticking to the incision or abrading it.

"The interesting thing about circumcision," Jack said, "is that the baby doesn't cry in response to what you're doing, even though there's no narcotic. He doesn't like being held down, he doesn't like being cleaned with the cold antiseptic, he doesn't like to be poked, but the incision he hardly seems to notice."

Sam MacGregor, now the image of his dad, had no complaints. Reswaddled, he soon was heading back to the nursery, where, in the Plexiglas bassinet with the label declaring "I'm a boy!," he would get a little shut-eye.

A little while later, a nurse brought Sam to his mother for his feeding. As Susan cradled him in her arms, he avidly pressed his face to her breast. Already the bonding between Susan and her child was far along. She had held him, caressed him, smelled him, explored him, listened to him, gazed at him, kissed him. Sam already seemed to be responding most readily to his mother's voice, and within weeks he would give her his first true "social smile."

• • •

Saturday morning. Above the desk at the Postpartum nurses' station was a blue sign saying: "DISCHARGE TIME: 9 A.M." The letters of the sign were big and emphatic, as if to deal with mothers who, reluctant to give up the luxury of all day in bed with room service, were clinging to their mattresses and refusing to go home.

According to the memoirs of Martha Ballard, a midwife in eighteenth-century Maine, the postpartum period in her day was considered over when the mother went back into the kitchen, usually the same day she gave birth. "Back in the kitchen," in fact, was the phrase used for the end of lying-in. Another test was the mother's ability to make her own bed.

Susan was ready. Her bag was packed. She was waiting for Sam to be brought to the room and for Tracy to arrive with the car and a fresh outfit for her to wear home. Dr. Gruenwald, a partner of Susan's pediatrician, Dr. La Conti, had been there earlier that morning and in the course of ten minutes had gone over the basics of baby care with her. Dress the baby normally, he said, the amount of clothing you'd wear yourself for the temperature that day. Some people, he said, overdressed their babies, but babies adapted to the temperature just as grownups did.

Susan looked out the window and down onto the parking lot, thinking she might see Tracy's Saab arriving. She hoped he'd figured out how to install the baby's car seat. She thought of what they'd said in the childbirth classes: that more babies were killed in auto accidents than by all the birth defects combined. You sort of thought, well, I can hold the baby in my arms and protect it. But in a head-on collision between two cars each going only ten miles an hour, the G forces make the baby weigh the equivalent of 150 pounds, enough to tear it from an adult's arms.

Tracy arrived and asked where the baby was. Susan explained that Dr. Bonamo had to come and discharge her first. She dressed and then sat in the armchair.

"Does your bottom hurt from the Rho-GAM shot?" Tracy asked her.

"It doesn't hurt at all." The baby, it turned out, like his father, did have Rh-positive blood.

A nurse wheeled Sam in. "No point your not having him with you," she said. "I'm sure Dr. Bonamo won't mind." She left the room.

The moment had come to dress Sam for the first time. A first for Sam, a first for Susan; she had never dressed a baby before.

"He's going to *love* this little outfit—if Mama can get it on him," Susan said. "See your little T-shirt?"

Sam began to whimper. "Oh, come on," Tracy said to him affectionately. "You're okay."

"How do we get him in this thing?" Susan said. She had worked Sam's head through the T-shirt's neck, but getting his arms into the sleeves seemed impossible.

"We'll have to figure it out."

Sam's umbilical stump, now purple from the gentian violet antiseptic applied in the nursery to prevent infection, popped out from under the shirt. Susan tugged the shirt back down. Sam looked up at her, mouth in a miniature O, and she couldn't resist picking him up and hugging him. "Oh, you smell so good!" she said. Sam squealed.

Yellow socks. Tracy did one; Susan the other. It was hard to do, like threading a worm onto a hook.

"It's the first time Sam's ever had real clothes on," Tracy said as he worked.

"You're doing a very nice job on that sock," Susan said.

"Is that a surprise?" Tracy said, feigning hurt.

Sam wagged his arms, and his little aged fingers, still wrinkled from all those months of marination, wriggled and closed and wriggled again. "Now if we can get these booties on," Susan said, "we'll be set."

She put a sun hat on Sam's downy orb. The hat promptly drooped over one ear. "That hat is really funny," Tracy said. Sam was not amused. His expression was that of a banker who, for a charity event but against his better judgment, has allowed himself to be garbed in a clown suit.

The nurse appeared. "Still no Dr. Bonamo?" she asked.

On cue, Jack came through the door. "How's your baby?" he asked. "How's the nursing going?"

"It's okay," Susan said. "He latches on and then he stops. I'm not too sure what to make of it."

"Well, it's his first time, and it's your first time. If you don't let him know that it's new to you, he's going to think you're the boss."

"He's a gourmet," Tracy said. "He takes a couple of tastes, he stops, he savors it, tries it again."

"For him, it's nouvelle cuisine," Jack said. "How do you feel?"

"Pretty good," Susan said.

"Basically your instructions are that there are no specific instructions. Just take it easy. You shouldn't drive for about a week. I want to see you back in the office in about six weeks. Up until that time, you probably shouldn't have intercourse. When you decide to start, make sure you use some kind of birth control."

"That would be handy," Susan said, laughing.

"All right," Jack said. "I think you've got this routine down. The next six kids will be a snap."

"Ho, ho," Tracy said.

"Thank you for everything," Susan said with feeling.

"Enjoy him," Jack said. "I'll sign all your papers." He brought a sheaf of forms out of his pocket and starting signing. "All the best," he said. "See you soon." And suddenly this man who had been such a presence in the MacGregors' lives for eight long months, so intimately a part of this immensely important event, was gone.

There was a light rapping at the door, and the transporter entered, pushing a wheelchair. Susan handed Sam to Tracy. She went over to the chair and turned and sat, and Tracy handed Sam back to her. "I'll go get the car," he said.

When they got to the lobby, the transporter placed the chair in front of the doors, in a row of wheelchairs also waiting for cars. Sam dozed. The light coming in from the outside was dazzling. It looked like a very hot day.

The green Saab pulled up to the curb. "That's my husband," Susan said, and the transporter guided the wheelchair out onto the sidewalk. Sam had left the hospital, left another womb, entered the great outdoors, entered the world. For the first time, sun fell on his face. Susan shielded his eyes.

When Susan and Sam were aboard and strapped in, Tracy got behind the wheel. He led the car around the sweeping curves of the exit lanes and out onto Old Short Hills Road. Tiger lilies were blooming in the verges, tall, bending with orange blossom.

As the car drew near the house, Susan glimpsed bright colors through the trees and then saw a large cluster of balloons on the lawn in front of the house, tethered to a brick. The balloon in the middle said "It's a boy!"

They entered the house, Tracy carrying Sam, and climbed the steps to the second floor. Susan showed Sam his little room and changed his diaper and wrapped him in a cotton blanket.

In the MacGregors' bedroom was the white wicker bassinet that Susan had had as a baby. Before Susan had left for the hospital, she had placed it by her side of the old brass four-poster, the bed in which Sam had been conceived, so that at any moment during the night she could reach out and touch her child.

She gently lowered the baby into the bassinet. He whimpered once, burped, yawned, and fell sound asleep.

There lay Sam MacGregor, the 260 millionth living American, plus or minus, and one of sixteen thousand born on that June twelfth. He weighed no more than a gallon of wine or an unabridged dictionary, but that weight was destined to multiply almost thirty times. There was a 90 percent chance he'd be right-handed, a 10 percent chance he'd be dyslexic, about a 95 percent chance he'd desire women (in due course), a 10 percent chance he'd have perfect pitch.

As a male, if the statisticians were right, he would be 36 percent less likely to read books regularly than the girl who'd been in the next St. Barnabas bassinet, have twice as much body mass devoted to muscle, be three times likelier to admire the way he looked naked, and be half as apt to clean his navel weekly.

And for all that, where was Sam? Not in the statistics but in the yet-to-be disclosed nature he'd picked up somewhere along the way, an eon ago, perhaps. He was a man of distinguished lineage, a direct descendant of the first human being, and a creature with unmapped possibilities. A gift already given but wholly to be received.

He was incredibly intricate. Once the human brain was held up as the marvel of intricacy, or the eye. Now scientists were way down into the human genetic structure—and going deeper. The miracle kept expanding. Sometimes the human organism, with its abstruse interplays of the chemical, electrical, and mechanical, seemed like a Rube Goldberg contraption—one of those silly machines that, in order to accomplish a simple task like blowing out a candle, employed an elephant that, tickled by a feather, would drop a bowling ball onto the end of a plank, thereby catapulting the ballerina into a pool of Jello, and so on. So many contingencies, so many things bearing on other things, improbable sequences that had to take place precisely. But to Rod O'Driscoll and Jack Bonamo and Doreen De-Graaff and Bonnie Bergman and the others at St. Barnabas who encountered creation daily, it seemed ineffably brilliant, way out beyond any med school curriculum, a light year beyond the comprehension of the brain it had manufactured, though not the heart.

New parents were somewhat insulated from the full miracle. Although they were living it, it was too overwhelming, too spectacular to hold in the mind constantly—the fashioning of this awesome complexity in so short a time: life. One grew accustomed to miracles. It was in the little tasks of caring for a child that the wonder became reality.

Epilogue

A week after Sam MacGregor was born the O'Driscoll-Bonamo practice moved a million miles, from the first floor of 95 Northfield Avenue to Jack's obstetrical-gynecological paradise on the second. It was like leaving an ancient hamlet that had grown up helter-skelter but was nonetheless a real community, enshrining the lives that had been lived there, then taking up residence in a triumph of modern city planning.

The new place was stunning—soft colors, subtle textures, indirect lighting, furnishings of high quality and low flash. The desk at which patients announced themselves was more like an altar, with Doric columns at either side. "I can hardly wait to see Jack's face," said Mary Jo, to the amusement of Barbara, Eleanore, and Louise, "the first time a kid throws something sticky at the wall."

There was no waiting room; Jack let it be known that this elegantly appointed area was to be called the reception room. "Waiting," he said, had bad connotations; "reception," on the other hand, sounded . . . receptive. Downstairs, women making their initial OB visits had been given their free samples and instructive literature in garish pink plastic bags carrying the name of a drug company; upstairs there were pearl-gray bags bearing the practice's handsome new logo.

Now there were six examining rooms instead of three, and three consultation rooms instead of one. It all anticipated the day soon to arrive when there would be three doctors instead of two. Dr. Jerry Ciciola, who as a resident had helped Jack deliver Marsha Phelps last February, was now a full-fledged obstetrician and had been invited to join the practice.

Anyone new to the world of O'Driscoll-Bonamo would think it all wonderful, and they wouldn't know the half of it—the foresight that had gone into the planning of the doctors' and nurses' spaces, and how it benefitted the orderly flow of work and thus the patients. Old-timers, though, might not be blamed for occasionally missing the intimacy and idiosyncrasy left behind. The lunchroom was no longer an agreeably grungy nook where the staff could hole up and grouse about the doctors. Now it was a mere alcove off the back hall, with no door to shut. Gone was the old sofa you could lie on awhile if you had to. Now there were just cushioned benches flanking a Formica-topped table, like a booth at Burger King.

Still, friendships would eventually form and deepen around that table, and the staff would come to think of that alcove as their own, a sanctuary. All of them were soon declaring that the new offices were ten times better to work in.

Like many a great creator, Jack had been tempted to push it just one step too far. He was offended by the idea of cluttering his sleek main hall with those five bulletin boards covered with disorderly patchworks of curling baby photos. He'd left them down. But old patients getting their first look at the place immediately noticed their absence and complained. The boards went up.

•   •   •

Bea Perez quickly found a job with Blue Cross Blue Shield, telling doctors whether or not they could do the procedure they had in mind. It was work well suited to her temperament. Nobody ever stopped missing her.

•   •   •

Sam MacGregor celebrated his first birthday in Richmond, Virginia. AT&T had transferred his father there, and the MacGregors had reluctantly sold their blue-shuttered house in Maplewood and gone south.

Sam was turning out to be a big boy, rangy, with a pot belly. Already he was wearing clothes meant for two-year-olds. The pediatrician said that for height and weight he was in the 95th percentile.

At one year he was still nursing a bit, in the morning, but abruptly would roll away, laugh at Susan, and burp. He now preferred bananas and mashed peas, oatmeal and applesauce—and plenty of them.

He was independent. He had learned to take his diaper off and loved to be without it. He'd shuck it and then stand in his crib and bellow.

He was attentive and interested. At baby class at the Y he listened carefully to the little songs, and at church he'd look around, serious, checking everything out, especially the ten-year-old girl who sat across the aisle. He wasn't impulsive; he would inspect, digest, and absorb.

He was a people person. He readily crawled up to other children and looked them over. At the petting zoo he'd ignore the goat and head for the other kids.

He loved to be tickled.

He was, in short, a baby. Once again the process had worked just fine.

Acknowledgments

At first this book seemed impossible: I couldn't find an obstetrician to write about. Many didn't seem appropriate, and those few who did turned pale at the very thought of letting a writer hang around their offices for the better part of a year, watching everything they did including deliveries. They worried about what their patients might think; they worried about malpractice. And then, one day, following a tip from a well-satisfied patient, I reached 95 Northfield Avenue.

Rod O'Driscoll and Jack Bonamo did not worry, I think because both are calmly confident in their own skills. Their attitude was "This could be interesting, maybe even fun." They welcomed me in, and off we went. Never once did they try to censor me. Rod was the rock at the center. His character set the standard, and his prestige validated the book and brought me cooperation wherever I went. Jack was my shepherd. His immense command of medical information and his gift for narrative have enriched the book. These are two fine men, and they made the experience—at least for me—extremely interesting and very pleasant indeed.

My luck held when it came to their remarkable staff. They took me into their circle and helped me endlessly. Any reader of this book will know how indebted I am to nurse Bea Perez, a breathtakingly capable professional and a great person. Barbara Valente and Eleanore Steel were tremendously kind and, well, sweet. Genevieve Collins, Mary Jo Ward, Jane Rissland, and Louise Bacino were good friends of the project. It was awful to finish my reporting and realize I couldn't have sloppy joes in the back room and discuss last night's *L.A. Law* with this gang anymore.

I thank Susan and Tracy MacGregor most fervently for the trust and courage that let them open their lives and their childbearing to me. I hope the book reflects my full, affectionate regard for them. I thank Sam MacGregor for the privilege of chronicling his earliest moments. Long life to you, Sam.

My fond admiration to all the patients of the practice, those mentioned and those who were equally helpful but whose stories for one reason or another weren't included. I am thinking especially of Barbara Armenti, Karla Clark, Arlene Feldman, Lauren O'Sullivan, Rachel Ring, and Allison Sargent. Also Rosemary Cartright, Joyce De Masi, Ellen Foye, Debra Kovona, Marilyn Maute, Diane McGarrity, and Mary Ryan. As Rod would say: "Salt of the earth."

My thanks to the people of St. Barnabas Medical Center, particularly Ronald J. Del Mauro and Dr. James Breen. I am grateful also to Ellen Greene, Sue Weinstein, Norma Miller, and Diana Sullivan Durham and her sterling labor-and-delivery staff. Dr. Catherine Sladowski gave the manuscript an astute professional reading.

Richard Pine, my agent, made this book possible; it's as simple as that. Richard is much more than a skilled literary businessman; he has a good eye and a great heart. I will always remember his kindness to me. My thanks also to his dad, Arthur Pine, and to Lori Andiman and Sarah Piel of the Pine office.

Marilyn Abraham, editor-in-chief of Simon & Schuster's Fireside and Touchstone divisions, was the original source of publishing enthusiasm, but she didn't just acquire the book; she worked hard and long and insightfully on the manuscript. Together with her colleague, Rebecca Cabaza, she immensely improved it. When I think what it would have been without them, I shiver. Senior copy editing supervisor Isolde C. Sauer, a real pro, deftly steered the text through the rapids of production, and Dawn Marie Daniels, Marilyn's gracious, able assistant, did the book hundreds of behind-the-scenes favors.

Close friends A. Scott Berg, Campbell Black, David Hapgood, and Barbara Shulgasser, along with experts Laura Gordon and the canny Jane Taylor, were kind enough to read the manuscript at various stages and to make the perceptive suggestions I'd gone to them for. Allison Sitrin and Kathleen Stolarski did able research. Anna Chapman did an excellent job of copy editing.

I benefitted from the professional expertise of Drs. Donna Baird, David S. Blumenthal, Gideon Bosker, Alan Wilcox, and the estimable Jack Klatell.

I found the science writing of *The New York Times* highly informative, particularly that of Natalie Angier, Sandra Blakeslee, and Gina Kolata.

At the American College of Obstetricians and Gynecologists, Penny Murphy, Mark Graves, and Pam Van Hine were helpful, as was Nancy Blankenhorn of the New Jersey Historical Society.

Each of the following made a contribution to the book, for which I am thankful: Tonia Blair, Randi Boyette, Claire Brown, Lisl Cade, Mark Christiansen, Larry Davidson, Rhonda Erb, Carol Farris, Donna and Andrew Fitzsimmons, Arnold and Elise Goodman, Elaine Goodman, Richard Heller, John Kobler, Bob Loomis, Toma Lord, Kate MacEnulty, Anne Nelson, Gabriella Oldham, Elizabeth Olmsted, Tom Owen, Marie Postlewate, Mary Louise Price, Lauren Richman, Nancy Caldwell Sorel, Howard Stowe, and Sue Woodman.

My friends were sensitively supportive during the long labor, and I thank them for understanding when, month after month, I couldn't come out and play. My daughters, Elizabeth Congdon Montgomery and Pamela Congdon, were their usual loving, enspiriting selves; Lizzie gave the galleys a smart, invaluable scrutiny.

My wife, to whom I owe so much anyway, was a stalwart throughout this trek. I relied on her keen editorial sense as well as her equanimity. The dedication of this book is made with a full heart.

Topics

Where to find the main discussions of these subjects: